The Anti-ageing Beauty Bible

Josephine Fairley & Sarah Stacey

Illustrations by David Downton

Kyle Books

Contents

It's this simple: there has never been a better time to age. Every year, billions are poured into research into the creams, the vitamins, the age-spot-zapping lasers – even magic tummy-flattening pants(!) – and the light-reflecting make-up innovations that can help us look great for our age, whatever that is

There are fabulous role models out there, too, to give us all hope. Women we know as friends. Women we see in magazines, or on screen, from Helen Mirren (who wouldn't want to look that good in a bikini at any age?), Julianne Moore, Cate Blanchett, Susan Sarandon, Oprah Winfrey, Isabella Rossellini and Sophia Loren. (Even, God bless her, Joan Collins, who just keeps pushing back the threshold for what's considered 'old': first forty, then fifty, sixty, and now – who knows where it'll end…?) We know plenty of women who once would have been written off as 'middle-aged' at forty, who are backpacking, dating, even clubbing (a dance-step too far, for us, but why on earth not…?) up to their eighties.

If you're reading this book, we know one thing: you want to stay looking and feeling your absolute best, for as long as possible. (Without, necessarily, going under the knife or having invasive treatments. Although in *The Anti-Ageing Beauty Bible* we've some advice on that, too – even if personally we'd never help nature along quite so drastically for ourselves.)

The real challenge for so many women is that as the years go by, our confidence wobbles. We can lose our way. We don't look the way we always did, but we haven't worked out how to embrace this new phase. One key thing we've observed as we look around: women can start to 'fade away'. Complexions get paler. Hair colour, ditto. And if we're not careful, we start dressing to match, to reflect the fact we feel a bit low-key, a bit less va-va-voom – in muted shades that eventually make us look like a ghost of our former, younger, more attractive-feeling selves.

But it doesn't have to be like that!!!!! Women really don't have to do a vanishing act. We know, because we've talked to the experts – from globally renowned hair colour wizards to A-list nutritionists, facial massage gurus to experts who know how to keep our brains sharp, too. (Because it's all very well knowing which concealer's going to blitz your under-eye circles, but it really helps if you can remember where you put your make-up bag…! Not to mention the car keys, your glasses, etc.) And if you're bothered by the effects of gravity, we've talked to people who can help everything become that bit more 'pert' again – from faces to thighs, even foot arches!

Crucially, we've tapped into the wisdom of

You're *never* too old to become *younger*

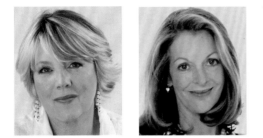

make-up professionals who understand mature faces, because they're facing the challenge of lines and wrinkles or 'sun spots' themselves, every day when they look in the mirror. Because make-up – applied well – can be your quickest way to drop a decade in little more than a flash. In fact, our advice to women who write to us for advice because they're contemplating a facelift is simple: get a makeover first. It is truly, truly, truly miraculous what the right foundation (with primer first), concealer, lipstick and brow pencil can achieve.

But which concealer, which moisturising lipstick, which age-defying foundation? (Not to mention which are the best anti-ageing eye creams, or shine-restoring hair masks, or body firming creams…?) As beauty editors that's what we're asked all the time, and the signature of our best-selling Beauty Bible series of books has been pointing you in the direction of the products which really, truly perform.

We've now had over 7,000 real women testing products – all aged from 35 to well into their sixties – who've put container-loads of anti-ageing products through their paces over a period of three months or more. There are super-whizz-bang, high-tech options, and all-natural choices (and our 'daisy rating' – see box right – helps you identify those).

There are dozens of new entries for this edition, but what our testers' incredibly consistent comments and scores (out of ten) confirm yet again is what we've known for a while: that there truly are many, many products out there which can help you look younger. Not as young as your 19-year-old daughter (let alone granddaughter), or the intern in your office. But radiant. Glowing. Not someone fading into the distance, but who's enjoying your life, looking and feeling the best you possibly can.

This book is exceedingly close to our own hearts – having a joint age of 125, as we sat down to put manicured digits to Apple keyboard. But yes, we do constantly get compliments about 'looking good for our age'. Which, frankly, are the compliments that any woman *d'un certain âge* wants to hear.

Through the pages of this book – organised as an A to Z of everything that our friends and readers have told us bothers them about ageing – we are about to help you feel your best. Look your best. And be your best, too. Life is no dress rehearsal and we only get one chance to enjoy this one.

The truth is that when your daily 'self-care' ritual is sorted – from the right skincare to the perfect make-up to haircare to at least a little bit of exercise – then you can do the things you still long to do, explore the passions you yearn to pursue, be the woman you'd really like to be.

Trust us: age really can be a thing of the past. With love,

Jo ~ Sarah
x

www.beautybible.com Don't forget: you can follow us on Twitter: @Beauty_Bible!

10 important things you need to know about make-up

While perusing 25,000 forms (yes, it nearly killed us) from the ten-women tester panels who trialled literally thousands of products for this latest Beauty Bible (which we believe is the definitive guide to ageing gorgeously), we realised there were some key myths and misconceptions about make-up. And also some key secrets that everyone simply needs to know – because make-up isn't cheap, and you want to get the very best value out of the cosmetics you buy.

So (with apologies to those of you who basically have a degree in make-up and know this stuff already), here goes.

A primer goes over moisturiser, under foundation. Used on their own, primers aren't moisturising enough. And if you're not sure why you need this extra step in your make-up regime, turn to page 89 to find out how primers will help you create the most flawless canvas ever for your foundation – and make it last longer.

Apply eyeshadow and other eye make-up before your base, though. That way, if it 'sheds', it's easy to clean up and won't spoil your foundation.

For eyeshadow, it also helps to own a 'blending brush'. This is quite simply the best way to make sure all the edges of your shadow are seamless. Jemma Kidd recommends dipping the blender brush in a little translucent powder and buffing over eyes to soften. ('The idea is to "sheer down" the colour, not remove it,' she advises.) All brush ranges feature a 'blender' brush, and if you can't identify it – well, that's what sales consultants are for.

The time to apply light-reflecting concealer (or a brightener) is before foundation. If applying under eyes, use the brush/wand to trace a triangle down from the corners of the eye to meet in the middle of the under-eye zone, and then blend with brush or ring finger. On eyelids, start in the inner corner by your nose.

Apply flaw-correcting concealers over foundation. Once you've evened out your skintone, you may not need so much.

Dry, dull-looking skin makes you look much older than you are. Youthful skin isn't powdery and one-dimensional; it's radiant. So we swear by this tip from Laura Mercier to achieve that, fast: 'Use the tiniest bit of a light moisturiser patted around the outer

eyes and along the top lip over your make-up. It makes skin look fresh, not dry, and it's a great de-ager as it stops make-up settling into any fine lines.' (You can do this during the day to refresh make-up, too.)

You really don't have to live with dry, cracked lips. But lip balm is only half the answer. Lips respond beautifully to buffing: press a wet flannel on to your lips, then use it to gently rub away flakes and roughness. And then slather on your balm or lip treatment (we've lots of good ones on page 137). Your lip pencil will glide on more smoothly, too: even the creamiest of these can be drying.

There's a quick way to deal with eye-make-up smudges. Don't ask us why make-up seems to flake and speck more now we're older – but it often does seem to, and during a busy day you don't have time to start again. Cleansing buds infused with make-up remover all seem to have disappeared for some reason but better still, we find, is to roll a Q-tip in a very little bit of foundation, then roll it back and forth over the eye zone. It removes smudges – but doesn't leave skin 'naked'.

Remember: self-tanner will always look patchy unless you exfoliate and moisturise first. It really is that simple, and not buffing and hydrating skin is the number one reason why we get negative comments from our testers about some fake tans. (OK, this isn't strictly make-up. But we have lots of testers who need to understand this!)

And whatever else you do, get a regular makeover. It's easy to treat make-up like a trusty recipe – finding something that works and clinging to it long after it's stopped doing what it once did for you – so we recommend regular makeovers. These are free (or at the very least, redeemable against purchase). There is no better way to discover what make-up can do to counterbalance the fact that skin has become thinner, thirstier and more transparent, or its tone has altered and faded. A good in-store make-up pro – we particularly recommend the make-up artists at Laura Mercier, Bobbi Brown, Giorgio Armani Beauty and on the By Terry counter in Space NK branches – can also help show you tricks to deal with lips that are thinning, eyes that are drooping and a chin or nose that is becoming 'longer'. As the ads say, Just. Do. It. (Please!)

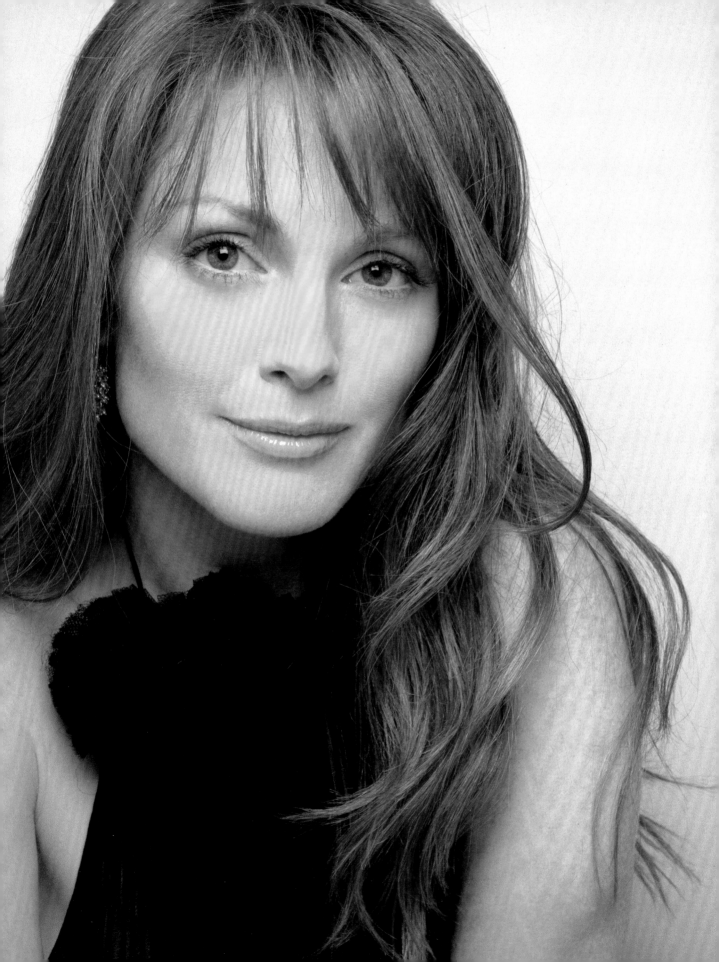

Cosmetics: your top 10 products

Before you consider a facelift, buy these Make-up Musts

We have four words to say when friends and readers tell us they're considering 'having work done', or even Botox. 'Have a make-up makeover.' Make-up really can work miracles. And showcased here are the ten make-up essentials that we know can melt away the years – blurring lines, delivering radiance and making skin look dewily fresher, smoother and younger. We feel strongly that cosmetic surgery (and even cosmeto-dermatology) should be a last resort. Trust us: by ensuring that your make-up kit features these ten categories of cosmetics, you really can drop a decade – with the wave of a magic (concealer) wand.

1 A make-up primer. With silicones (to smooth the skin) and light-reflective pigments (to 'blur' the appearance of fine lines), a make-up primer also helps solve the problem of make-up that 'disappears' into thin air, which can be a particular problem for drier, mature complexions. (For specific recommendations, see page 89.)

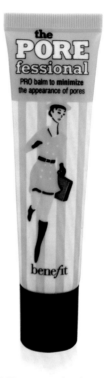

2 A 'line-smoother/ pore-filler'. Real magic, these. Again, they feature silicones and sometimes even nylon particles, and can be applied as required to deep grooves, finer lines and open pores. (We favour the type with a teensy nozzle, for targeted application.) They simply 'sit' on the skin's surface, and can be patted into the skin to create a truly velvety surface. Lines? Pores? Now you see them. And now, with these, you don't. (Our testers' favourites are on page 95.)

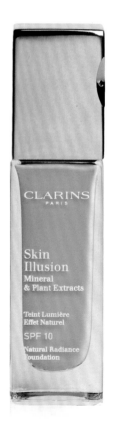

3 An anti-ageing foundation. Many foundations now have age-defying properties. These can work in several ways: through the addition of skin-caring ingredients, plus moisturisers to ensure skin looks 'plumper'. This new generation of 'anti-ageing' foundations also harnesses the power of 'optical pigments'. (Want to know which ones are worth investing in? Turn to page 90 for our testers' experiences.)

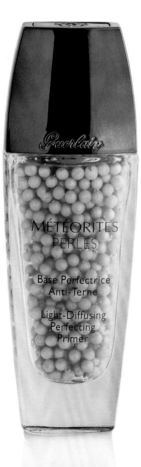

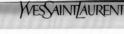

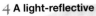

4 A light-reflective concealer. We probably get more anxious queries addressed to www. beautybible.com about dark circles than any other beauty woe. As well as effective lifestyle tips (on page 54), we bring you the low-down on the wand-style concealers which go a long way to disguising the darkest circles, and can lessen the appearance of deep grooves and lines. (For Beauty Bible award-winning concealers, go to page 91.)

5 Cream blusher. Lots of reasons to love this. First, the texture 'melts' into skin, so doesn't look dusty (which is always a risk, as we age). That makes it fairly goof-proof, too. But another reason cream blush should nudge the powder option out of your kit once you hit 35 plus is that it adds another layer of moisturising protection against the elements. (Which versions did our testers rate? See page 23.)

6 Lip pencil. Does double-duty, at this phase in life: it not only defines lips (the contours of which can become blurrier with the years), but it helps prevent lipstick from 'travelling' into feathered lines. (For the best, see page 135.)

7 Lip gloss. Recent research showed that the plumpness of lips is a way that we (subconsciously) gauge an individual's age. Lip gloss is the fast-track to a juicier pout: a smoosh on the lower lip makes them look instantly fuller. (But because not all lip glosses are created equal, you'll want to read our panellists' opinions, on page 134.)

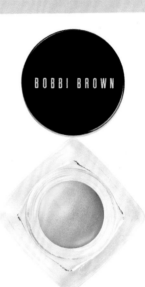

8 A bone-coloured cream eyeshadow. You can shade your eyes with a rainbow of colours, but our prescription is always to use a neutral eyeshadow as a base, first. Why? Because it evens out the skintone of the eyelids, which tends to darken and redden as we age, while at the same time creating a velvety-smooth, even base for shadow – whether that's another cream version (turn to page 70 for our testers' favourites), or powder.

9 Brow colour. Because 'not fade away' should be your beauty mantra, at this time in your life – and because defined, groomed brows help give your face much-needed structure. (The most outstanding brow pencils on the market are listed on page 64.)

10 Waterproof mascara. A boon, as we age, because waterproof mascara stays put through hot flushes and survives watery eyes. It's a fact: eyes get touchier and well up more as the years roll by. (It's hard to find a good version – one which neither gives you panda eyes by teatime, nor requires industrial-strength remover – so our testers tried them all on your behalf. See page 73 for those that 'wowed'.)

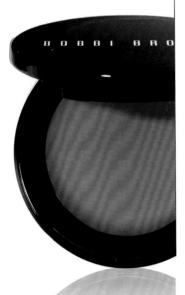

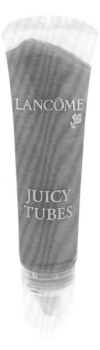

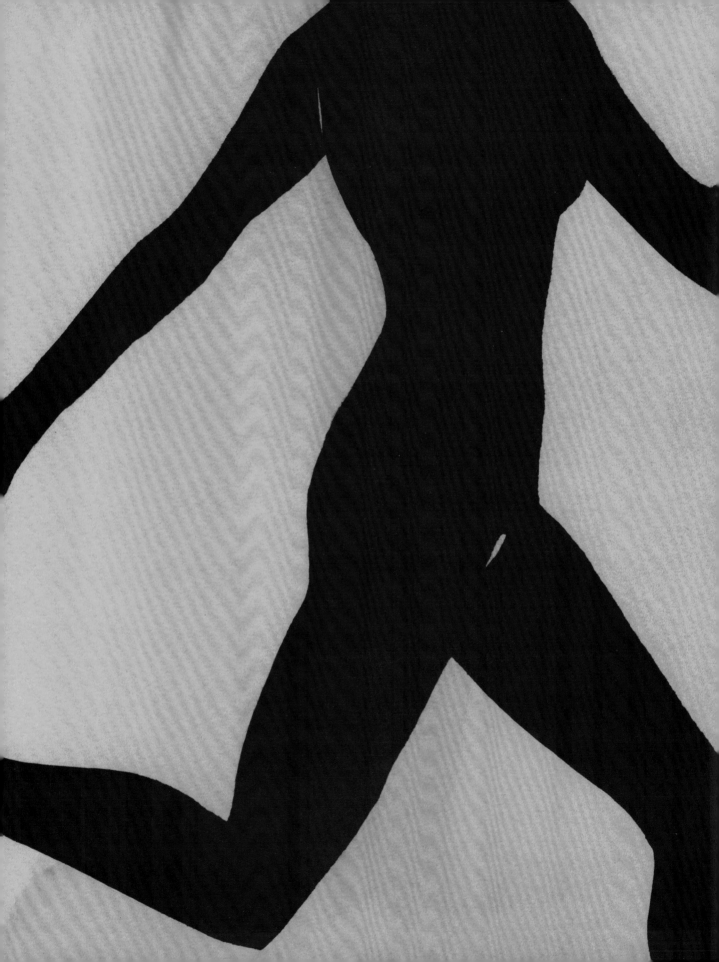

LOVE
the BODY
you're in
...and it will
LOVE YOU
right back

Be more active
(your body will love you for it)

A simple programme of daily exercises will help tone your body – and make you feel happier, too. So counteract the force of gravity by following our 10 easy steps to a firmer, fitter, more confident you…

As the T-shirt slogan goes, 'Gravity sucks'. Because after 35 (if not before), bodies start to head south. At the same time, our bodies get stiffer and less flexible. Some people embark on a major blitz to counteract this – the gym, jogging, Pilates, whatever. But the best strategy to start with is simply to become more active, all the time – then you can add your favourite exercise, as we suggest below. Being more active boosts the rate at which the body burns calories. It firms you up and (done properly) stretches you out. And it also produces feel-good hormones called endorphins so that your mood, as well as your body, feels less saggy.

So if you're standing disconsolately in front of a long mirror in your undies and wondering what on earth you can do to shape up and/or slim down, take heart. Embarking on a simple daily programme of little shifts will really make a difference to your body (and at the same time, to how you feel about showing it – on the beach, to a new lover, or in that Little Black Dress that used to fit but doesn't now). Best of all, you can start in your very own bed. (Although probably better alone, in this instance…)

1 **When you wake up,** lie straight and flat in your bed, take a few slow, deep breaths (in through your nose and very slowly out through your mouth), then lift your arms above your head and point your toes, feeling the stretch right through your body on both sides. Stretch your whole body, then each side, and finish with your whole body again.

2 **While the kettle boils,** tense your buttock muscles ten times for ten seconds each time. The more you practise this, the firmer your bottom will become, so practise whenever you're standing: waiting at the bus stop, stirring a pan, queueing to pay in a shop, etc.

3 **While you brush your teeth** for the recommended three minutes morning and evening, squat down with your back against the wall or door. (It feels weird, but it's a great stretch.)

4 **When you're watching TV,** hide the remote control and when you get up to change channels, do ten squats to tone your upper thighs. As you squat down, with your back straight, push your weight down through your heels so the front of your thighs work harder.

5 **Tone up your arms and bingo wings** by pushing light weights above your head: do ten pushes at a time, as many times a day as you can. No weights? Use cans of baked beans. (We love baked beans – to eat! – especially with a slurp of olive oil and grated Parmesan.)

6 Lose five pounds by improving your posture…
• Stand up straight, as if the crown of your head is suspended from a thread in the ceiling/sky.
• Let your shoulders sink down and back: feel as if your shoulder blades are meeting at the back.
• Do a few shoulder rolls both ways while you are sitting at your desk or on the train.
• Walk like a cat (think model on catwalk…), hips swinging forward with your big toe leading.

7 Walk briskly everywhere you can, swinging your arms (put belongings in a backpack – the kind that fastens across your front is easiest if you carry a lot). Look for hills and climb stairs rather than using the lift. Get in the habit of striding out for at least 15 minutes in the evenings to help you relax. You should aim for 10,000 steps a day – easy to calculate if you have a pedometer.

8 Every time you get up from a chair, consciously pull your belly button in towards your spine to work your tummy muscles. If you are picking up things from the floor, bend sideways while pulling in your tummy to help smooth your love handles.

9 Finally, do exercise you enjoy. Whether it's walking or swimming, dancing or yoga, riding or fencing, if you look forward to it you are far more likely to stick with it and get a feel-good double whammy. Aim for at least 30 minutes, five days a week.

10 Make all of this a habit. It takes 16 to 21 times of repeating an activity for it to become a habit – so in less than a month, all this can become second nature. And by then you should look very luscious in that Little Black Dress.

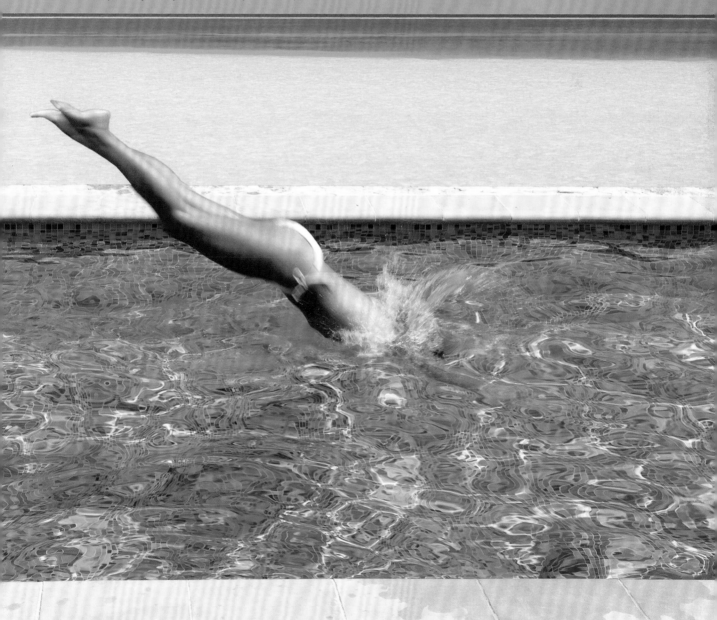

First, find your MIRACLE

For this new and revised edition, we've tested 148 new anti-ageing 'miracle' products on our ten women panels, who've put hundreds and hundreds of 'dream creams' through their paces. This process serves to confirm what we've known for years: that there really are creams and serums that lift the years from your face. But the challenge is this: how on earth do you find out which ones…? Well, there's no need for (expensive) trial and error – because our testers have done the research for you. Excitingly, this latest round of testing revealed more very high-scoring products than ever before, with three new entries.

The diligence of our trials means that we get support for what we do from the whole beauty industry, who happily supply products for our trials – from high street/ supermarket anti-agers right through to the priciest creams on the market. Our ten-women tester panels were under strict instructions: use the treatment on one side of your face, observe and note any immediate improvements, then after two weeks, and finally, at the end of the tube or jar. (NB: Many of our testers started out cynical – and were converted.)

OK, so no cream is going to make you look 17 again, waving a wand to magic away every line and wrinkle. But the scores here are high. So: there really ARE products which, as well as softening and smoothing your complexion, can help plump out deeper lines, make smaller ones disappear, firm skin tissue – and turbo-charge the glow. (For more 'miracles' – in the form of specific night treatments – please see page 156, while miracle serums are on page 172.)

Now, just before you dive in… While, as we've said, we tested all price ranges for this book, the simple truth is that all the top scoring ones are pretty pricey – even after this latest extensive round of testing. But on page 19 you will find a rundown of more moderately-priced creams (around £25 for 50ml at current prices).

Something for every age-defying beauty, we think…

Anti-ageing miracle creams: our award winners

REVIEWS

Temple Spa Skin Truffle Total Face Rejuvenation

 9.31/10 A truly stupendous score: the highest we've ever had for an all-round, all-singing-and-dancing miracle cream, in 18 years of Beauty Bible testing. (Not that Sarah's surprised: she's long been a Skin Truffle-ette.) Diamond powder, gold and silk clearly do illuminate the skin from first application, testers report; other key ingredients include black truffles, grapeseed champagne, purifying strawberries and lush cocoa butter, in a cashmere-soft formulation.
Comments: 'Oh, this is a wonderful cream: I'm so in love with it you can look out for the announcement in *The Times*! Skintone is brighter and all my nasty lines – even the deeper ones – appear to have lessened' • 'face looks younger and not a needle in sight' • 'skin looks glowy and dewy, forehead grooves smaller – and husband says I look great' • 'the best anti-ageing moisturiser I've ever used – fantastic miracle product; skin looks like I have a luminising primer on, even when not wearing make-up' • 'gives a definite glow to the skin with improvements in brightness, softness, crêpiness, fine lines' • 'noticed a difference in texture, smoothness and brightness within days' • 'gives an "instant lift" to skin' • 'my husband and my mum both said I looked really healthy – fine lines were rendered invisible and I really loved the radiance'.

Philosophy The Microdelivery Peel

 9.31/10 Not a miracle cream but this at home peel, now a joint top-scorer, is definitely a miracle product for resurfacing and replenishing the skin, effectively smoothing, brightening and evening the tone, according to our testers who all received compliments. The two-step process, which Philosophy recommends using weekly, involves mixing granules to a 'thick sugary syrup, almost like icing, which smelt gorgeous and citrusy', then applying a gel that forms a light foam and gives a warming sensation. Philosophy founder Cristina Carlino pioneered lunchtime peels among other doctor procedures and this is her home version. NB You must apply sunscreen diligently.
Comments: 'I could not stop using this and have already bought more; after first use, my skin was smoother and brighter, after two weeks, pores were smaller, crêpiness improved, skin much brighter, fine lines and wrikles slightly better' • 'skin really silky, plumped and more even, definite improvement in fine lines, frown lines and crêpiness' • 'amazing results, fantastic product that really lifted the appearance of my skin' • 'I was concerned that it might be abrasive however it was very gentle and husband complimented me' • 'I followed the directions for sensitive skin after experiencing a little irritation, and then had none; made skin visibly younger. I loved it.'

Kiehl's Super Multi-Corrective Cream

 9.19/10 This 'Super' cream from a long-established US company exploits three powerful natural actives – Jasmonic acid, beech tree extract derivative and fragmented hyaluronic acid – in a cutting edge formula to address the problem of damaged older skin, which takes over 30 hours to repair, compared to six hours for young skin. Kiehl's own consumer tests showed signicant improvement in wrinkles, elasticity, firmness, texture, pore size and radiance within two weeks, with a double whammy in four. Our testers were wow-ed too.
Comments: 'This product is amazing, thick but light, luxurious, smells divine and the side I trialled it on is so soft, plumped up, radiant and hydrated – and fine lines smoothed. I am now a Kiehl's convert' • 'love this product, which has made a real difference, texture now very smooth, no sensitive redness which I had been suffering and

AT A GLANCE

Temple Spa Skin Truffle Total Face Rejuvenation

Philosophy The Microdelivery Peel

Kiehl's Super Multi-Corrective Cream

Pevonia Timeless Repair Cream

L'Occitane Immortelle Divine Cream

Decléor Excellence de l'Âge Sublime Regenerating Cream

Emma Hardie Age Support Treatment Cream

Filorga Time-Filler

If you know you have
sensitive skin and you
want to try a powerful
anti-ageing treatment,
go carefully. Start by
using the product two
or three times a week,
and build up from
there. Alternatively, do
a 'patch test' (using
the crook of your
elbow or the skin just
behind the ear), and
check for any redness/
irritation/flakiness
24 hours later. If that
happens, you may be
one of the people who
simply can't tolerate
some ingredients –
and if you do suffer a
reaction, it is always
worth taking the
product back to the
counter (although
the beauty industry
will probably have
hit-men trained on
us for suggesting
this). Sometimes a
sympathetic sales
consultant feels
empowered to give
you a refund, confident
that you'll be back
again in future. (Which
you certainly won't be,
if they don't.)

corrected dehydration and unevenness; I have a pink glow on my cheeks instead of brillo pad redness' • 'wrinkles seem greatly reduced, make-up glides on a lot better and gives more of a dewy look, colleagues say how fresh I am looking' • 'you only need a very little; skin looks bright, alive and healthy; friends says how well I look'.

Pevonia Timeless Repair Cream ✳

Best known through its widespread spa distribution, Pevonia's age-proofing award-winner also features luxe ingredients like caviar, pearl and something called 'Escutox', alongside green olive squalene, brightening lemon peel oil, chamomile – and an SPF8 (not enough for protection in all but the dingiest months, we'd counsel). It's got a pretty fragrance – a touch of honeysuckle, we'd say, to further enhance application pleasure.

Comments: 'My face literally felt as if it was drinking it in: after application, one half of my face felt supple and soft and looked rested' • 'a Holy grail find' • 'after two days, let alone two weeks, I was in love with this product: my skin's brighter, softer, smoother and it has helped with fine lines and skin tone' • 'didn't want to see the bottom of the pot! I love this and hope if I hint strongly enough my husband/sons might be generous enough to buy me some more' • 'love this: have never used anything before with such a dramatic effect on my skin – after six weeks my face was starting to look lop-sided – seems to be acting like a facelift on the side I'm using it on' • 'fabulously soft skin, much better under chin' • 'bigger wrinkles in particular were reduced; I have some large grooves which seemed to improve' • 'skin firmer and plumper, even forehead grooves less prominent – and big thumbs-up from my husband!'.

L'Occitane Immortelle Divine Cream ✳

This truly 'divine' high-scoring award-winner has gone on – justifiably – to become a global anti-ageing bestseller and a new anti-ageing 'classic' since the first edition of this book. (Jo's a massive convert, too.) It's helped put L'Occitane firmly on the map as a serious skincare brand, with its fabulously aromatic formulation (featuring lavish quantities of Corsican Immortelle, 'the flower that never dies'), together with myrtle and other key anti-agers. Enriched with 34 per cent plant oils, Divine Cream is formulated to boost cell regeneration and 'increase cellular

vitality', which translates to enhanced radiance.

Comments: 'Love the texture and smell, it took a little while to sink in but it was worth the wait; skin instantly looked brighter and much smoother and plumped; after two weeks, fine lines around mouth much less noticeable and skin much more supple, and the improvements continued: my husband said my skin was looking nice and for him to notice is quite remarkable' • 'my skin hasn't looked so good for a long time, so much brighter I look as if I've had a good night's sleep; crêpiness, fine lines, grooves all reduced – a fantastic product and I got lots of positive comments' • 'lovely thick product with fabulous smell, absorbed very well and skin felt so hydrated and really supple; definitely boosts the skin; but do give it five or ten minutes before applying make-up' • 'complexion was more plump, less drawn, less sagging, with really nice bright glow, eyes glowed too and normally ruddy complexion reduced'.

Decléor Excellence de l'Âge Sublime Regenerating Cream

A day cream (Decléor like their customers to use oils at night), this meltingly-smooth cream-textured cream works to enhance firmness, smoothness, hydration, and to even out skintone. As you'd expect from an aromatherapy brand, fragrance is an important part of the pleasure factor, although this is powdery/creamy (with notes of sandalwood, amber and peach) rather than 'botanically-scented'.

Comments: 'I was dubious as this cream looked too rich and thick for my oily combination skin but it is amazing, after five weeks skin looks luminous, almost glass-like, firmer, smoother and springy to the touch – rejuvenated' • 'fine lines reduced, deeper grooves too, and crêpiness? There is none! This cream really makes me look better and younger, lots of people have commented' • 'immediate discernable improvements, skin felt softer, less dry, fine lines plumped out and after two weeks, skin looks more youthful, fine lines less visible, skin around eyes and lips less dry and crêpey, overall more radiant and fresh-looking – works wonders on an ageing face' • 'skin looks brighter and love the texture and scent'.

Emma Hardie Age Support Treatment Cream

From a wonderful facialist who started off 'lifting and sculpting' faces with her hands and then launched her Amazing Face range (which is amazing) comes this new nourishing moisturiser plus treatment cream for older faces. Deliciously scented and stuffed with naturals including marine and botanical extracts plus avocado peptides, it's designed for am and/or pm and promises to reduce signs of ageing and reddening of the skin (it has an anti-inflammatory action too), increase luminosity as well as protecting it from environmental pollutants and preventing collagen loss.

Comments: 'It absorbed quickly and skin felt velvety smooth immediately; after two weeks, skin looked full and healthy and felt super soft, as well as more radiant; I felt positive and uplifted when I used it' • 'skin looked brighter for sure, smooth and softer' • 'definite improvement on deeper lines around the sides of my mouth; definitely makes me look as if I have had a good night's sleep, when unfortunately I haven't' • 'compliments from my daughter who is a hard critic!' • 'surprised how quickly I saw results in hydration and clarity; I use a lot less make-up which is always a sign that my skin looks more even – a great confidence booster' • 'seems to put back what life's taken out'.

Filorga Time-Filler

 A couple of products from this French super-haute-tech brand have snuck into this book. We're not surprised as Filorga's already a beauty editors' firm favourite. But the extravagance of the promises made for this rich gel-like cream is pretty off-the-scale: 'filler-like', 'Botox-like', 'peeling-like' are some of the adjectives used, with suggestions it will plump up wrinkles with a combination of high-weight hyaluronic acid, antioxidant vitamin E, and Synake: an ingredient Filorga insist is able to block the receptors responsible for muscle contractions. Hype or not, testers liked what they actually saw for themselves.

Comments: '10/10 for this lovely moisturiser that ticks all the boxes. Skin felt smoother, softer and plumper overnight; after two weeks I had to use it on both sides as the first side looked so good. Can't praise it enough…' • 'I also applied to my chest and body, it just smoothed the lines out' • 'noticeable improvement after two weeks: fine lines around eyes have nearly disappeared, also enlarged pores on my cheeks, my skin looks plumper, brighter and younger' • 'a really great product, now part of my skin care routine, not too expensive, economical to use and I am really pleased with the improvements to my skin'.

Beauty Steals

In general, 'miracle creams' tend to be pricey, partly reflecting the research and development and, more often, the high cost of the ingredients. But our testers did award high marks to these products, which we believe really do qualify as beauty steals for budget-watching times.

Nourish Argan Skin Renew

 Created by organic skincare expert Dr Pauline Hili, this range ticks all the 'green goddess' boxes – ethically sourced, organically certified, vegan – Nourish sets out to be a happy marriage of nature and science. A significant score for this pot of deliciousness which features rose of Jericho, frankincense and a bunch of skin-nourishing botanicals, as well as argan oil.

Comments: 'Skin immediately more hydrated and plumped, after two weeks much more glowing, brighter and more even toned' • 'amazing brightness! I looked much more awake; by end of testing skin was tauter, smoother and generally younger looking' • 'I love the smell and even the funny texture now – my skin is brighter, smoother, clearer – younger!' • 'a visible improvement: I was very impressed'.

Argan Organics Regeneration Skin Smoothing Face Serum

Equally successful with our testers was another argan-based product, this time a serum (though testers thought it more like an oil), which also offers rosehip, evening primrose, macadamia and pumpkin oil with an anti-ageing blend of essential oils. This hand-made Scottish range (a favourite of Judy Murray, which Sarah likes too) was founded by scientist and mother of three Aileen Smith, whose farming family had a long interest in herbs.

Comments: 'Skin immediately looked soft, smooth, healthy and luminous, after two weeks more plumped out; a little goes a long way so great value' • 'subtle improvement in skin brightness and crêpiness, eye area a bit less puffy, I really like this product – price is brilliant' • 'skin is softer, healthier-looking and more even'.

Manuka Doctor Api-Nourish Repairing Skin Cream

We've always been fans of this bee-based range, and testers agree. This light day cream (more like a serum said some testers) features a natural anti-ageing cocktail of purified bee venom, Manuka honey and royal jelly, together with vitamin E, and claims to make skin more radiant within four weeks. Our testers support this… NB One tester experienced temporary slight tingliness and blotchiness on first use.

Comments: '10/10. Sinks in very easily and quickly, make-up goes on easily – skin softer and smoother which helps a youthful appearance. I really like the texture and ease of use' • 'skin felt firmer and looked more even after two weeks, great non-greasy moisturiser for normal to oily skin, also evened out my pigmentation' • 'skin much brighter-looking, firmer around the eye area, smoother and lines softened generally, big reduction in wrinkles and grooves'.

βPlump up your cheeks!

If you're looking pale and wan and your cheeks (like the rest of you) are beginning to head south, you can create a brighter, more uplifting appearance in next to no time…

Every woman with a thinnish face knows that when you're tired or under par, you're liable to look a lot less than radiant – peaky, sad and, at worst, like Lady Macbeth's rather haggard first cousin (as Sarah knows all too well…). As the years go by, the upsides of a slender form mean your cheeks tend to drift downwards with the rest of your body. But there are immediate ways to give your cheeks (and thus your whole face) a lift – plus some mid- to long-term strategies which we promise can transform you.

For instant lift, apply a 'pop' of blush to your cheeks (see overleaf for more). And marvel at the mirror…!

Pinch your cheeks. No blusher? Gently pat and pinch your cheeks for a few seconds until they glow rosy pink. Better still, if you have five or ten minutes, do some star-jumps.

Pop on some earrings. Sparkly, shiny or lovely fat pearls, in colours that flatter your skintone – and never, ever dangly. If you can, find ones that wing their way upwards, taking your face with them. (Sarah's favourite pair are rather Art Nouveau-ish wings in blue, green and amber-y faceted glass.)

Sweep your hair up. Brush your hair back and up, clip it on top, pop in pretty combs, roll into a pleat… Anything to take the eye of the beholder upwards.

Try milk! Drinking it, that is – which is a suggestion given to us by Beverly Hills make-up artist Valerie Sarnelle. One of her starry clients (there's a galaxy flashing in and out of her elegant salon) – a *femme d'un certain âge* with divinely plumptious cheeks above her slender form – told Valerie they were due not to cosmetic fillers but milk! We suggest organic full-fat milk from grass-fed moos because it should have more conjugated linoleic acid (CLA), which may help your facial muscles. (Cheeks are the 'meatiest' part of your face, and increasing muscle mass will make them look fuller.) Milk will definitely give you magnesium – great for your mind as it's a natural tranquilliser, and helps with teeth, bones, muscles and sleep, among lots of other things. (We love magnesium!)

Apply skincare products upwards. Whenever you apply skin cream, oil or lotion, always stroke upwards from your chin to your cheekbones, then out to your temples. Facial therapist Suzie Mitchell suggests: 'Put a little facial oil or cream in one palm and rub your hands together, then smooth over the face, neck and bosom. Rather than fingertips, use the big muscle in the cushion at the base of your thumb, always working upwards. Start by fanning out over and round your neck, then work round and up your jaw and cheekbones to the temples, then across and up your forehead to your hairline. Repeat, covering the whole face for five to ten minutes. The oil or cream will be absorbed, skin velvety, and your face look rosy and "lifted".'

Pop some supplements. Consider supplementing with omega-3 essential fatty acids, hyaluronic acid (HA) plus Sun Chlorella. The first two keep skin cells

For *instant* lift, apply a 'pop' of *BLUSH* to your cheeks, and *MARVEL* at the mirror!

FACE-PLUMPING EXERCISES

NB: We recommend doing these exercises in private…!

1 Put a finger in your mouth, close your lips round it and suck on your finger for five to ten seconds, as hard as you can while sucking in your cheeks. It's like a child making a fish face. Release, and repeat 15 more times. This will help strengthen your cheek muscles and enhance the circulation and oxygen flow to your face, so your cheeks look more pink and full. It also helps prevent lip lines.

2 Tone your cheeks by placing your fingertips on top of your cheekbones. Now inhale and tilt your chin down towards your collarbone; exhale and push the skin and muscle fibres of the cheekbones upwards. Then open and close your mouth five to ten times, feeling the muscles tightening as you do so. Do this three times a day or as often as you can.

3 Place your index finger and middle finger on each cheek and then slowly rub in a circular motion. This will stimulate the muscles, which will thicken them up and cause them to look fuller. (It also makes your cheeks rosy!)

at optimum lipid (fat) and hydration levels, and we also suggest Sun Chlorella A, a Japanese brand, to keep your gut happy; it really does show on your face, due to the two pairs of stomach meridians which run down the face – one pair down the sides to the chin, one pair from under the eyes to the chin. If your tum's upset, your face gets longer and more gaunt; keep your gut in good shape and you won't believe the difference! Sarah's skin plumped and peachified almost incredibly when she started taking Sun Chlorella, which she anticipates taking for life. (Also see the Supergreens Facelift Diet, page 176.)

Sign up for a course of facial acupuncture. And have regular maintenance sessions (see page 155).

TIP

Supermodel Carmen dell'Orefice recommends doing any inverted (upside down) yoga pose, such as Downward-facing Dog, to bring colour to your face. If you don't practise yoga, simply plant your feet a hip-width apart then try touching your toes. Hang there for a few seconds as the blood pours to your head.

Keep regular appointments with the dentist. Teeth and gums need to be in optimal shape to support your facial bone structure.

And if slimming down rather than plumping up your face is your problem, see our section on facial contouring, on page 44.

Blush becomingly

A subtle hint of pink blusher applied to the cheeks will bring a youthful glow to your complexion (and we mean subtle – you certainly want to avoid an alarming doll- or clown-like appearance). And it's uplifting too. Here's how to make it work for you…

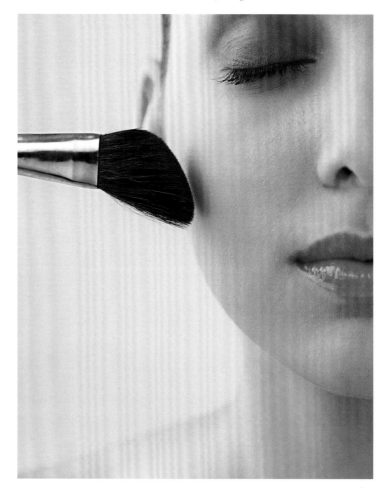

Choose a transparent rose blusher. 'By mid-life you are naturally losing that youthful "rosiness",' explains Terry de Gunzburg, 'and you want to recreate that. That doesn't mean turning into a babydoll, but finishing with a hint of blush: a nude rose or a transparent rose, even a pinkish coral, high on the cheeks. Even if you have "couperose" [rosacea/redness], it's very important, but in that case use a beige-y rose. Blusher gives an instant "lifting" effect.'

If you prefer powder blushers, try Chanel Joues Contraste in No 15 Orchid Rose. We're mostly cream blusher girls but less dry skins may be fine with powder. This looks really muddy in the compact but in fact it's a whisper-light soft rose that Mary Greenwell uses on everyone on the planet, with (as we now realise) good reason.

Use the right brushes. Of course cream blushers can be applied with fingers, but we find the best way to apply cream blusher (and to get longer-lasting results) is with a foundation brush; just 'feather' it into the skin with the lightest touch. Jo uses the flip side of her regular foundation brush, but if you do the same, you need to be religious about washing your brushes once a week or the blusher shade starts to 'pinkify' the foundation (to be avoided at all costs). For a powder blusher, apply an angled blusher brush with the short side on top, laid against your

cheekbone, to wrap the colour around without overloading it. Try them out in store to find one with a handle that suits your grip – personally we don't like too-short handles, but they might suit you.

Remember: nobody blushes brown. Because many women with high colour are scared that pink blusher will draw attention to that, they're tempted to use bronzer instead of blusher, so that it won't pick up the redness. Don't go there. Instead, use foundation to tone down that redness and then – as above – a very soft pinky shade on the top.

And never forget that less really is more. You need a whisper of colour not warpaint.

Cream blushers: *our award winners*

We trialled many new launches for this edition of the book (making almost 50, in all), requesting suits-all-skintone shades – usually a mid-rose tone. The challenge we set our testers: identify the brands which deliver a healthy flush that looks subtly, naturally glow-y – but crucially, stays put too

REVIEWS

Bobbi Brown Pot Rouge for Lips and Cheeks

9/10

This does double-duty: use as a cheek tint – as our testers do – but it is also designed to use on lips. (Bobbi's memory of her grandmother using lipstick on her cheeks inspired this product.) It's creamy but sheer – with a matt finish – and now comes in a mirrored flip-top compact for on-the-spot application. Nine shades; our lot got Pale Pink this time. Here are testers' thoughts.

Comments: 'Loved this: can be adapted to suit the effect you desire and stays put all day' • 'naturally glowing, long-lasting – didn't need reapplying all day' • 'first time I've used a cream blush – love it, and the fact you can use it on lips too' • 'so easy to apply with fingers – very smooth, no dragging, with a colour that appears natural and bright' • 'gives a fantastic glow – like the healthy cheeks I used to have 30 years ago'.

Bourjois Cream Blush

8.67/10

Historical fact: Bourjois' first baked powder blush was created in 1868. Now their latest rose-scented formula (in a mirror-lidded compact) offers cream-powder technology: it goes on as a cream then becomes a silky powder on your cheek.

Comments: 'sheer with slight shimmer that makes it look slightly dewy – perfect blush for summer; lasted all day' • 'I experimented with brush and fingers – preferred the latter; used lightly for a healthy glow in the daytime then a bit more for a more obvious blush for evening – a real find and prime price' • 'fabulous texture and very easy product to apply'.

AT A GLANCE

Bobbi Brown Pot Rouge for Lips and Cheeks

Bourjois Cream Blush

Liz Earle Healthy Glow Cream Blush

L'Oreal Nude Magique BB Blush

Elizabeth Arden Ceramide Cream Blush

♡ WE LOVE...

In Jo's kit you'll find several favourites: Liz Earle Colour Healthy Glow Cream Blush in Nude, and a divine compact from Aerin Lauder's signature Aerin range: Multi Color for Lip and Cheeks, in 01 Natural. As well as Liz Earle's offering (above), Sarah is devoted to Charlotte Tilbury Beach Stick Moon Beach Lip to Cheek Dewy Colour Pop, which is perfect for summer.

Liz Earle Healthy Glow Cream Blush

8.5/10

Small user-friendly palette, with mirrored lid, makes applying a swoosh of healthy colour the work of seconds. The creamy, semi-sheer formula, with skin-nourishing vitamin E, is designed to be used with fingertips.

Comments: 'I hated cream blushes 'til I tried this – it's a make-up must-have and I am never without it' • 'effortless to apply, blend and a joy to use: colour so natural and lovely, and didn't dry or age my skin – or emphasise pores' • 'also used it on my lips – a dream product'.

L'Oreal Nude Magique BB Blush

8.17/10

It's 'Magique' because this transparent blush magically adapts to each and every skin tone. So there's no need to choose your shade because the universal tint chooses you.... Smart.

Comments: 'Colour looks impossibly clown-pink at first but becomes a sheer gel with a hint of extremely natural pink when you blend it on the cheeks' • 'a brilliant product and I really like the tube' • 'SUPER! My cheeks look divine, with such a healthy glow and softer – I ADORE this fabulous product'.

Elizabeth Arden Ceramide Cream Blush

7.67/10

We normally request brands to send products in just one shade for our trials, but Elizabeth Arden sent a selection of Honey, Nectar and Plum blushers – and testers found them all pleasingly natural-looking. Skin-caring ceramides are a key ingredient for this brand, here helping to deliver a silky, dewy finish – and this is also enriched with vitamins A, C and E, in a mirrored brushed gold-effect compact.

Comments: 'This product gave a very natural glow without that harsh blusher line that you sometimes see' • 'I'm a new mum who's had about two hours' sleep for the past 10 weeks and this blush perked up my skin beautifully' • 'I now use this every day and have binned the powder blush!' • 'made my cheeks look like I've been out in the fresh air: a soft, natural glow' • 'useful mirror' • 'colour and finish long-lasting even on hot days' • 'a good product to perk you up whenever you're looking tired'.

'When you're *younger*, you want to be PERFECT, but *later* you learn that perfect isn't really that INTERESTING'

Susan Sarandon

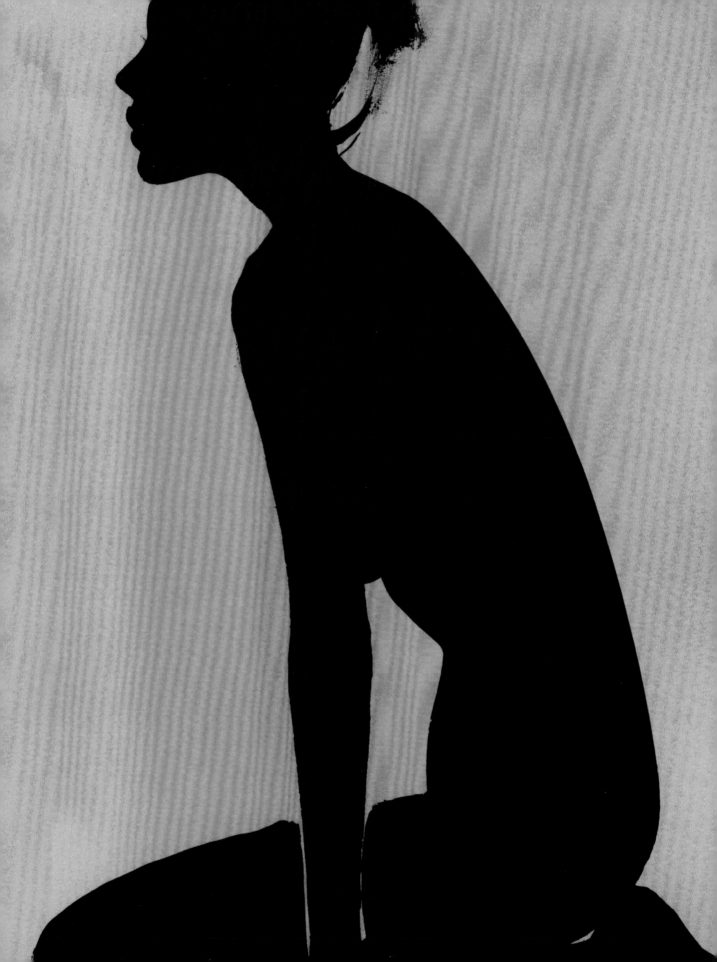

Body: how to look better naked (*truly*)

We have a sneaking admiration for nudists of mature years, who throw caution (and just about everything else) to the wind, and go naked. (And even play badminton or volleyball *au naturel*.) Are we about to do the same? Not for all the tea in Fortnum's…

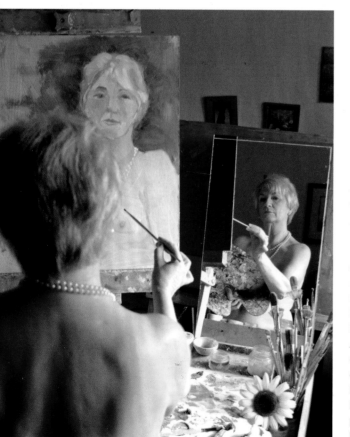

Bodies, like our faces, show signs of gravity and sun damage. And often they're more neglected than our faces: swathed in layers of clothing for much of the year puts crêpey skin, bingo wings and even saggy knees out of sight – and off our beautycare radar. Even when it's roastingly hot, we see many women hiding under kaftans and sarongs feeling self-conscious about a body that's less than Elle Macpherson-esque.

But the naked truth is that nobody is ever going to judge you as harshly as you judge yourself. Just think of that little mental dialogue when you shop for a swimsuit: 'Omigod, look at my backside.' Contrast that to the thoughts running through a man's head when he catches sight of you naked: 'Whoo-hoooo!'

However, there are ways for every woman to feel a bit more 'Whoo-hoooo' about her own body. Overleaf, you can read about creams to slather on which, according to our testers, really can help body skin be more resilient, more velvety, more bare-able (and stroke-able, too). But there's a lot more that you can do to look better naked – which in turn, makes you feel better in your clothes. We just love that French phrase: '*être bien dans sa peau*' – literally 'to be good in your skin' – meaning 'to be content with yourself', which we think is definitely worth aspiring to. So, here are some suggestions that we're confident will make you feel that bit more comfortable in your own skin…

Stand up straight. Good posture not only makes you look an inch or two taller, but magically takes an inch or two off your mid-section, by un-sagging it. We've explained this on page 15, but it's so vital that here it is again! Imagine lifting your ribcage as if there was a string going up from your breastbone to the ceiling. At the same time, gently pull your shoulder blades back and down. It's pretty easy to remember to do this every time you catch sight of yourself in a mirror, but you want to make more of a habit of it than that. For enhancing posture permanently, nothing beats Pilates (though yoga and the Alexander Technique come pretty close), through which you become much more aware of how you're standing, sitting and moving. And strengthening the core muscles in the tummy (the aim of Pilates) and the obliques creates an invisible 'corset' around the body, flattening your abs with absolutely no need for Playtex or Spanx.

Soften your water... and you'll soften your skin. Hard water is really drying, leaving skin looking and feeling papery. If you aren't sure whether your water is hard or soft, try the soap test: if your soap lathers extremely well and is hard to rinse away, it's soft. If it lathers only moderately and leaves skin rapidly squeaky-clean upon rinsing – or if there's a chalky residue on your shower door or curtain – then it's hard. You can actually buy a gizmo which fits into your shower to help remove the minerals, softening the water you use for washing your body. (See DIRECTORY, or simply Google 'shower water filter'.) The lower-tech alternative for dealing with the effects of hard water is to keep baths and showers short – under five minutes, if possible. Use a mild soap and use it only in areas of skin folds – underarms, neck, feet and, er, 'bits'.

Quit smoking... We can give you a gazillion reasons why you'll be better off not smoking, but in this case it's because the swirl of smoke around your body has an ageing effect on skin, bombarding it with free radicals – which break down collagen and elastin. There's some suggestion that smokers have a more negative body image, and the more a woman smokes, the worse she feels about herself.

...and get moving. On the other hand, the act of exercising actually makes you feel better about your body (never mind the physical improvements), according to a study from the University of Florida.

Get rid of 'goosebumps'. Shy to take that summer cardie off because of your bumpy upper arms? Blitz with a twice-weekly scrub. If that doesn't beat the problem, you may have an inherited skin condition called keratosis pilaris (KP), for which a consultant dermatologist recommends using a product called Dermol 500, with Vaseline Intensive Care Lotion to remoisturise afterwards. In fact, we recommend body-scrubbing to everyone as a preparation for any anti-ageing body lotion/butter/oil: a top-to-toe rub-down with a sugar- or salt-and-oil-based scrub, followed by moisturiser, is an instant skin makeover.

Tackle dry shins. Skin over the shins is particularly prone to dryness and can even develop cracks that look like a dry river-bed. Also, observes beauty therapist extraordinaire Nichola Joss, 'We're generally unaware how much waxing and shaving can dry out the skin.' There's another good reason for keeping shin skin supple: later in life, this is where leg ulcers can develop – hard to shift and unpleasant to live with. Prevention is very definitely better than cure, here. We cannot recommend too highly that you try This Works Skin Deep Dry Leg Oil, which we love because it's absolutely miraculous for easing the itchiness and

TIP

If you're heading for a 'red carpet'-type event, you might want to consider this advice from Kylie Minogue: 'My real skin tip is that I use all-over body make-up, which makes a real difference because you get this even, lovely finish everywhere. When you hit forty, you need a little more help.' Recommended products are Per-fékt Body Perfection Gel, a gel-mousse that slides on to give a natural build-upable coverage and smooth airbrushed glow, and Prtty Peaushun Skin Tight Body Lotion, a natural product with light-reflecting particles devised by Hollywood make-up artist Bethany Karlyn, which helps even out skin tone and enhance muscle tone. MAC does a range of body make-up, including Face and Body Foundation, which is water resistant and available in a wide range of colours.

tautness of dry shins. You could also follow Nichola's advice: 'Use a body oil first because it penetrates deeper into the skin, then double up with cream on top to hold the moisture in.'

Apply a self-tanner. According to all the beauty pros we know, the very fastest way to look slimmer is with a body self-tanner, which helps create the illusion of a slimmer body (a little like the way darker clothes do). Self-tanner can also help conceal the dimpling and puckering from cellulite. If you're self-tan-phobic, we recommend one of the gradual options which can be massaged into the skin in circular movements, just as if you were applying a body lotion: favourites with Beauty Bible testers include St Tropez Gradual Tan Everyday Body, Crème de la Mer The Face and Body Gradual Tan, Palmer's Cocoa Butter Formula Natural Bronze and Dove Summer Glow Nourishing Lotion.

Use camouflage. If you're self-conscious about red veins on your feet and legs, you have three options: make-up, sclerotherapy or lasers (see page 203). Sclerotherapy (generally using local injections of saline) has been tried-and-tested over the years and it's a fraction of the price of lasering (for questions to ask before venturing into either of these procedures, see page 46). But for occasional pin-baring, Nichola Joss recommends concealing veins (or other blemishes) with Laura Mercier Secret Camouflage concealer, which works as well on legs as it does on faces: she advises applying with fingers as the warmth helps the make-up 'meld' into skin for a seamless finish. It's pretty budge-proof, too. (And see also our suggestion above about self-tanner: flaws of all kinds are infinitely less visible when the rest of the leg is 'sun-kissed'.)

Gloss up. Polish off your body make-over with a spritz of 'dry' (ie, non-greasy) body oil on shoulders and bosom (we love Melvita L'Or Bio Sparkling Oil), and a slick of varnish on toes and hands.

Anti-ageing body treatments: *our award winners*

The women we know are finally waking up to the fact that, yes, skincare should extend below the neck-line. In fact, right down to your toes. Firming, smoothing and moisturising ingredients can deliver rapid results, improving dull, papery, flaky (and even saggy) body skin – and with it dramatically boosting body confidence

AT A GLANCE

Emma Hardie Natural Lift & Sculpt Body Butter

Liz Earle Nourishing Botanical Body Cream

Decléor Aroma Sculpt Divine Rejuvenating Cream

This Works Skin Deep Dry Leg Oil

Pevonia Botanica Ligne Tropicale De-Aging Body Balm

Bombshell Body Show-Off Body Lotion

Crystal Clear Velvet Skin

We tested lots more new entries for this latest edition, dispatching creams, butters and oils which made a big difference to the resilience, smoothness and touch-me-softness of arms, legs, bums and tums. (Though if it's cellulite you want to blitz, see page 38.) So which texture – lotion, oil, cream, serum – and fragrance (or not) should you go for? We suggest choosing whatever you'll enjoy most – because as our testers found, that's what inspires regular use. And goodness, how they enjoyed these – with three outstanding new entries.

REVIEWS

Emma Hardie Natural Lift & Sculpt Body Butter ✻

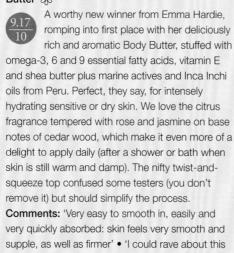

9.17 / 10 A worthy new winner from Emma Hardie, romping into first place with her deliciously rich and aromatic Body Butter, stuffed with omega-3, 6 and 9 essential fatty acids, vitamin E and shea butter plus marine actives and Inca Inchi oils from Peru. Perfect, they say, for intensely hydrating sensitive or dry skin. We love the citrus fragrance tempered with rose and jasmine on base notes of cedar wood, which make it even more of a delight to apply daily (after a shower or bath when skin is still warm and damp). The nifty twist-and-squeeze top confused some testers (you don't remove it) but should simplify the process.
Comments: 'Very easy to smooth in, easily and very quickly absorbed: skin feels very smooth and supple, as well as firmer' • 'I could rave about this all day long; quite possibly my favourite body product ever and I am an ex-beauty therapist; loved the luxurious smell, skin tone also appeared more even' • 'left a constant improvement with regular use, even great on sunburnt and/or freshly shaved skin with no irritation' • 'expensive but goes a long way' • 'best for night time – skin looked instantly moisturised and glowing with a nice sheen'.

Liz Earle Nourishing Botanical Body Cream ✻

9.07 / 10 High scoring new entry from this multi-award winning range, originally launched by beauty editor Liz Earle, who is still very much involved with the whole UK operation. As with all the products this concentrated hydrating body cream contains lots of natural actives, including softening shea butter and avocado oil, plus antioxidants in the shape of natural source vitamin E and beta-carotene, and is fragrant with essential oils of orange, lavender and rose-scented geranium.
Comments: 'A delight which far outstrips many more expensive products; divine smell and does as much for your mind as it does for the condition of your skin. I used it on one shin with my usual lotion on the other; the Liz Earle'd skin had no scaliness and dryness, which I usually suffer from' • 'because skin is so well-hydrated it tends to look plumper which is always a bonus' • 'noticeable improvements in skin condition: lower leg dryness and itchiness has disappeared and skin on my upper arms has improved so much I've even worn vest tops this summer' • 'lovely smell which my man loves as well as how it makes my skin feel'.

Decléor Aroma Sculpt Divine Rejuvenating Cream

A scrumptious cream from the well-known aromatherapy-powered brand, featuring an aromatic cocktail of essential oils (rose, chamomile, lemongrass, lemon, grapefruit, frankincense, myrrh), plus shiitake mushroom extract, tamanu and macadamia oils. Pearlescent particles deliver a lovely instant radiance, while the cream is designed to have a draining, firming and even a 'lifting' effect, making it ideal (so Decléor promise) for use after weight loss, as well as for general anti-ageing.

Comments: 'I would give this 12/10 if I could; I used to be a bit slapdash but the improvement is so noticeable that I apply every morning' • 'skin no longer flaky, tone has improved, and I got a compliment on how smooth my legs are' • 'fabulous fragrance, my skin feels so much fresher and softer, and looks almost shimmering' • 'I have to confess that I only did the trial on one side of my body for two days: the instant difference in skintone made me switch to using it all over'.

This Works Skin Deep Dry Leg Oil ❄❄

Shins start out with few oil glands, but as we age they can become super-dry and paper-thin. And there's a health issue there: poor circulation and a fragile skin barrier can increase the chances of 'leg ulcers' in later years: painful, hard to budge and depressing. This blends over a dozen rich plant oils – including jojoba, macadamia, evening primrose, plus rose oil, tuberose and sandalwood (hence the heavenly smell) – to nourish skin deeply. Not just thirsty shins, but all over…

Comments: 'I've always had rough, dry patches on knees and elbows but they're much smoother now, with an overall healthy glow that makes me feel happier to wear clothes that expose more skin' • 'lizard legs now non-flaky and look younger' • 'delicious aromatherapy smell' • 'skin appears totally revitalised and it's perfect to use on your whole body' • 'although it's an oil, it doesn't seem to get everywhere (as other oils do)'.

Pevonia Botanica Ligne Tropicale De-Aging Body Balm

Gosh, this is luscious: a really rich, creamy product. 'Micro-emulsified' shea butter delivers its truly voluptuous texture, alongside pomegranate and acknowledged

anti-ageing tropical botanicals, plus 'tegospheres with Retinol'. Hey, we're beauty editors, and we don't even know what those are – but the bottom line is that it truly seduced testers with its feel and exotic, tangy fragrance.

Comments: 'A dream: light, smooth, creamy; my upper arms benefited most – they're less bumpy and more toned' • '10/10: overall skintone better' • 'used to suffer dry, flaky skin on lower legs/shins, and dry arms that appear finely wrinkled when pinched: the treated side seems to "bounce back" more quickly and looks firmer and plumped-up' • 'so luxurious, and smells divine' • 'improvement in skintone after a couple of days'.

Bombshell Body Show-Off Body Lotion

The Bombshell range was created by Lulu (yes, singer Lulu), to sit alongside her fab anti-ageing skincare (a QVC bestseller, BTW). It's enriched with skin-repairing avocado oil, shea butter, vitamins C and E and antioxidant white tea – plus white truffle for a luminous, dewy glow, and comes in a sleek, user-friendly tube.

Comments: '10/10 for this lovely light silky lotion! Lovely light fragrance; made my very dry skin instantly soft and supple, with a subtle sheen' • 'my skin is now soft and smooth and more youthful instead of dry and flaky' • 'legs felt smooth and very silky straight away' • 'skin elasticity was improved and dryness on knees and elbows greatly so' • 'a touch of super quick luxury that lasts all day'.

Crystal Clear Velvet Skin

This is a serum-style product from a high-science range, which features peptides at generous levels, plus crushed precious stones. They deliver a lustre, as well as mineral benefits. It's non-greasy, melting texture ensures Velvet Skin sinks in fast – making it ideal not just at bedtime, but when you need a body quick-fix. (And we find we often do!)

Comments: 'Top marks for this divine smelling creamy body lotion; dry areas felt nourished immediately. I love the smell, the luxurious feel: skin looks healthy and glowing' • 'made my crocodile skin silky smooth and plumper' • 'melts into skin and disappears almost immediately leaving skin nourished, smooth and silky' • 'after a few days, the veins on my legs were less noticeable and this continued as I used it' • 'even the harsh chill of a Scottish winter couldn't diminish the silky smooth effect; also soothed skin after waxing'.

Body scrubs: *our award winners*

When you want fast body improvements, we say: reach for a scrub. These are pretty darned miraculous for transforming dry and rough skin in about 30 seconds flat. (Especially when the exfoliating particles are suspended in an oil base that delivers a softening, sensual 'slick' on the surface, to nourish as it sinks right in.) What's more, if you then choose to layer another body oil, lotion or cream on to body-scrubbed skin, the ingredients will work their cell-plumping magic more effectively because you've buffed away the dead surface cells first

AT A GLANCE

Ila Beyond Organic Body Scrub for Energising and Detoxifying

Soap & Glory The Breakfast Scrub

Pevonia Tropicale De-Aging Saltmousse

REN Moroccan Rose Otto Sugar Body Polish

Liz Earle Naturally Active Skincare Energising Body Scrub

Dermalogica Exfoliating Body Scrub

So: our Beauty Bible recruits trialled several dozen body scrubs, including several more for this latest edition – and these were their super-smoothing favourites, with some truly stellar scores plus a new entry this time round. Several also earn at least two daisies for naturalness. (See page 7 for more about our daisy rating.)

REVIEWS

Ila Beyond Organic Body Scrub for Energising and Detoxifying ❀ ❀

 Ila's the Sanskrit word for 'earth', and this all-British luxury spa brand – founded by an aromatherapist who set out to fuse holistic wellbeing with beautiful skin – prides itself on being all-natural, too. Hand-blended in the Cotswolds, the scrub's based on Himalayan mineral salts to detoxify and restore energy, with a sense-awakening essential-oil blend of organic rose geranium and juniper. Congrats to Ila for a truly outstanding score (very few products ever exceed an average of 9/10 from our testers).
Comments: '10/10! The skin on my legs looked dull and tight, overall my skin lacked lustre; after using this it shone, smelt fragrant, was smooth and very moisturised – and didn't need any body lotion; after a few uses skintone visibly improved' • 'I looked like a pork sausage before it's been cooked! But instantly my skin really glowed,

with a lovely sheen, and after using twice a week it looks more toned and less pasty' • 'gorgeous smell of rose geranium' • 'luxurious packaging and nice-sized pot, slightly drier than other oil-based scrubs, with nice grainy bits of salt which dissolved in water, now have silky soft thighs and arms'.

Soap & Glory The Breakfast Scrub

 Another off-the-wall name – and another serious performance from Marcia Kilgore's so-affordable brand. Thick, luscious and almost gloopy as an uncooked banana muffin (and with something of the same scent!), this serves up skin-calming oats, alongside luscious shea butter, honey and almonds – and all sprinkled generously with maple sugar.
Comments: 'I have the skin of a reptile but now it feels a lot smoother; little white spots on upper arms appear less obvious and some have gone completely' • 'not only did it smell absolutely heavenly, it was extremely effective and after just one use I noticed how soft my skin was – may actually persuade me to exfoliate more!' • 'didn't feel I needed moisturiser afterwards and smells amazing: buttery/maple syrup fragrance' • 'loved this product – self-tan went on much more smoothly' • 'I was absolutely amazed how after just one use, my skin felt so different – like a baby's; I just kept running my hands up and down my legs in disbelief; my beauty therapist asked what I'd done

as patchy bits of rough skin had completely disappeared'.

Pevonia Tropicale De-Aging Saltmousse ❀

9.27/10

Question: what's a 'Saltmousse'? Answer: a salt scrub with a slightly mousse-y texture (and in this case, a quite scary tangerine colour!). Pevonia's award-winner features sea salt harvested from the Brittany coast, in France, blended with minerals, vitamins and enzymes. The 'Tropicale' refers to the use of papaya and pineapple enzymes (which have an exfoliating action in their own right), and it has an 'exotic fruit sorbet' aroma, as a result.

Comments: 'Gorgeous and fruity and I wanted to eat it' • 'it smelt gloriously dreamy – very fruity and fresh' • 'it was like a breath of sunshine to the skin' • 'this has converted me to the benefits of body scrub: skin feels soft and moisturised and elbows much smoother' • 'skin looks as if it has come alive again! It was like a breath of sunshine to skin that had been covered by winter clothes' • 'when I showered it washed away easily, unlike other scrubs' • 'can see improvement in rough, dry knees and elbows' • 'you get addicted to this product – an even bigger tub would be great!'.

REN Moroccan Rose Otto Sugar Body Polish ❀ ❀

9.27/10

Oh, we love it when this happens… Yes, this product has featured previously in *The Green Beauty Bible* – but we sent it out to ten different testers specifically for this book, who awarded the scrub virtually the same impressively high score as when previously trialled. With Paraguayan cane sugar, skin-conditioning olive and almond oils, kola nut and tea extracts – and the heady fragrance of rosa Damascena oil (you lot really are suckers for rose scents), we're elevating this to the Beauty Bible Hall of Fame.

Comments: '10/10! Not really messy, easy to rub in, beautiful rose smell, good texture like soft sugar, washed off quickly leaving nice soft film on body; lovely to use in bath – rose-scented water – or shower' • 'left skin very smooth and moisturised, no need for body cream on my very dry skin; bumpy skin on upper arms has gone after a month of using regularly' • 'like a spa treatment! Skin more even in tone now, I loved this – the best scrub ever!' • 'moisturising lasts for days, skin silky and much softer and clearer, particularly around my thighs and buttocks, and bumpy arms reduced – fabulous'.

Liz Earle Naturally Active Skincare Energising Body Scrub ❀

8.87/10

What universally seduced testers with this product was the rev-you-up, sense-awakening smell (a combination of sweet orange, grapefruit, geranium, peppermint, eucalyptus, pine, rosemary, patchouli and petitgrain). With a more liquid texture than other scrubs in this category, this could almost qualify as a skin-buffing body wash.

Comments: 'Very impressed: skin felt smoother, no need for body lotion' • 'I like the eucalyptus scent; the texture's not too abrasive and it feels like a body wash as well as a scrub' • 'it's like a spa treatment and using it leaves the whole bathroom smelling like your own spa' • 'skin looked brighter after first use; lumps and bumps also improved over time' • 'application very pleasant: easy to rub into skin, helped by a slight foaming action' • 'kept the flaky patches at bay on my legs and I saw an improvement in the amount of ingrowing hairs I had; the top of my arms looked less bumpy and I have fewer flaky patches there too' • 'left skin feeling really "alive" and fresh due to the menthol and peppermint'.

Dermalogica Exfoliating Body Scrub

8.81/10

Dermalogica's high-tech products have many unswervingly devoted followers, who now include Beauty Bible recruits to this body scrub. Creamy and lightly foaming, it gently buffs skin without scratching, deploying ultra-fine date seed, olive and fig fruit powders, together with rice bran. In addition, there's papain – an enzyme from papaya, which helps 'digest' skin cells – and antioxidant green tea. But the feature our testers particularly commented on was the smell, a sense-awakening fusion of sandalwood, orange, lavender and rosemary.

Comments: 'Overall my skin looked smoother, brighter and healthier, with a reduction in dry patches, particularly on elbows, knees, thighs and upper arms. A no-nonsense, no gimmick product, which does exactly what you want it to do' • 'marked improvement in my skin over a month, slight flakiness all over has totally gone, skin much softer, smoother, less red and I really love the fresh invigorating scent' • 'I just fell in love with this product – skin feels really soft and moisturised, even my very dry legs; it left bits in the bath but you expect that!' • 'as a bonus, my hands were much softer from applying it'.

♡ WE LOVE…

Well, first we'll tell you what we personally don't love: those body scrubs based on crushed nuts and seeds, which drift to the bottom of the bathwater and make you feel like you're sitting in a tub of grit. (Not such an issue if you shower, but we're mermaids.) Now for Jo's favourites: ESPA Detoxifying Salt Scrub, Temple Spa Sugar Buff, and ylang-ylang and rose-scented Organic Pharmacy Cleopatra's Body Scrub all have a place on Jo's bath-side. Sarah's bathroom features a cornucopia, with current favourites being Sanctuary Spa 4 Day Moisture Oil Scrub, Clinique Sparkle Skin and He-Shi Exfoliating Bodywash, as well as the REN Moroccan Rose Otto Sugar Body Polish that did so well with testers. For something a little different, Dermasuri is a magic mitt, made of some high-tech fibre that rubs and rolls all the dead skin away. Simply brilliant.

We must, still must, improve our busts…

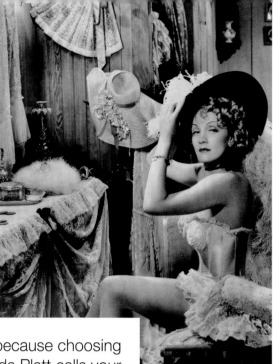

And we CAN! Starting now, with the right bra – because choosing the right 'underneath' (as fashion guru Amanda Platt calls your bra), is as crucial to looking great as what you put on top

When you can't rely on youthful perkiness, you need a better bra to give you uplift. Undies have become increasingly important in our lives. To put it plainly, at this stage in life you need a bra that's not only pretty but does its job impeccably (and don't forget equally well-fitting knickers). We'd always urge you, if possible, to go to an expert: the difference it can make is staggering. And it's not just a question of looking good: your bra can affect your health.

Think of your bra as a suspension bridge. You may never have linked your bosom and engineering, but according to chiropractor Tim Hutchful, it really is like a suspension bridge! 'You need a well-engineered bra so your shoulders don't end up doing all the work. Bras that don't fit affect the shoulders and chest and usually cause pain as you get older.' Poorly-fitting bras can lead to all sorts of physical problems, including head-, neck-, shoulder-, and/or back-aches (back pain is common among large-breasted women). Too tight a bra can even restrict your breathing.

Most importantly, wear the right size. Amazingly, about 80 per cent of women are wearing the wrong-size brassiere. In one study, most women with shoulder pain found it lifted completely when they removed their bra. (Though the researchers didn't try kitting them out in the right-size bra to see what happened then…) Add to this the fact that our bosoms lose firmness with age and you can see why it's vital to confront the bra issue if you want your *poitrine* to look alluring and feel comfy. Be aware too that, however carefully you handwash them (and never tumble dry), bras lose their oomph as they get older, so depending on how often they're worn you should replace them every six months. (If necessary please shuffle your budget – it's really worth it.)

Become a savvier bra-shopper. There are more types of bra than we've had hot dinners (well, nearly) but whether you choose wired (or not), padded or plain, demi-cup or full, black lace, crimson satin or classic white cotton, there is basic advice that's common to all styles. Plus, for energetic exercisers, you can now find a range of sports bras that is specially designed to keep your bosom stable rather than bouncing with every movement (think of the way a ponytail bobs up and down as you run, play tennis, even do yoga). So…

● First and most importantly, says June Kenton,

BRAS AFTER BREAST SURGERY

June Kenton of Rigby & Peller, who has had a mastectomy herself, is passionate about the concerns of women who've had this surgery. 'Getting a prosthesis and bra after mastectomy is often treated in the same way as getting a pair of crutches, but it should be about fashion, not a medical appliance,' she says. The key is to find a bra which fits the other breast perfectly before choosing a prosthesis. 'Get bras to fit your "good" side then fit the prosthesis so it matches,' she advises. (Find more advice at www.rigbyandpeller. com, and other specialist mastectomy lingerie suppliers.)

owner of Rigby & Peller (the legendary lingerie emporium in London), 'Be really grown-up and have a proper expert fitting. Try on lots. Move around, sit down, stand up, lift your arms – make the bra work for you. Then choose the style which performs best.'

● The two crucial measurements are cup size and band size (the bit at the bottom) – so make sure the fitter measures those each time. The perfect position for your breasts is midway between your shoulder and your elbow. The most common problem is wearing a bra too small in the cup and too big in the band at the back. Most women wear their bra bands too high (see next point), so their measurements are wrong. Often the key is to get a deeper cup and a smaller band. This usually eliminates the dreaded 'back sausages' too.

● The band should sit evenly around the chest, ie, the back shouldn't be higher or lower than the front. It shouldn't ride up but stay parallel to the floor.

● Breasts should be supported primarily by the band around the ribcage, not the straps.

● Breasts shouldn't bulge over the top or sides of the cup, even with a low-cut style such as a balconette.

● The nipple should be in the centre of the cup.

● The cup should fit smoothly, and not wrinkle, be loose, or cut in at the top so you get a bulge (called 'double-cupping' in the trade).

● The centre piece of the bra should lie flat against the chest.

● If it's underwired, the wires should go under the bust contour and follow it snugly – not cut in or rub.

● Straps should not dig in or slip off the shoulder. Choose straps that are comfortable and make you feel supported. Generally that means wider straps – but they don't need to look bulky.

● A well-fitting bra shouldn't leave marks on your skin – and that means the straps too.

BOOST YOUR BUST... AND BANISH BINGO WINGS!

There are very simple actions that will help firm your bosom – and arms too. Fitness trainer Andy Wadsworth suggests the following for bust uplift, followed by a couple for debagging the dreaded bingo wings! But most important of all for the bustline, he says, is your posture: stand tall, keep your shoulders down and wide, lift your chest. Don't round your shoulders or slouch.

1 **Palm push:** standing or sitting, extend your arms in front of you at chest height, elbows bent as if you are hugging a tree (or a person...). Now push your palms together with force. Hold for ten seconds. Repeat ten times. Do this as often as you can. Watchpoint: keep your shoulders relaxed, pushing your shoulder blades down and together.

2 **Floor press-up:** do full press-ups on the floor if you are strong (and used to this type of exertion); if not, keep your knees to feet (you're on tiptoes) on the floor and press-up the rest of your body. Once you can do 20 knee press-ups, try doing a full press-up. Aim to build up to three sets of ten press-ups.

3 **Wall press-away:** stand facing a wall, then extend your arms at chest height a bit wider than a shoulder-width apart, so your hands touch the wall. Bend your arms and let your body fall towards the wall, then push away by straightening your arms. Aim for three x ten repetitions.

4 **Chest press:** lie on the floor (or bench or fitness ball), with a weight in each hand (either a 2kg weight or a full bottle of water). Raise your arms up in the air above your chest. Aim for three x ten repetitions.

5 **Butterfly:** standing with feet a hip-width apart and with a weight (as above for Chest press exercise) in each hand, start with hands at about 45 degrees to the floor; then lift the weights up in an arc to meet in front of your chest. Aim for three x ten repetitions.

FOR BINGO WINGS...

6 **Tricep dip:** sitting on a chair or the edge of the bath, with your feet under your knees a hip-width apart, grasp the sides of the chair or bath while you lift your bottom from the seat and let it drop down and forward; keep your elbows behind you rather than out to the side. Straighten your arms to come up. Move down and up without pausing for three sets of ten, building up to 20.

7 **Overhead triceps press:** put your hands behind your neck with a weight in each (as in exercise 4), then push them up above your head in a straight line. Go up and down smoothly without pausing for three x ten repetitions.

PS Any activity that uses your arm and chest muscles will help tone and firm: Jo swims and does yoga, Sarah brushes big horses, mucks out stables – and finds that scrubbing the bath with both arms is an amazing workout for arms and tummy!

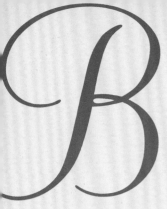

Bust treatments: our award winners

You've found the perfect-fitting bra to give maximum support – now lavish your bust with treats that not only leave the skin feeling soft and smooth but, amazingly, claim to make your breasts feel firmer and more pert… So you can reveal your décolletage with confidence

AT A GLANCE

Liz Earle Superskin Bust & Neck Treatment

Lulu's Time Bomb Trouble Shooter Neck, Jaw and Chest Cream

Elemis Pro-Collagen Lifting Treatment Neck and Bust

Temple Spa Bosom Pal

Motherhood, gravity, going bra-less when you were a carefree twentysomething – they all take their toll on the bust area. Add to that the effects of gravity over the decades and none of us is as pert as we once were – although good underwear, fitted properly, can be nothing less than a miracle-worker (see page 32 for more). Frenchwomen swear by the perkifying effects of cold water (once upon a time, Clarins even made a device that blitzed boobs with icy water – and rather effective it was, too), but nowadays there are more treatments than ever which allege that they'll firm and uplift breasts, not simply leave the skin soft and silky. (Any body lotion would achieve velvetiness in the boob zone, frankly.) So do these targeted bust treatments achieve the near-impossible and deliver real uplift? To find out, we've now dispatched considerably over two dozen products to testers, and are featuring two new award winners in this latest paperback. NB: Testers were instructed to use the product for four weeks on one breast alone and note any difference.

REVIEWS

Liz Earle Superskin Bust & Neck Treatment ❋

8.29/10
A favourite of Jo's (see We Love…), this light serum, which is designed for mature, crêpey or very dry skin, due to age, menopause or sun exposure, is packed with plumping and smoothing botanicals. These include the African kigelia tree (sourced from a community-based sustainable forestry project in Malawi), organic rosehip and cranberry seed oils and pomegranate extract. A new round of testing

catapulted this into the top spot, with some very high scores: it was formerly the fourth highest scoring product.

Comments: 'Immediate pleasant tingling sensation and my skin felt much smoother and softer; a little tacky at first but soaked in well and after two weeks the skin on my test breast looked more hydrated, plumper and felt silky, also my décolletage appeared less crêpey' • 'really loved this product: by the end of the tube, breast looked much plumper with noticeably smoother and more luminous skin, more youthful but sadly not firmer, but this is difficult with a larger bust' • 'something amazing happened after two weeks: I am 35, my boobs are 65 after breastfeeding two kids and I had given up on them but this proved me wrong – it is a miracle in a bottle. I was used to them looking like a prune and they looked smooth with the stretch marks disappearing'.

Lulu's Time Bomb Trouble Shooter Neck, Jaw and Chest Cream

7.94/10
It doesn't actually mention the word 'bust' on the packaging, but Lulu (yes, that Lulu) and her team submitted this for our 'boob treatment' trials, and it slipped straight into the top slot. (NB: All this team also noted neck/décolletage improvements.) Ingredients include vitamin E, pea extract, sunflower and shea butter extract; it has a fabulous, waft-you-to-Provence lavender scent, which encourages diligent application – and that's half the battle, with bust treatments. Like every product, these are only effective with regular use.

Comments: 'Prior to use I felt my bust skin was starting to develop a crêpey look but this not only made me feel as if I was receiving a luxury salon treatment, seeing results serves to confirm these

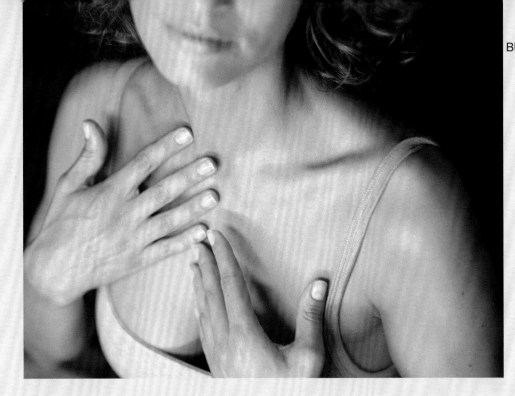

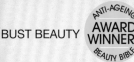

impressions' • 'skin on my bust is now soft, smooth and supple – and also good for droopy jaw-line and crêpiness' • 'smells lovely – like lavender-y baby powder, but nicer' • 'loved this – it's done what it says it will, improving both my bust and neck/jaw area, which are more toned and soft to the touch' • 'surprised by its effectiveness and will buy again' • 'from bust to neck, skin looks fresher and more youthful, with improved texture and tone'.

Elemis Pro-Collagen Lifting Treatment Neck and Bust

7.63/10

The Pro-Collagen range has gone down a storm with our testers over the years – and a new addition to Elemis's Beauty Bible Award-winning line-up is this powerful treatment, featuring Padina Pavonica (Pro-Collagen's signature 'wonder' ingredient), sea buckthorn, royal jelly and propolis. If you're looking for a product that does double-duty on the entire chin-to-bra-zone, you might also like to know that Elemis's own research show a 33 per cent reduction in crêpiness with regular use of this cream/gel.

Comments: 'This product really did what it claimed to do: skin felt firmer and more elastic on the treated boob; after four weeks, I saw a reduction in crêpiness – I don't have a lot but it was noticeable' • 'skin felt very soft and smooth, it absorbed very quickly – no tackiness – and smelt lovely: lines are a little less defined' • 'my bust has improved in tone and like my neck looks smoother, shinier and much younger: one of those rare products that does what

it says' • 'after a month, my husband could clearly see which side I used the product on: texture is smoother, younger-looking, better moisturised, more toned and firmer also my bust has a better shape' • 'this works: it really does make a difference but you need to give it a couple of weeks before the results start to show: skin smoother, less crêpey, with renewed firmness and elasticity'.

Temple Spa Bosom Pal

7.63/10

Temple Spa have wowed our readers with their Skin Truffle – the highest-scoring miracle cream all-rounder in all of Beauty Bible's history – and have a notable new entry in this edition with this aptly-named bust-booster, designed for use morning and night to target loss of elasticity post-pregnancy, weight loss or general, gravity-induced ageing. It features what they call a Cell-Active-Form Complex derived from plant ingredients, together with vitamins.

Comments: 'The treated side of my bust appeared more toned and firmer after two weeks' • 'after four weeks, skin had dramatically improved: it looked and felt supple and toned around neck, décolleté and bust. I felt less self conscious about wearing a v-neck and noticed a vast difference when I wore a low cut frock' • 'sun damage to décolleté improved, difference in skin tone and clarity between treated and untreated breast was noticeable' • 'after four weeks, definite improvement in firmness and elasticity, no noticeable difference in volume, which was good'.

♡ WE LOVE...

We don't really 'do' bust treatments. But Jo does slather Liz Earle Superskin Bust & Neck Treatment on her décolletage, for suppleness. (At Jo's suggestion they renamed this as '& Neck' because it's so great for that – see page 153 for more.) And Sarah always slathers moisturiser and oil on the upper bosom zone.

Give cellulite the brush-off

Tone those thighs and de-dimple that derrière. (Because there's a lot you can do to smooth out cellulite)

Dimples may be appealing on babies (and handsome men), but on your thighs and backside? Not so charming. So the bottom line on cellulite – hallelujah – is that there's much that can be done to improve it (and thus, in turn, your body confidence). You may never conquer the problem completely – but a combination of nutrition, body-brushing, exercise and localised massage can make a visible difference…

Scrub off the dead skin cells. As well as dry-skin body-brushing (see right), do use a scrub on your backside, thighs and hips, because any cellulite product you apply to the area is going to penetrate better if it doesn't have to make it through dead skin cells. Targeted body exfoliation also brings about incredibly rapid improvements in skin texture: in our experience it can take less than a week of daily blitzing to combat 'goosebumps' in the cellulite zone and thereby transform skin smoothness.

Body-brush the bumps bye-bye. The skin is a vital (and often overlooked) organ of elimination and nothing is better at stimulating localised circulation than daily brushing. It wakes up a sluggish lymphatic system – and many women have told us it works astonishingly well to improve digestion and aches and pains as side benefits.

First, find your brush: most diligent body-brushers choose a brush with a strap that slips over your hand, and has a removable long handle to get at your back, etc. There are plenty of options on the high street but do just test them on your skin first. The brush shouldn't be scratchy: if it makes little white scratch marks when you brush the back of your hand with it, it's too hard.

We recommend total body-brushing rather than targeted brushing of the affected area, because you get the all-over lymph drainage and circulation-boosting benefits – here's the how-to:

● Body-brush dry skin, not damp or wet, and never areas that are bruised or irritated, or your breasts.
● Begin by standing in a comfortable position. Place one foot on a higher surface, such as the edge of the bath or a bed.
● Start by brushing the soles of the feet from toes to heel. Move on to the top of the foot and then upwards, with smooth, long strokes – always in the direction of the heart.
● Give extra attention to the skin between the knees and the waist, going over the cellulite area several times. Don't ignore the lymph nodes in the groin. Upwards, upwards, upwards.
● Next, move on to the top half of the body: palms of hands, backs of hands, sweeping towards the armpits (plenty more lymph glands there). Now do your shoulders and back – you'll probably need your long-handle brush here.
● Continue the sweeping movements on the front of your torso, going a little more lightly as the skin can be very sensitive here. (But miss out your breasts and nipples.)
● Brushing should be firm and vigorous, but shouldn't hurt. A rosy glow is fine; red or irritated skin isn't.
● Three to five minutes is ideal. Realistically, two minutes is OK. But the key is: do it daily, and if you can only manage even one solitary minute every morning, that's infinitely better than a once-a-week longer blitz.

Give your fat a mini-massage. Dermatologist Dr Elizabeth Tanzi explains: 'Fat doesn't have a lot of blood flow, so kneading the skin helps increase circulation – and in turn, lessens the appearance of lumps.' Massage with your knuckles, moving up the fronts of your thighs, across your rear and then up the back of your thighs. (If this requires a little contortionism, so be it.) Alternatively, book regular massages with a deep tissue masseur

or practitioner of manual lymphatic drainage (MLD): these can help both to improve circulation and to drain away any excess fluid, which can exacerbate the appearance of cellulite.

Take exercise! As usual, more is better…it works. And you might want to try FitFlops, the footwear range with the inbuilt gym in the sole, for its proven leg-toning benefits.

Eat more veggies and high-fibre foods. They'll help in the war on dimples (and benefit your whole body): loads of veggies and salads (green leaves, onions and garlic); fruit (especially deep reds and purples – so make the most of berries and dark grapes); some wholegrains (brown rice, oats, and anything sprouted); olive oil and herbs. Also go for good-quality protein: oily fish and shellfish, eggs, poultry, tofu and natural live yoghurt. When you're out and about, choose a freshly-squeezed veggie juice or berry smoothie over tea and coffee, and take snack-packs of seeds and nuts (especially Brazil nuts and almonds). Basically, let 'fresh' be your watchword.

And it's about what you don't eat, too. Avoid processed and preserved foods, sugar, refined salt, 'fungal' foods (which means mushrooms, vinegar, blue cheese). Some people find that giving up gluten helps, too, and we also suggest you avoid caffeine and alcohol as much as is realistic. (NB: We do appreciate you're not a nun.)

Take goji. Dermatologist Dr Howard Murad (who's written an entire book on the subject) calls goji 'the cellulite assassinator' (it comes as berries and also juice). We've long espoused an inside-out as well as an outside-in approach to cellulite, and pharmacist Shabir Daya has put together a Cellulite Busting Kit (see DIRECTORY), incorporating the latest guidelines to help minimise the look of cellulite. This includes a food state multi-nutrient, vitamin B50, omega-3 essential fatty acids, glucosamine sulphate and goji berry juice.

And give yourself a break. We know women get incredibly angst-y about cellulite, but we would encourage you to relax a bit about the problem. Cellulite is never as apparent to others as it seems to our own so-critical selves (we've never yet met a man who even quite knew what cellulite was, let alone complained about it on a woman) – and other people see the 'big picture' (your sense of humour/great cooking skills/your laugh). And if all else fails – well, that's why sarongs were invented.

> FAT doesn't have a lot of blood flow, so *kneading* the skin helps INCREASE circulation

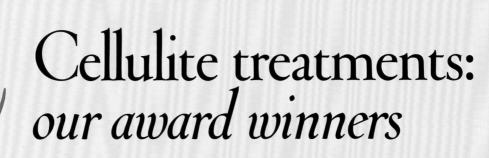

Cellulite treatments: *our award winners*

It's a fact that even if you've been mercifully dimple-free until mid-life, the breakdown of collagen and elastin, which leads to wrinkles, bags and sagging in the face, can become all-too-apparent on the hips, derrière and (especially) thighs – in the form of cellulite. Certainly, diet plays a role, as does exercise, and we always advise body-brushing, which is our own secret weapon. And now there's an abundance of cellulite-blitzing products. Do they really work? Our research with younger readers showed that yes, some definitely do. But we wanted to know – can they rise to the challenge of a more mature body? Now well over four dozen cellulite products later – each dispatched to ten testers who 'fessed up to *peau d'orange* – here's the bottom line

AT A GLANCE

L'Occitane Almond Milk Concentrate

Clarins High Definition Body Lift Cellulite Control

Thalgo Crème Thalgomince

spaFind Inchwrap Super Cellulite Cream

REVIEWS

L'Occitane Almond Milk Concentrate ❀

8.33/10 This classic from the bestselling Almond range has been reformulated so we retested it with good results. The delectably lush cream is a pleasure to apply, leaving skin satiny-smooth. It is rich in almond milk and oil (with a slightly marzipan-y smell), together with almond proteins and silicium to activate collagen synthesis. They suggest Almond Concentrate, which was previously an Award winner in the Body Treatment category and now retrialled for this, can be used on thighs, hips, stomach – but also the bust area, too.
Comments: '10/10: cellulite was improved and skin soft and smooth, looked a lot better, wobbly thighs firmer: perfect!' • 'I absolutely love this: my skin is so much nicer and the smell has grown on me: I haven't lost inches but my skin is firmer and smoother and brighter' • 'immediate softness, and after six weeks dimples reduced slightly on treated thigh, appearance of cellulite is less noticeable' •

'great as a rich body moisturiser and skin felt slightly firmer after six weeks, may have had better results with diet and exercise or body brushing!'.

Clarins High Definition Body Lift Cellulite Control

8.28/10 From a brand that has produced notable cellulite-banishers in the past comes this new light gel/serum formulation, based on recent scientific discovery about the nature of fatty (adipose) tissue. It claims to target both early and stubborn cellulite with a combination of four patent pending natural actives – and extracts of scabius, geranium and cang zhu, which contain caffeine, a long-used ingredient in cellulite products. They emphasise the importance of massage and the Clarins Anti-Cellulite Self Massage Method is available to follow online.
Comments: 'I loved the distinctive minty medicinal smell and it sank in very well; after two weeks even my husband noticed the improvements – my skin is so much better and lines and crêpeyness softening and merging, sometimes disappearing altogether'

ANTI-AGEING AWARD WINNERS BEAUTY BIBLE

• 'I have lost a lot of weight over the last few years and this cream certainly tightened things up. I'm shocked at how well it's done as experts always say these products don't work' • 'my skin is so much softer and it feels really great' • 'tighter, tauter, smoother skin and my husband has commented that my skin looks firmer and slimmer; however it is time consuming and you have to be very committed to get the best results' • 'skin felt tighter and lifted, looked smooth and dewy, cellulite less visible; easy to use with no fuss, no mess' • 'a brilliant product that is now one of my staples'.

Thalgo Crème Thalgomince

Thalassotherapy spa brand Thalgo actually prescribe this for massage twice daily, so that key ingredients – horse chestnut, caffeine complex, plus a plant extract they call 'Adipo-reset'(!) – are able to get to work round-the-clock. It's rich and creamy, enveloping skin 'like a slimming patch', Thalgo tell us, and though it's designed to complement two specific salon cellulite treatments Thalgo offer, our testers trialled it as a stand-alone product, observing impressive results. Several gave it nine or ten marks out of ten.

Comments: 'Lovely light but rich cream, which sunk in immediately; I used it on one leg which was instantly smoother and softer, and after six weeks cellulite definitely less noticeable, orange peel almost gone, firmer, and smoother than it has been for years; lost half an inch around my thigh – loved it' • 'very luxurious product with wonderful aroma, really feel good and my cellulite was a little improved' • 'after six weeks, skin looks and feels smoother and firmer – really loved using this treatment' • 'cellulite markedly reduced, thighs much less uneven and lumpy; when you pinch the skin, the orange-peel effect is much less obvious, plus thighs look and feel much firmer and tighter: expensive but I will be buying more – I love this and recommend it unreservedly' • 'silvery stretch marks and orange peel were much improved'.

spaFind Inchwrap Super Cellulite Cream

This at home spa range is based on formulas that blend natural de-ionised water with pure Dead Sea minerals and organic plant extracts. This product also contains Iso-Slim Complex, which includes soy isoflavones, caffeine, carnitine and spirulina and is, they say,

♡ WE LOVE...

Jo was cellulite-free until she hit 50. Then, she observes: 'I suddenly understood what all those "resort wear" sarongs were created for...' She regularly uses a cellulite brush discovered in Germany with copper bristles. She is a recent convert to Legology Daily Air-Lite Daily Lift for Legs, wonderfully lemon-scented, which makes the whole leg zone feel 'light as air'. Sarah's dimples are relatively shallow – possibly due to riding and walking for miles every weekend – but she scrubs thighs regularly, applies body lotion most nights and skin-brushes virtually daily while her tortoise-like hot water system heats the shower.

TIP

Double up your daily application of product morning and night. You may get through more, but the active ingredients will have twice the opportunity to tighten and drain. If you just apply once, do it before bedtime: loose night clothes are less likely to rub the product off again than tight daytime clothing.

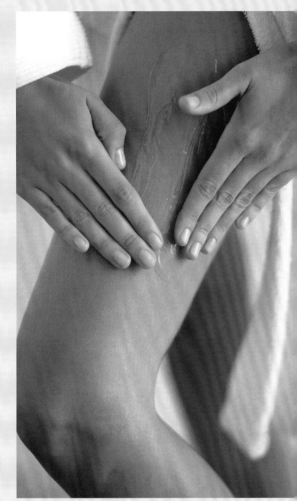

clinically proven to reduce cellulite and increase skin elasticity, even to boost natural collagen production to help 'lift' skin.

Comments: 'After six weeks cellulite appeared less dimpled, tighter and smoother, skin tone more even; the action of a daily massage may have improved the texture but hey! All improvements gratefully accepted' • 'rich cream which was easy to massage in but needed quite a bit to cover the area, easy to follow instructions; by the end of testing skin felt smoother, half an inch reduction in thighs and they do feel firmer: love the product and will buy the whole range' • 'amazing improvement in skin texture; great improvement in firmness and skin tone; never saw my hips and thighs look like this before. I could hardly believe what I was seeing in such a short time'.

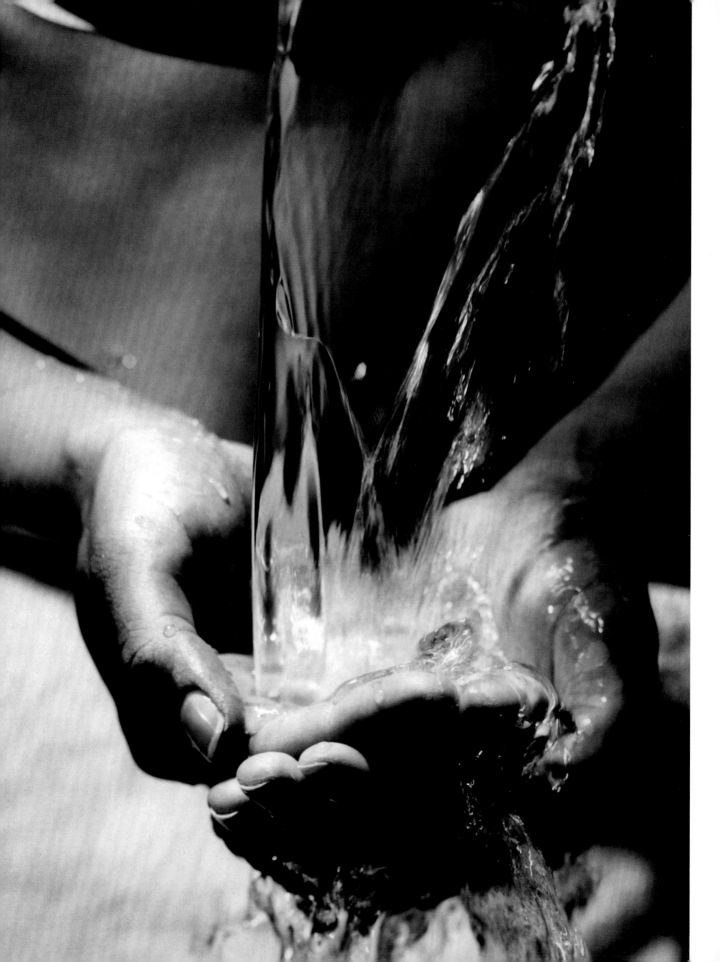

Turbo-charge your cleansing regime

We are the Queens of Clean – always have been – but we know many, many women who are so bored by cleansing they skimp (and even occasionally skip) this important part of the anti-ageing ritual. You can spend hundreds of pounds on an anti-ageing cream (if you really must…) but it's money down the drain if you aren't cleansing properly

The reason is simple: unless you've got rid of the daily build-up of dead skin cells, your anti-ager is just going to sit there. Doing not very much at all. Quite expensively…

Cleansing in this specific way – as espoused originally by Eve Lom and then Liz Earle and now many, many happy and fresh-faced followers – is, in our experience, the most effective way to swoosh away the day and 'prep' skin for everything that comes next.

Step 1 Massage your cleanser into dry skin – balm, lotion, cream, whatever your preference. (Ideally at this stage in life you will have progressed from foaming cleansers, which in general are too drying for mature complexions. And if you're still using soap and water? Stop. Right. Now.)

Step 2 When we say massage, we mean massage. Ideally, use a pressure-point massage, making firm, small circular movements starting at chin-level and working up the cheeks to the eye zone, then shifting along the jaw-bone towards the ears (a distance of around 1.5cm), mid-cheek, cheekbones. And then the same on your forehead. Sweep your fingers more gently around the eyes in a circular but outwards direction. But – important BUT – if you can't be bothered to follow that precise prescription, just general firm massage of your face using circular movements will work wonders for melting make-up, improving circulation and decongesting the skin. You can do this for as long as you like. We recently talked to a Frenchwoman who explained that in France, it's not unusual to spend ten minutes on cleansing. We award ourselves Brownie points if we manage two, but really, the longer you knead your face with your fingertips the more it will reward you for it.

Step 3 Take a hot, wet cloth – a muslin cloth, or a flannel (Sarah prefers that). Press on to the face to remove the first load of cleanser and debris. Rinse under hot water (warm-to-hot water if you are prone to broken veins), then be a bit more vigorous as you swipe away more of the cleanser. (NB: Never rub at areas where you have those aforementioned vein problems.) Repeat, until you feel you've swooshed away all remaining cleanser.

Step 4 Rinse the cloth again and wrap a corner of the flannel or cleansing cloth over the tip of your index finger. Rub at areas where skin and make-up build up – particularly in the crease around the nose, the cleft of the chin, and the sides of your face. If you do this, you may never need to use a specific exfoliator. (We rarely do.)

Step 5 As a final step, try swishing the flannel/cloth in cool water and press it on your face. (Jo does this while imagining the day and all its stresses are trickling away down the plug-hole. It isn't compulsory, but she finds it a relaxing technique…)

And overleaf, see the run-down of specifically anti-ageing cleansers. But we say: they'll all work best if you use this technique.

Cleansers: our award winners

A good cleanser is in itself a wonderful weapon against ageing. Unless you get the gunk off your face at night thoroughly, you're wasting your money on age-defying moisturisers and serums – because they simply sit on cellular debris and the day's make-up, with no chance of performing miracles. Now, though, there's a new category of cleansers that claim, in themselves, to offer anti-ageing benefits

AT A GLANCE

Emma Hardie Amazing Face Moringa Cleansing Balm

Elemis Pro-Collagen Cleansing Balm

Elemis Pro-Radiance Cream Cleanser

Aurelia Miracle Cleanser

Balance Me Cleanse and Smooth Face Balm

Alpha H Age Delay Cleansing Oil

Frankly, we've been a bit cynical about that: a cleanser is meant to be swiped or sluiced away, so how can it do anything more than cleanse and maybe brighten…? This book, however, gave us the opportunity to put several dozen 'anti-ageing' cleansers through their paces, to find out whether you really can cleanse the years away. These scores (and new entries) suggest the answer is a resounding 'yes' – because this section now features the highest-scoring product ever trialled in all of Beauty Bible history!

REVIEWS

Emma Hardie Amazing Face Moringa Cleansing Balm ❀

9.61/10 We're blown away by this: super-facialist Emma Hardie's botanically-based cleanser has romped home with the highest score for any product that we've put through its paces in 18 years of Beauty Bible trials. Based round moringa seed oil, wild sea fennel and vitamin E, it has a deliciously uplifting fragrance – orange, neroli, jasmine, rose and mandarin – which (as testers comment) makes the make-up-melting experience a total pleasure. NB: Our panellists used it in tandem with the special Emma Hardie Amazing Face Dual Action Buff and Polish

Cleansing Cloth – and we recommend you do the same: it's like an 'e-cloth' for faces, and very effective indeed.

Comments: 'Left my skin clean, very moisturised and happy' • 'the best cleanser I have ever used; it removes all traces of make-up (except my waterproof mascara) and the cloth is easy to clean' • 'oily, very rich and feels wonderful going on. An amazing multi-tasker' • 'my skin is much smoother and it has a moisturising and brightening effect that reduces the appearance of ageing' • 'stopped break outs in their tracks and my glowing skin certainly gave me a youthful appearance'.

Elemis Pro-Collagen Cleansing Balm ❀ ❀

 9.38/10 This new entry is a luxurious-textured make-up melting balm, with its own cotton cloth, which has romped into second place, just above its stable companion – testament to a range that our rigorous consumer panels just love. Based on wheat germ and oat, starflower and elderberry oils, rose and mimosa waxes, anti-ageing Padina pavonica and Elemis signature blend of essential oils, you massage in, then apply water – so it turns into milky veil, which you remove with the cotton cloth provided. NB It's not suitable for sensitive eyes.

Comments: 'I absolutely LOVE LOVE LOVE this. Rich without being greasy and perfect texture.

Really anti-ageing, it has improved radiance, tone, softness – I can't live without this' • 'I use less facial oil and moisturiser as my skin is already "fed", my pores don't look so pronounced' • 'am converted to this and it lasts for ages' • 'VERY impressed: removed all traces of make-up and left my skin very soft, silky and moisturised. Amazing, fabulous product.'

Elemis Pro-Radiance Cream Cleanser

 Elemis suggest massaging this richly-nourishing, antioxidant-powered cleanser directly into skin, or – if you like a lather – to mix with warm water first. Active 'anti-ageing' ingredients include moringa seed peptides, 'super berry' açai and burdock, while shea butter moisturises, in addition to melting make-up. It comes with a cotton facial mitt, to be used with warm water for optimum cleansing.
Comments: 'I really love this product – I thought my face was clean when I first used it but when I removed this cleanser with the cloth provided, I was shocked at the make-up that had remained on my face; it also left my skin moisturised' • 'a fabulous cleanser, thick but easily spread, removed all traces of make-up, even eyes and a waterproof lip stain' • 'this cleans effectively, doesn't dry skin, and leaves it looking brighter' • 'I looked forward to the ritual of using it, and skin felt so soft and velvety after that it makes you feel uplifted'.

Aurelia Miracle Cleanser ❀❀

 Chockfull of BioOrganic plant and flower essences, this multi-award-winning range (which won our Best New Brand Award in 2014) features scientifically proven natural probiotic and peptide technologies so it's a perfect marriage of science and nature. Their creamy aromatic cleanser, which contains omega-rich baobab, firming Kigelia Africana and antioxidant-rich hibiscus, comes with its own bamboo muslin cloth to buff away dead skin cells. Testers were wow-ed.
Comments: 'Dreamy consistency and very easy to use – left my skin clean as a whistle, soft plump and moist' • 'removed all traces of waterproof make-up easily; my foundation goes on better after using this; loved the recyclable packaging' • 'this has jumped into being my top cleanser, and lasted for four months, used twice a day; my skin adored

being massaged with this and I can leave my contact lenses in, leaves skin brighter, clearer and with a youthful glow'.

Balance Me Cleanse and Smooth Face Balm ❀❀

One key action of an anti-ageing cleanser is to brighten skin – which Balance Me's does beautifully by buffing away flat, dead surface skin cells with the teensiest, gentlest particles of complexion-friendly oatmeal. The oil base blends antioxidant-rich Arctic cloudberry, shea and cocoa butter, rosehip, camellia, virgin coconut and kukui nut oils, deliciously fragrant with essential oils from Roman chamomile, lemon and red mandarin – all designed to be swiped away after 30 seconds of 'polishing', with a muslin cloth.
Comments: 'Fantastic product: lovely to use, cleanses quickly, gently but thoroughly and leaves skin feeling soft, plumped and moisturised' • 'noticed blackheads disappearing from my nose with each use' • 'my skin's never been as good as this in my whole life' • 'would recommend to anyone with a dry, parched skin like mine'.

Alpha H Age Delay Cleansing Oil

Zingily fragranced with tangerine peel oil, this balm-like oil cleanser features grape seed and sea buckthorn oils plus other water-compatible oils (coconut and vitamin E), which combine to melt and trap the stubborn waxes and pigments in modern cosmetics, including waterproof mascara. After massaging in, you add a little water so it emulsifies and lifts away grime, excess sebum and dead skin cells. It comes in a tube so is easily transportable. NB Despite the name, it doesn't contain alpha-hydroxy acid.
Comments: 'The perfect cleanser for me, gently removed waterproof make up, and better than my usual eye make remover for mascara and eyeliner. My skin felt fresh and clean, soft and wonderfully supple' • 'one of the best cleansers I have ever tried – love the very fresh smell' • 'my skin was completely clean and looked younger, softer and glowed' • 'amazing, luxurious-feeling cleanser; after massaging in for some weeks, I saw improved skin clarity and texture, less congestion and definite improvement in moisture levels'.

Jo is possibly the last woman on the planet to be converted to Liz Earle Cleanse & Polish, after she was given a tip to add a few drops of Superskin facial oil per dose, for extra nourishment. (Previously, she never found it 'rich' enough.) She alternates this with the new and gloriously-scented Elemis Pro-Collagen Cleansing Balm. 'I do like to switch between cleansers to avoid the boredom factor. My golden rule? A cleanser must smell gorgeous, to entice me to use it...' (Those last two cleansing choices are both pricey, but a bottle lasts at least six months – even without switching!) Sarah's default cleanser is always Liz Earle's Cleanse & Polish, which not only cleanses admirably but also, unlike many cleansers, does not irritate her sensitive peepers. However, a recent discovery is MV Organic Skincare Gentle Cream Cleanser, from an Australian range that is fast becoming her desert island favourite.

Learn to contour and sculpt your face

Over the years faces lose definition, with saggier and more padded cheekbones and jawlines. Here, make-up expert Mary Greenwell shares the secrets to creating a more sculpted, slimmer look

A little extra weight as we age can be flattering to the face. There's an old saying: 'After a certain age, you have to choose between your face and your a**e', and it's true. A little fat on the face plumps out the lines from within (as you'll know if you've seen, say, a fiftysomething friend lose a lot of weight – and watched what happens to the depth of her wrinkles).

However, the flipside is that as faces fill out they lose definition. Cheekbones and jawlines get more padded, pouchier and saggier. Even beauties like Grace Kelly and Catherine Deneuve look heavier-jawed, with less gloriously-winged cheekbones. Here, international make-up pro Mary Greenwell – who's made up many a gorgeous older face in her three-decade career – gives us the secret of 'contouring', for a slimmer-looking, more sculpted face. (And it's not the conventional wisdom.)

Always even out your skintone with primer and foundation first. Contouring on to bare skin, even if moisturised, could look dingy. Prepping properly gives the best effect plus staying power.

Use a fawn-y eyeshadow or a mineral powder. The traditional wisdom is that you should use bronzer for contouring but both Mary Greenwell and Terry Barber, director of make-up artistry at MAC (whose products Mary recommends for contouring) say, simply, don't! 'Look at the colour of the shadow under your chin,' says Mary. 'It's fawn. To mimic that, you need something with no red in it, and zero sparkle or shimmer.' Terry recommends

> If you *long* for a slimmer-looking face, *contouring* is an *art* worth mastering

MAC's new-generation powder called Mineralize Skinfinish Natural, in a shade a couple of notches deeper than your skintone. It's 'satiny matt to give a moisturised finish', and will add definition without creating dull 'theatre' shadows. Terry advises a two-step approach: 'Add a hint of bright, fresh rose or apricot quite high on your cheekbones, then sweep the deeper colour in from your temples, under the lower half of your cheekbones.'

Use a blusher brush to apply the shadow (an angled one is good). 'Think "shade" here. Sweep the brush across the eyeshadow and tap the handle on a hard surface to remove any excess. To refine the jawline, sweep the brush along the underside of the jaw from edge to edge,' says Mary.

Don't forget right underneath the jaw. 'If you look at someone's chin and jaw, you'll notice that a real shadow goes all the way back to the angle at which the underneath of the chin meets the neck. So should the contouring. Apply lightly, and then add more until the jaw is more defined.'

Give yourself cheekbones, too. 'The principle is the same for under your cheekbones as under your jaw: same product, same brush. Start at the hairline by your ears, and sweep the shadow under the cheekbone. For a truly natural effect, you can apply a whisper of blusher (or blusher and bronzer) to your cheeks, as you normally would, on top of the contour powder.'

Spend an evening practising at home in front of the mirror. Ideally, use a 'triptych' mirror or angle a couple of mirrors so that you can see yourself from the side. If you long for a slimmer-looking face, contouring is an art worth mastering.

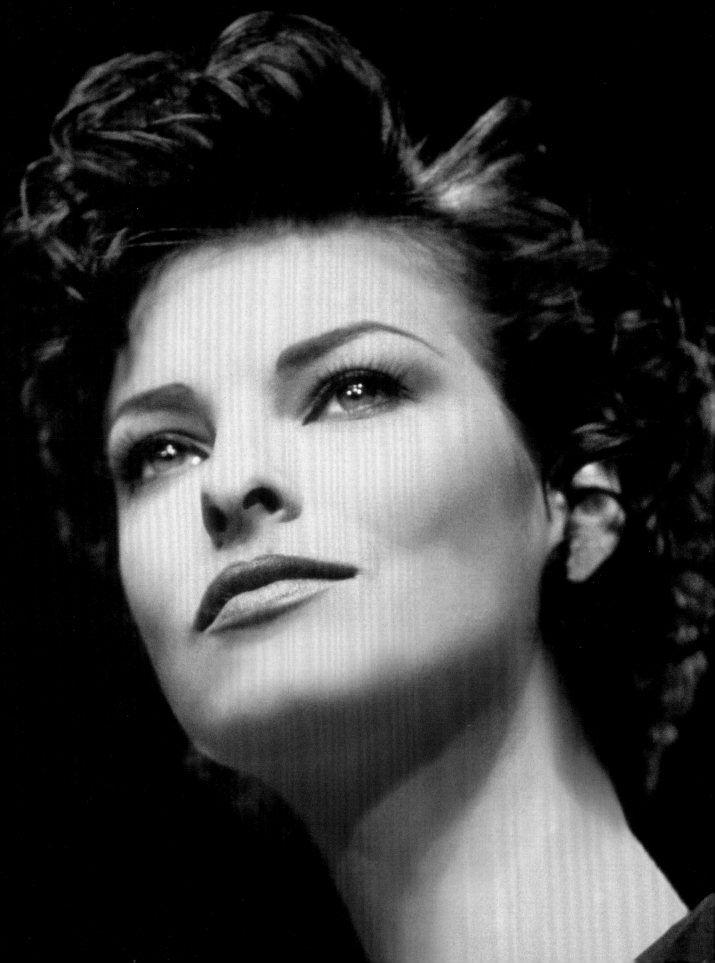

Before you sign up for cosmetic fillers, read this!

If you're considering filler injections, laser treatment, a peel, Botox or even a facelift, it's essential to get as much information as you can first. Cosmetic surgery expert Wendy Lewis tells you all the questions you need to ask to help you get the best possible result

Whenever we want the lowdown on cosmetic procedures and clinical treatments, we turn to Wendy Lewis – aka The Knife Coach, who runs the truly independent Global Aesthetics Consultancy in the UK, Europe and America (as well as writing books, which we list at the back of this one). There is nothing Wendy doesn't know about who's the best, what's new – and the questions that every single woman should ask, not just before undergoing major surgery, but even having what may seem like a minor procedure such as Botox.

As Wendy says, there are – amazingly – people who sign up for fillers, Botox, lasers, peels and even full-blown facelifts without giving the issue much more thought than if they were shopping for a new face cream.

We can't tell you whether you should have a filler injection, or whether you really need a facelift. We believe this is very much a matter of personal choice (though ours is not to). But it is vital to know the right questions to ask before you take the plunge – to optimise your chances of a successful treatment and a good outcome.

Get real. Although some of the most popular procedures are non-surgical, none of them are non-medical. They should be performed in a clinical environment under good lighting and under the direction of a qualified and medically-trained professional. For example, wrinkle-relaxing and filling injections should only be done by a medical aesthetics practitioner, which in the UK includes doctors, nurses and dentists.

Have an initial consultation. Make an appointment with one or preferably two healthcare practitioners. Insist on having adequate time with the individual who will actually be carrying out the procedure – not an assistant or sales person. Your relationship with the person who will be doing your treatment is most important, and he/she is not interchangeable.

Ask serious questions (see box right).

Ask for detailed printed information on every procedure you are considering. Every doctor should have his own materials, pre- and post-treatment instructions, or at least brochures from companies whose products he/she is using, and there should be more consumer information on the websites of all of these brands. However, be aware that no honest or responsible practitioner can guarantee a specific result – we are all individuals and everyone responds differently.

Ask to see photographs of other patients. You should be able to look at real photos of clients who have undergone the procedure/ technique carried out by this specific practitioner. This is most important: there have been instances where one doctor may be showing patients another doctor's results, or labelling the filler company's 'before-and-after' photos as his own work. The caveat: be aware that you can expect to see only photos of the best-case scenario and judge from there – no one will show their worst results. It is impossible to predict the

TIP

Before treatment, Wendy recommends:

● **Avoid aspirin products (Nurofen, ibuprofen), blood thinners or vitamin E** for one to two weeks before treatment to prevent increased bleeding and bruising.
● **Don't have a treatment on an empty stomach** – you may get dizzy or faint.
● **Ice packs before and after** can help with pain and swelling.
● **Bring concealer** with you to cover up bruises or needle marks.

exact result that you may get from a procedure, but photographs offer a good guideline for what is reasonable to expect.

Check out the practitioner's qualifications, experience and training. Find out what professional organisations he/she is a member of and visit their websites for confirmation if needed. Check online to see if the practitioner has had any legal cases brought against them, and what the outcome was.

Tap into your intuition. How do you get along with the person who is going to be wielding the needle? You should feel you can trust him/her with your face and/or body. If you don't get a good vibe, move on. There are many practitioners and clinics to choose from.

Have a good look round. Is the clinic clean and orderly? Does he/she employ professional assistants and nurses? Ask to see inside the room where the procedure will take place, and satisfy yourself that it's the proper clinical setting necessary for a medical treatment. Also look at the other patients in the waiting room – do you like the way they look? And do you like how the staff and even the doctor look? If not, run a mile!

See DIRECTORY for organisations where you can research your practitioner and/or clinic.

WENDY'S VITAL QUESTIONS TO ASK

● What is the medical name of the treatment the practitioner is recommending?
● How long has it been on the market?
● How long has the practitioner been using it?
● What is the name of the manufacturer and where are they located?
● What clinical studies have been done?
● What is the source of the filler material – is it natural, animal or synthetic?
● What are the possible side effects?
● Could I be allergic to it?
● What does a reaction look like and how long does it last?
● What can be done if I have a reaction?
● How many treatments will I need and how often will I need to come back?
● How much will each treatment cost?
● If I don't like it, what can be done?
● Can I still have other treatments (fillers, wrinkle relaxers, lasers, peels) later?
● Is this the best laser technology/filler/injection to accomplish my goals?
● What are the alternatives?
● Does it have a CE mark (ie, comply with European Health and Safety legislation)?
● Is it approved by the US Food and Drug Administration (FDA) and UK Medicines and Healthcare products Regulatory Agency (MHRA)?
● Is it licensed for cosmetic use?

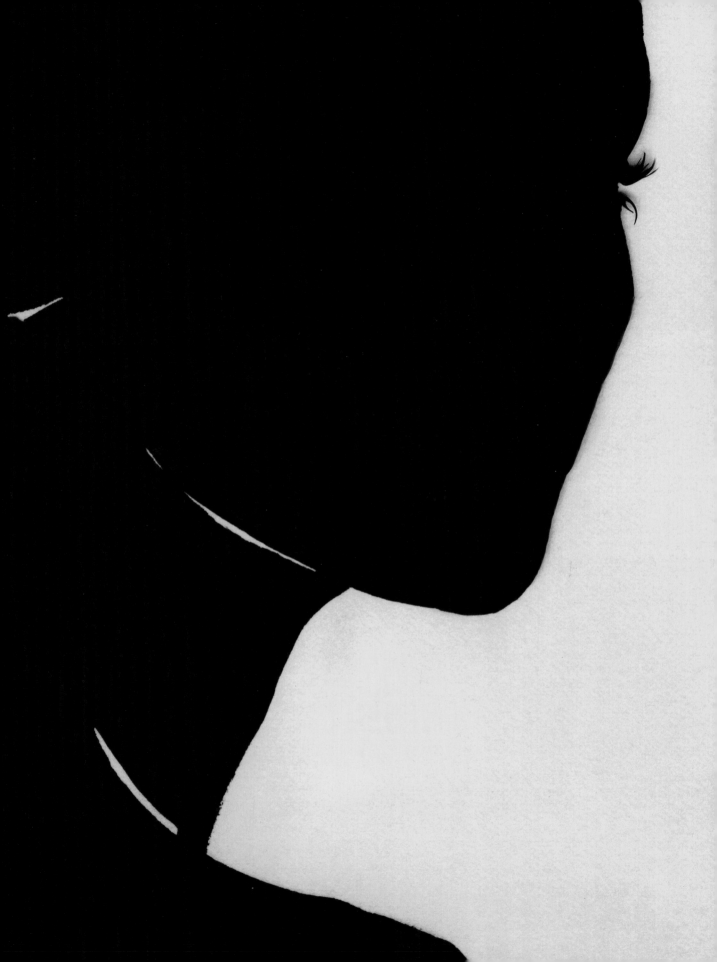

'I NEVER want to lie about my age. The actresses I *admire* are all women who have not fought growing older, but EMBRACED it – like Sophia Loren or Audrey Hepburn'

Penélope Cruz

Keep your eyes on the prize

For eyes, read 'angst'. They can be top of many a woman's list of beauty woes, as the years roll by. Think: puffy bags. Think: dark circles. Think: 'laugh lines' (that's the nice way to describe them). And then there's the challenge of applying eye make-up when a) skin's just not as smooth as it was, and b) you can barely see what you're doing anyway…

But leaving vanity aside (temporarily!), what should be absolutely paramount is eye health. Beauty may be in the eye of the beholder, but the bottom line is that we all want to go on beholding everything. So before we give you a rundown of products over the next few pages which will help with the beauty challenges, and share some fabulous make-up tips, here's how to optimise eye health – and help prevent eye-lines at the same time.

Don't frown! Forgive us for stating the obvious but how do you think frown lines get there…? Exactly. But looking after your eyes isn't just about a smooth forehead: taking very good care of eye health in general is absolutely vital as we get older. So…

Wear big sunglasses. Choose glasses which are UVA/B protective. And slap on a broad-brimmed sunhat, not just for the sake of your skin and hair but also, very importantly, for your eyes. Just look at the way people screw up their eyes and face in bright sunlight… Even in not-so-bright conditions, wind is a damage-doer too – and sunglasses provide great protection from dust, specks of dirt and the eye-drying effect of a mistral. Remember, they're also instant glam!

Take reading glasses everywhere and *wear* them. Sarah recently looked at a photo of herself trying to decipher a Christmas cracker joke and nearly choked as she saw the two deep lines scored down her forehead. Motto: must take specs – in chic case, possibly hanging round neck – with you at all times. (Jo keeps a pair in every room of the house, which is also very much appreciated by presbyopic friends.) If you are caught out and about without them, get someone to read to you – the menu, the programme, whatever. (One super-elegant friend takes a lorgnette out and about…!)

Have regular eye tests. The right specs help you read, work at a computer screen, drive safely and prevent frown lines and headaches. Testing can also pick up any other conditions such as glaucoma, which damages the optic nerve and may cause blindness if untreated. Every two years is a minimum when you're over forty, and every year if you have glaucoma in the

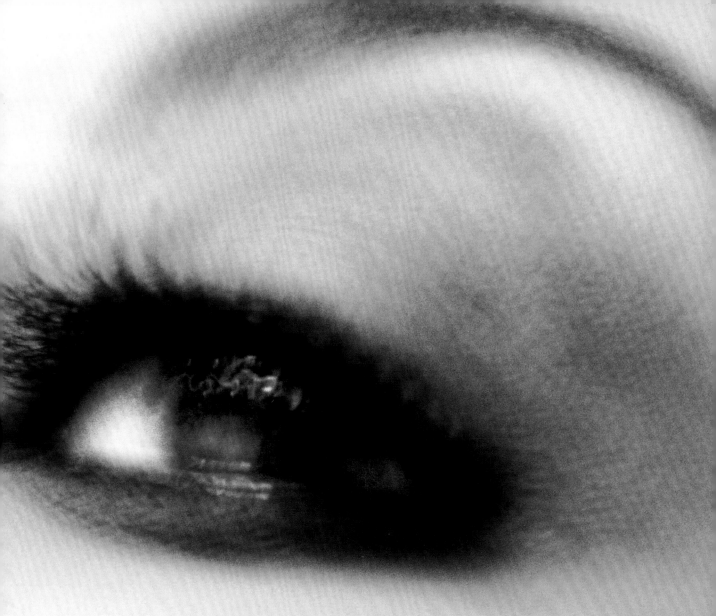

family. NB: Women over sixty in the UK can claim free eye tests and will usually get a discount on spectacles. (Remember to get at least one pair of prescription sunglasses, too.)

Attend to dry eyes. OK, it's age again! Like our skin, eyes get drier as we get older, especially if you work at a screen and/or in an office with aircon. If your eyes are itchy, sore, red, stick together on waking and, more seriously, you have any blurred vision, consult your family doctor or talk to your optician. Hopefully, it will just be a case of applying drops once or twice a day. (Sarah swears by Viscotears, a thin gel/ointment you can apply any time – but beware it can blur your sight for a few moments.)

Invest in a good, strong reading light. According to consultant ophthalmologist Professor Charles Clark, 'This can improve vision enormously, slow the deterioration of sight – and reduce frowning!' Obviously, this isn't just for reading but for any close-up fine work, such as tapestry (which Sarah does – very slowly – in the dark winter evenings; Jo knits!). We like the range of lamps from www.seriousreaders.com, which have options for everything.

Consider a supplement. The 'Age-Related Eye Disease Study', sponsored by the US National Eye Institute, reported that two nutrients – called lutein and zeaxanthin, which are both found in healthy retinas – may help your vision and protect your eyes from the age-related condition called macular degeneration. A product called Brite Eyes Formula by LifeTime Vitamins is based on bilberry and eyebright, which contain these nutrients, plus a range of other helpful ingredients. Fish oil, which contains omega-3 essential fatty acid, may also help vision. But you should still eat lots of green, red and orange vegetables and fruit (full of lutein and zeaxanthin) plus at least two portions of oily fish weekly, if you're not vegetarian.

Anti-ageing eye creams: our award winners

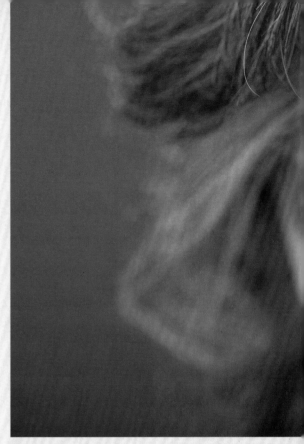

Because eyes are so expressive – conveying joy, or sadness, or anger – the skin around them wrinkles faster than anywhere else on the face. The skin beneath the eyes also contains less collagen and elastin than the rest of the face. And as a triple whammy, this fragile skin is fine as eggshell – only one quarter as thick as that on the soles of your feet. (Precisely because it's so thin, moisture evaporates very easily)

But – hallelujah – we do know, from years of trials on real women, that there are plenty of products out there to make a difference to those expression lines. We've now dispatched over 130 different products to panellists for this book series, requesting them to try them on one eye only. There were some truly spectacular performances – and two new award winners in this latest edition.

AT A GLANCE

Elizabeth Arden Prevage Eye Advanced Anti-Aging Serum

Liz Earle Superskin Eye & Lip Treatment

Dr Hauschka Regenerating Eye Cream

Murad Intensive Wrinkle Reducer for Eyes

Elemis Pro-Collagen Advanced Eye Treatment

REVIEWS

Elizabeth Arden Prevage Eye Advanced Anti-Aging Serum

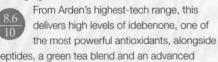

From Arden's highest-tech range, this delivers high levels of idebenone, one of the most powerful antioxidants, alongside peptides, a green tea blend and an advanced moisture complex, designed to target puffiness and dark circles as well as lines. In general, because serums sink in faster, you can apply this type of eye treatment to lids in addition to the whole eye zone: they don't 'travel', and so avoid irritation.
Comments: 'After a few days I could see the difference and my "crow" lines seemed softer; I was also amazed by how well it worked on my puffy eyes and I had to start using it on both, as there

was a noticeable difference' • 'fine lines, wrinkles, dark circles, crêpiness all reduced and it seemed to "lift" the area' • 'lines reduced; I was pleasantly surprised – I've used lots of eye creams and this is the best so far' • 'skin around the eye zone a lot smoother' • 'eye make-up went on really well afterwards, including foundation and brow pencil – a real winner' • 'I know it's not cheap, but worth it: I'll definitely be buying this'.

Liz Earle Superskin Eye & Lip Treatment

Like all the Superskin range this is formulated for more mature or very dry skin, to apply morning and night before moisturising. Ingredients include organic pear seed extract, shea butter, plus cranberry, rosehip and borage seed oils. Although our testers were asked to trial it as an eye treatment, they loved its double-duty beauty bonus for lips too.
Comments: 'I liked the pump and the very light consistency, which absorbed really easily, wasn't greasy, left no residue and didn't irritate my very sensitive eyes; left skin round eyes looking instantly brighter, hydrated and plump. I can't recommend this enough' • 'after six weeks fine lines are less noticeable, wrinkles less prominent, eyes brighter and puffiness reduced also dark circles: was told I

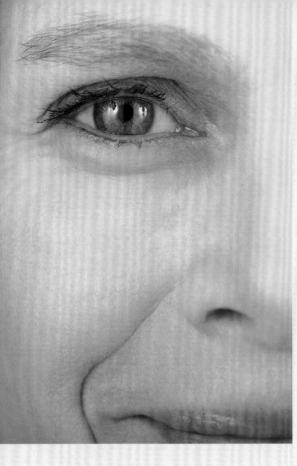

looked "bright eyed and bushy tailed" by a colleague' • 'fabulous multi-tasking treatment' • 'one of the best of the many eye creams I have tried; skin texture looks smoother and fine lines improved – I will absolutely buy it' • 'fine lines have not disappeared but skin looks a lot smoother on the 'test' eye'.

Dr Hauschka Regenerating Eye Cream

8.43/10 Another pump dispenser, which our testers liked, with this product from a dedicated organic and biodynamic German brand, which we have loved for decades. The light cream features a protective, toning and replenishing bunch of botanicals, including red clover, acerola berries and sea buckthorn, with birch leaf, quince seed and borage to refine pores and shea butter. The brand recommends using this fast-absorbing cream in the morning as a primer for eye make-up
Comments: 'Nice creamy texture that went in well – only need a tiny amount; skin felt smooth and moisturised and instantly brightened up eye area on the treated eye; noticeable reduction in dark circle and lines, which continued over six weeks of use' • 'my sister noticed reduction in dark circles and wanted to try herself; much better than my usual product and no irritation' • 'skin looked "perked up"

with overall brightness round the treated eye area; positive comments – a delight to use and you can really see a difference in the eye I used it on' • 'I used this after being on holiday in the sun and it definitely helped to remoisturise skin round eye area' • 'no flakiness when I applied make-up over the top'.

Murad Intensive Wrinkle Reducer for Eyes

 8.43/10 Dr Howard Murad's was one of the pioneering dermatologist brands in the skincare world, founded in 1989, and this features a breakthrough ingredient derived from the superfruit durian, alongside powerful antioxidants including goji berry, plus anti-inflammatories and moisture-boosting hydrators.
Comments: '10/10: fabulously hydrating, improved wrinkles, lines, puffiness, dark circles and crêpiness, made eyes look brighter and seemed to "lift" the area; my partner said the "test" eye looked better' • 'fine lines improved, deep lines less deep and defined, eye area looks younger, eyes much, much brighter and tired bags almost gone. I can see a real difference in the left eye. One of the best products I have used in a long time!' • 'finer lines definitely improved and skin more elastic and smoother, wrinkles less prominent, crêpiness of eyelids improved and disappeared after four weeks, puffiness definitely down, dark circles not gone completely but am hopeful. Several people said I look well'.

Elemis Pro-Collagen Advanced Eye Treatment

 8.43/10 Throughout this book the phrase 'Pro-Collagen' appears time and again: this line is an amazing Elemis performer, with the newly launched gel eye treatment finding instant favour. Key active include amino acids and a 'Macro Cellular Complex' (including water-retentive mushroom polysaccharides and wheat proteins), plus nourishing linseed extract, in a 'weightless' formula that gives the eye zone the appearance of dewiness.
Comments: 'Eye area felt really moisturised and conditioned after using, and it sank in immediately; fine lines improved significantly even though I wasn't using an eye cream on top, it even helped with puffiness and eyes looked brighter' • 'one drop for each eye is plenty, so it lasts for months, eyes felt hydrated all day' • '10/10, this was wonderful, fine lines were smoothed out instantly and wrinkles less prominent, dark circles gone. Made me look gorgeous and several years younger'.

♡ WE LOVE...

With sensitive eyes, Jo tried dozens of anti-ageing eye treatments but is now unswervingly devoted to the ever-so-slightly coffee-scented This Works No Wrinkles Tired Eyes, which is slightly illuminating to eliminate dark circles and signs of fatigue, but also (she believes) has helped with lines. Sarah's eyes rebel against many products, but when her eyes are super-sore, she strokes on Trilogy Very Gentle Calming Serum, a tip from a biochemist friend.

TIP

Use your ring finger for applying eye creams, as this has the lightest touch and is least likely to pull the skin. Starting at the inner corner, dot the cream from just below your lashes to the outer corner of your orbital bone, patting it into the skin. Do the same above the eye. NB: Serums and gels can be applied to the lids – but not creams; put them no closer to the eye than the top of the crease, where you can feel bone beneath your finger.

&Lighten those dark circles

Fact: we get more anxious questions about under-eye circles to www.beautybible.com than almost any other subject (except eye bags and crow's feet). In a survey by Clinique of 13,000 users, about 53 per cent cited dark circles and puffiness as their number one concern. So here's how to make shadows, well, a shadow of their former selves

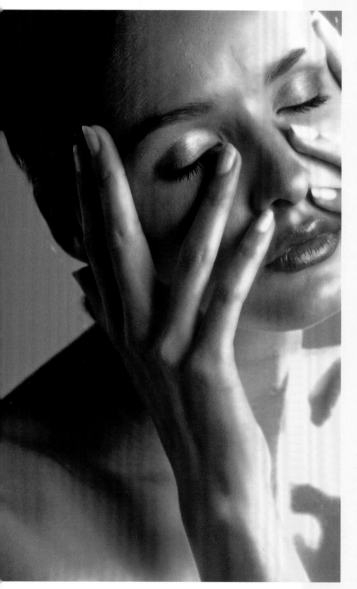

Conceal, conceal, conceal. Overleaf, you'll see the top light-reflective concealers, in our testers' considered opinions. If there's a shade choice, pick a yellow-based concealer if your dark circles have a purple or blue cast; go with a peachy colour if they are browner in tone. Meanwhile, women with darker skintones may find that light-reflective concealers just don't work for them – so you'll want to know that Guerlain Precious Light and the legendary YSL Touche Eclat come in darker shade options. And Bobbi Brown actually created her Corrector concealer specifically for dark circles, with the darkest shade being Very Deep Bisque, from the wide range of 16 shades.

Try Traditional Chinese Medicine. In TCM (as it's known in the holistic realm), dark circles can be linked to an imbalance in kidney energy – which can be helped by acupuncture. With TCM, as with all complementary therapies, seek out someone who is qualified and registered (see DIRECTORY for more details).

Drink plenty of water. For some women, dark circles can be a sign of dehydration. Another good reason to sip those eight glasses a day.

Consider using a cream targeted at 'sun spots'. For some women, dark circles can be linked to hyperpigmentation (see box opposite), in which case it may be worth trying one of the age-spot-lightening creams which performed best in our trials (see page 190). Don't apply so close to the eye that there's a risk of the product 'travelling' into the eye itself, as these can contain potent ingredients that might sting.

Try a D-I-Y Ayurvedic eye mask. Ayurvedic beauty expert Monisha Bharadwaj swears by a recipe for tackling dark circles handed down by her family. 'Crush five mint leaves in a little water with a pestle and mortar. Strain the juice and add to one teaspoon of almond oil and half a teaspoon of honey. Stir until completely mixed and apply a tiny amount under the eyes before going to bed.' Works wonders, she swears.

Clear your nasal passages. As nasal congestion is a common cause (see box right), clearing the respiratory tract may help. If it could be an allergy, try a supplement such as Aller-DMG, and also a barrier product (balm, cream or spray) in your nose which helps to prevent allergens being inhaled. A steam 'head bath' (also brilliant for your complexion) clears nasal passages a treat: fill a bowl with very hot water, add a few drops of essential oil such as eucalyptus, peppermint, rosemary, cover your head with a towel and steam gently for five minutes.

Try an antihistamine. If you think your underlying problem could be an allergy to an airborne substance (as in hayfever, or an allergy to something in a fragrance or cosmetic), an antihistamine could be a simple solution.

Eat dark-circle-busting foods. Certain antioxidant-rich foods may help to strengthen capillaries: edible eye TLC comes in the form of blueberries, cranberries, bilberries, blackcurrants, onions, peas and beans, as well as green and black tea.

Follow the dark circles blog! Believe it or not, there is an entire community on the net, written by dark-circle sufferers and focusing on women's experiences with many of the creams and non-surgical treatments on the market targeting this beauty challenge – www. mydarkcirclesblog.com is pretty commercial (and US-based), but it will at least reassure you that you are far from alone.

WHAT CAUSES DARK CIRCLES?

There are multiple causes for dark circles (medically called periorbital hyperchromia), according to medical research.

Genes They can be genetic, affecting any skin colour and type, but Asian and Afro-Caribbean races and southern Italians are particularly prone to them.

Hyperpigmentation The browner type of dark circles, rather than the bluish-hued type, could be the results of post-inflammatory hyperpigmentation due to sun damage or hormonal fluctuations, notes dermatologist Dr Nicholas Perricone.

Older, thinner skin As we age, we become more prone to permanent dark circles – simply because, as skin thins, the blood vessels in the under-eye zone show up more. Airborne allergens cause blood to pool in the vessels under the skin, worsening the appearance of any dilated blood vessels.

Nasal congestion Famously, they're linked with lack of sleep, but consider this insight from beauty guru Liz Earle: 'The most common cause of dark circles is nasal congestion. When your nose is bunged up, veins that usually drain from your eyes into your nose become dilated and darker.' Ask yourself if you tend to get them with hayfever during the summer, or ongoing colds in the winter. Equally something in your beauty regime could be the culprit (we have often found the finger pointed at a new mascara or eye cream, which may also cause puffiness).

Stress Dr Perricone also blames stress: 'When your body is in fight or flight mode, your brain, like every other organ, leaches every single molecule of oxygen it can from the blood, so a darker, more deoxygenated blood flows through your veins. This dark blood is most visible in the transparent skin under our eyes, and is what causes the appearance of these discoloured veins.' (The skin under the eyes is the thinnest on the body.)

Drugs Some drugs, including the contraceptive pill and HRT, can darken the eye area by dilating blood vessels.

Smoking Women who smoke – which affects micro-circulation long before it leads to heart and lung problems – can be prone to dark circles, too.

'I choose *NOT* to hang on to this **ideal** of looking 20 years old but **understand** that I have a wealth of EXPERIENCE to share. I make the *best* of what I have, but I don't long for who I *used* to be' Elle Macpherson

Concealers for dark circles: *our award winners*

At our age, a woman needs a (small) wardrobe of concealers. Here, you'll find the best candidates for disguising dark circles under eyes, which also work well on pigmentation

AT A GLANCE

YSL Touche Eclat

Lancôme Teint Miracle Perfecting Concealer Pen

Clinique Airbrush Concealer

Guerlain Precious Light Rejuvenating Illuminator

TIP

Don't only apply light-reflecting concealer under the eye: a couple of dots at the inner corners of your eye, near your tear ducts and on the bridge of the nose, instantly makes eyes look fresher.

Three out of our top four are light-reflecting so they also blur lines – stroke them in grooves and wrinkles too, to see the effect of the 'optical pigments'. Light-reflective concealers can also be used to highlight the brow bone, or accentuate a pout, when stroked along the top lip; they can do double-duty as an eyeshadow base, too. Of the many, many choices now out there, our testers help you by narrowing it down to these top picks. (And for concealers to hide those other flaws, such as veins and redness/scars, turn to page 91. For products to help puffiness, see page 60.)

REVIEWS

YSL Touche Eclat

8.55/10 We make no apologies for the fact that this classic concealer has appeared in previous books – because we sent it out to be trialled all over again for *The Anti-Ageing Beauty Bible*, and Touche Eclat (aka Radiant Touch) romped home in first place with a fah-bu-lous score, just as it did before... Created by Terry de Gunzburg (who now has her own By Terry range) in 1992, it was the first of its type. And its legions of fans still think that this pump-action, pen-style concealer – with its built-in brush and light-reflective, line-blurring formula – is unrivalled. Our testers were assigned No 1 (Luminous Radiance), which has slightly peachy-pink hints. (NB: Great news for women with darker skins: as of fairly recently, Touche Eclat is now available in a much wider range of shades. Hallelujah.) A Hall of Fame product, if ever there was one.

Comments: 'Perfect for dark circles – the best product in my opinion! Didn't cover completely but blended them in and made them less noticeable' • 'looked very natural; I always carry one in my make-up bag' • be careful not to overdo or it can look too pale' • 'blended in well over a moisturiser or cream foundation but not as good over a mineral base; great cover-up job on thread veins round my nose and sun spots under eyes; ideal quick fix before morning school run' • '10+++ for this brilliant camouflage for dark circles, also great for lines on my forehead' • 'my magic wand – I thought it was all hype, but how wrong I was! It's easy to use, gives an amazing effect – so many comments about how well I look!!!'.

Lancôme Teint Miracle Perfecting Concealer Pen

8.43/10 This light-reflecting silver wand-style concealer comes in four shades (our testers had the lightest, 01), and is very lightweight in texture. Though designed to be used with Lancôme Teint Miracle Foundation, our testers trialled this alongside/over/under their regular base, with great results.

Comments: 'Looked more awake on mornings when I was tired and hadn't slept much' • 'blends easily and gives decent coverage without caking – I sometimes use it now when I'm not wearing any other make-up as it looks so natural' • 'I never bothered with concealers in the past, considering them a waste of money – but I love this and don't think I'm going to be able to live without it when finished' • 'this product fools people into thinking

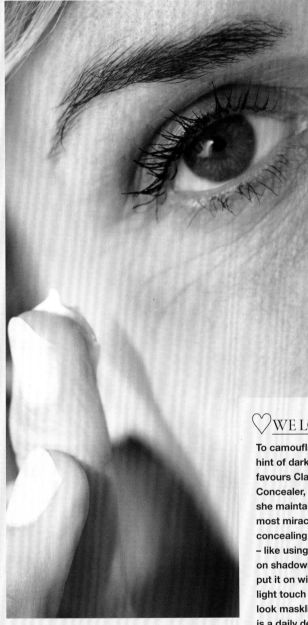

hide shadows and dark circles, and also to illuminate the eye area – and your complexion. So a real multi-tasker which you can apply on bare skin or over foundation, then pat lightly into skin.

Comments: 'Excellent! Light, moisturising product that blended in very easily and looked very natural, covering pesky dark circles and disguised wrinkles. I have dark circles and have tried MANY concealers but not this one, which is better than other illuminating pens I have tried including the really famous ones' • 'great under eyes – best one I've used – and hid the redness round my nose well too, giving coverage without caking' • 'I was so surprised at the coverage for such a light product, it uplifted the blue/black circles round my eyes without caking' • 'I love this product and recommend it completely! Looks very natural indeed and I would absolutely buy' • 'the bonus is that it evens out redness on my T-zone too…'.

Guerlain Precious Light Rejuvenating Illuminator

8.4/10 Like Touche Eclat, this comes in a sexy gold wand, with a brush at the tip to sweep on a formula enriched with Gold Radiance Pigments and Precious Rejuvenating Complex. Which means that… Precious Light claims to offer skincare benefits as well as the instant cosmetic boost. Myrrh – known for its invigorating and rejuvenating powers – is a key ingredient. In three shades – our testers had the lightest, 01.

Comments: 'Fantastic at covering up quite dark circles under eyes, also small scars; a pigmentation mark on my forehead became invisible' • 'very easy to apply, blended well; brightened up dark circles, small scars looked less obvious; good coverage' • 'a must for your make-up bag' • 'very clever at reflecting light away from my face – great product' • 'very effective product on my very pale skin; when I get tired it looks so obvious and this created a good complexion' • 'smooth consistency and didn't cake when built up thinly; made eyes look younger, also covered freckles and hyperpigmentation' • 'I used a lot on my dark circles but it didn't cake or crack, despite a whole evening of laughter and smiling'.

♡ WE LOVE…

To camouflage any hint of dark circles, Jo favours Clarins Instant Concealer, which she maintains 'is the most miraculously concealing concealer – like using an eraser on shadows, but do put it on with a very light touch or it can look masklike'. Sarah is a daily devotee of Liz Earle Light Reflective Concealer, which she uses in the dark corners either side of the bridge of her nose and the lower inner corners of her eyes, which are often blue-y. Also brilliant for the creases under eyebags.

you've had eight hours of sleep!' • 'disguised dark circles and definitely gave a more luminous look' • 'definitely lives up to its promise of providing radiance' • 'looked very natural after being applied and patted into the skin' • 'pleased to find this didn't cake at all, even after wearing it all day'.

Clinique Airbrush Concealer

8.41/10 This light reflective concealer, in a brush pen dispenser, comes in 11 shades, including two dark ones. It's designed to

Unpack those eye bags

Maybe you get them just sometimes. (We all do.) Maybe they're the bane of your life. (As for many of our readers.) The simple truth is: none of us likes excess under-eye baggage and, as we age, skin loses elasticity, so the eye area can be more prone to swelling. Here are the best fixes we know…

Sleep with an extra pillow. If you can get in the habit of sleeping on your back (not everyone can – and remember it is the sleep position most linked with s-n-o-r-i-n-g), then this extra elevation can help to prevent fluid from building up in the eye area overnight. (Most puffy-prone women find the problem's worst before lunch – good reason never to be photographed until the afternoon…)

Check out eye products containing caffeine. In our experience (and anecdotally that of our testers), some products containing caffeine as an ingredient can be especially helpful for smoothing away puffiness.

Or give your eyes a drink of tea. Since caffeine has proven useful for banishing dark circles, a low-tech solution is two tea bags (black, caffeinated, rich in natural tannins), kept in the freezer rather than the fridge and placed on the eyes to constrict blood vessels and drain fluid.

Try a roller-ball. It makes perfect sense to us that something which has a physical action can literally smooth away puffiness – and sure enough, metal roller-balls can prove amazingly effective. You literally roll them around the puffy area in a circular/outward motion, to disperse fluid. As a low-tech version, real silver/silver-plated teaspoons kept in the fridge can be used to 'tap' away fluid. Jo uses a little silver-tipped applicator – like a baby drum baton – that she got with a Crème de la Mer eye product, for the same task: 'miraculous', is her verdict. It's an expensive way to get your hands on one of the most brilliant eye de-puffers of all time… so failing that, go the teaspoon route.

Have a chilled, gel-filled mask on standby in the fridge. There are quite a few on the market, although we prefer the type that don't have eye-holes, as they offer more even pressure (and cooling action) on the whole eye area. (The Body Shop's Cooling Gel Eye Mask is excellent, or see DIRECTORY for other sources.) Lie prone, place mask on eyes for 10–15 minutes and let the cool gel work its soothing magic.

Eliminate your eye cream itself from the list of culprits. Sometimes a product which is designed to deal with lines and wrinkles can very annoyingly trigger puffiness. If you think there's any chance at all that your puffy eyes are product-related, stop using the potential culprit for five days and note any difference. If it's the cream, you'll know because you'll see an improvement. If it's not, your puffiness will be unchanged. Be aware that eye gels are less likely to 'travel' into the eyes themselves than creams; only gels or serums can be applied on the lids themselves, as there's a risk with any oil-based product of getting into the eye – and puffiness, as well as redness, is your body's sign of rebellion.

Reduce salt intake and drink less alcohol. Oh, we're a couple of killjoys, but if you're serious about this, cut down on salt and alcoholic drinks, both of which are notoriously linked with fluid retention. Ditto any foods containing MSG; you can ask in

WHAT CAUSES PUFFINESS?

As with dark circles, there's a long list of potential culprits and it can help to try to 'unpick' your personal trigger/s, so that you can take the lifestyle steps needed to minimise the problem. First (darn it): heredity – your genes may simply incorporate the DNA that leads to thicker fat pads under the eyes, in which case there may not be much you can do to tackle the problem. There is surgery available for fat-removal under the eyes, but if performed too early in life (or if too much fat is removed), this can lead to a really hollow look later on (not a good look). Second is water retention – which is linked with diet, sleeping habits, alcohol and even hormonal roller-coastering. Third, allergies can be responsible if you're allergic to pollen, pesticides, latex, certain foods, including grains and additives including MSG, cosmetics or fragrance. These can all trigger puffiness. And even the most smooth-eyed among us can get all pouchy with a cold.

Chinese restaurants for this ingredient to be left out, but it features in a lot of ingredient lists on processed foods, often by different names such as glutamic acid, vegetable protein extract, hydrolysed vegetable protein/HVP, sodium caseinate or even yeast extract. The safest way to avoid it is always to eat fresh, unprocessed foods. Foods which have a diuretic (water-banishing) effect include celery, cucumber, watermelon, radishes and parsley.

Do plenty of cardiovascular exercise. It revs up your circulation, which helps to eliminate excess water through sweating. In our experience, everything just 'flows' better when we've exercised – and a brisk 30-minute walk can work wonders for unpacking that eye baggage. A workout followed by a sauna or steam bath can flush out puffies almost miraculously.

Make like Linda Evangelista. Readers of our earlier books may be familiar with this trick, but it sure as hell is worth repeating: stroke an ice cube over the skin, working in an outwards direction. If you're prone to broken veins, wrap it in clingfilm first. Jo watched Ms Evangelista do this on a photoshoot and it was right up there with the miracle of the loaves and the fishes in terms of transformations. (Sarah has been known to order a bowl of ice simply to stroke round her super-sensitive, prone-to-puffies eyes.)

&Treats for tired & puffy eyes: *our award winners*

There are two issues that we get more emails about to www.beautybible.com than almost anything else. First, dark circles (which we help you to conceal on page 56) and, second, under-eye puffiness. Even if you've never had tired-looking eyes in your youth, the mid-years can be a time of excess eye baggage and shadows. Since bright, sparkling eyes make you look instantly rejuvenated, we're delighted to bring you the newly updated results of this trial – which proves that there are effective treatments to tackle these Big Beauty Challenges. Yes, in the blink of an eye…

AT A GLANCE

A'Kin White Tea and Cornflower Brightening & Tightening Eye Day Gel

Estée Lauder Stress Relief Eye Mask

Repêchage Cell Renewal Eye Rescue Pads

Decléor Aroma Solutions Serum Hydrotenseur Anti-Fatigue

TIP

'I keep a bottle of witch hazel lotion in the fridge for when I wake up a bit puffy around the eyes. Soak two cotton pads in it, place them on your eyes and lie down for a few minutes. It really takes away the tiredness.' – Mary Greenwell

REVIEWS

A'Kin White Tea and Cornflower Brightening & Tightening Eye Day Gel

8.08/10 This lightweight refreshing gel cream from an Australian natural skincare brand that has garnered several Beauty Bible awards for eye products and now gains the top score in this category. With white tea and alpha lipoic acid antioxidants, plus esculin to help stimulate microcirculation and cornflower to help smooth and refine skin texture, this can be used under make-up or to refresh eyes during the day.

Comments: 'Cooling gel that definitely makes eyes feel refreshed, eyes felt and looked brighter and – after some gentle patting, under eye bags looked a lot better' • 'gel wasn't too runny and not at all sticky or tacky, eyes felt very refreshed and looked bright, more awake; I suffer itchy stingy eyes in the summer and this was a great treatment: uplifting, calming, soothing and a pleasure to use' • 'puffiness less prominent, eye area felt a bit tighter, darkness and appearance of wrinkles reduced slightly' • 'I now apply this half through the day as my eyes get tired from sitting in front of a computer; I was amazed at the difference it made'.

Estée Lauder Stress Relief Eye Mask

8/10 These see-through gauze pads come in sachets (two pads per single-use sachet), to be pressed on to the under-eye zone while you relax for ten minutes and allow ingredients such as vitamin A palmitate, hyaluronic acid (for a moisture boost), aloe vera, cucumber, allantoin and bisabolol to soothe, hydrate and reduce redness.

Comments: 'A bit of a hero product this: puffy eyes from a cold visibly reduced, and my life-long dark circles much improved; also I am a big investor in eye creams and concealers and both work much better if I have used the mask before; when eyes are tired, tight and sore, the effects are very soothing, cooling and moisturising' • 'my sensitive eyes look brighter, fresher and more hydrated, made me awake again after a very hard day – brilliant when you want to go out after a long day' • 'love the cooling sensation, and made the dehydrated skin around my eyes look more plumped and moisturised – does what it says and is worth the money'.

Repêchage Cell Renewal Eye Rescue Pads

7.98/10 These are pads, too (from a Manhattan spa brand): circular cotton versions, infused with moisturising seaweed elements and no less than four types of antioxidant tea to reduce puffiness and tone the area. Again, ten minutes should do the trick.

Comments: 'Eyes felt clear and bright and skin smooth and moisturised; the packaging for these pads says these are a vacation for the eyes and it really is the case' • 'because I felt so refreshed I

ANTI-AGEING AWARD WINNERS BEAUTY BIBLE

Jo has plenty of beauty woes, but puffy eyes and shadows aren't really among them. However, when her eyes feel computer-weary, she reaches for she reaches for the pair of 001 EyeCicles she keeps in the fridge: 'these glass liquid-filled globes on "sticks" are amazing for smoothing away puffiness. Expensive, no question, but so effective.' Sarah does have puffy eyes – but no dark circles – and reaches for the ice cubes first thing in the morning, then strokes on Bright Eyes by Goldfaden MD, a natural US dermatologist brand, which brightens, lightens and de-puffs. A new find is Radical Skincare Eye Revive Crème, which is a fab eye-refresher.

needed less concealer around my eyes, and didn't pile on so much make-up; would absolutely buy' • 'really liked these pads which I kept in the fridge for extra de-puffing; using them in the morning after a late night was bliss!' • 'reduced puffiness and eyes did look brighter and renewed – very relaxing and great for a little pamper session'.

Decléor Aroma Solutions Serum Hydrotenseur Anti-Fatigue

7.78/10 This serum was formulated to smooth, moisturise and firm the eye area. Described as an 'intense treatment', it contains a high proportion of hyaluronic acid 'to

rescue to delicate eye contour area' and promises to help your eyes look as if they have had a good rest. NB one tester had a sensitivity reaction and stopped testing the product.

Comments: 'A lovely product that makes my under eye area look and feel more hydrated and will last for ages: though I will have to be careful not to drop the glass bottle' • 'eyes felt and looked brighter and under eye area less crêpey' • 'definitely felt puffiness had been reduced but not one to use when you are wearing eye make-up' • 'impressed at the instant lifting effect around the eyes – really cooling effect too, which definitely refreshes them'.

Don't let your eyebrows fade away…

Brows disappear – f-a-d-i-n-g away – if we're not careful. They may just get more sparse or go grey. Whichever, your face will quite simply lose definition – brows are the architecture of the face – if you don't either tint them (your hair colourist may be able to do this, albeit somewhat sneakily), or colour them in

TIP

Lots of clients ask expert Jenny Jordan about cutting unruly brows. She advises investing in a cheap pair of hairdressing scissors for this task. Brush brows upwards first, using a little soap on the brush to make them stick up. (It works a bit like a wax.) Then trim with the scissors – but not too close: brow hairs will fall downwards naturally and if you don't leave a bit, you may create 'huge' holes, she warns. Our advice: proceed with caution, but it can be done.

Brush on a mid-taupe/grey-ish powder shadow to colour your brows. This is most flattering for almost all brows, at this stage, to define them. Too dark and you risk that Cruella look. (Alternatively, use a pencil with a soft chalky texture – read about those which our testers got on with, overleaf.)

Extend the brow outwards, not downwards. Of course you need to follow the natural line of your brow, but by now many of us have lost the 'ends' of our brows (just plain vanished into the ether we guess) and if you need to recreate them with make-up, make sure the line wings out towards your temples, rather than down towards your cheeks. (Also see 'Plot your brow line', right.)

Brush your brows to groom them. By now, for many of us, brow hairs are literally all over the place – it sometimes seems as if they're all making a bid for freedom in different directions. A brow brush – or make-up genius Terry de Gunzburg recommends an old mascara wand that's been thoroughly washed – does the job beautifully. Brush them, apply colour, brush gently again. It makes for a much more natural effect. Legendary Hollywood make-up artist Valerie Sarnelle finishes off with her own Valerie Brow Tamer to keep them in place all day. London's brow goddess Jenny Jordan favours Tweezerman Browmousse, a gel which 'sets hairs in place without them getting crispy'.

And brush them again, if you use face powder. If you powder your face after you do your brows, you need to brush them one more time or (as expert Mary Greenwell notes), 'they can look dusty and dirty. And "clean" brows are really important at this time in life'.

Or you could try a stencil. This creates a stronger brow look than many women are used to. And we admit: when Valerie did our brows we had fits at first – they were so much more prominent than we were used to. But she's not known as 'the brow queen' for nothing, and the reactions from onlookers were so positive, we grew to love (slightly trepidatiously) the routine for special occasions. (In LA this means everyday…!) Valerie's range is simply called Valerie Beverly Hills, and her trademark Star Stencil Kit includes a foolproof stencil system for brow perfection. You choose the shape that's most flattering for you (from a wide range), then literally fill it in with a Brow Queen Pencil. Valerie teams 'significant' brows with a sheer wash of eyeshadow and lots of mascara, or even false eyelashes for a 'gorgeous, wide-awake look'.

Balance your brows with your eye make-up. More on your eyes means subtler brows; less eye make-up means you can play up your brows (as per Valerie's advice, above).

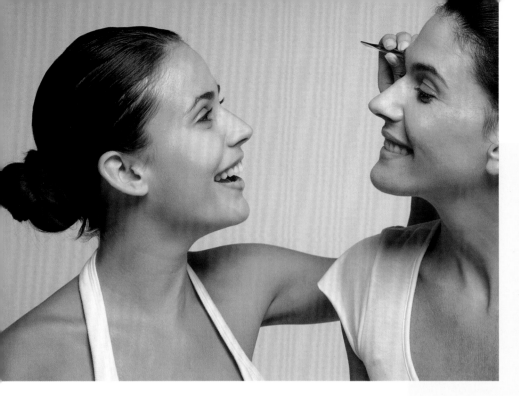

THE EYEBROW FACELIFT

There's no doubt that 'clean and tidy' brows are essential to a glossy, groomed look. If you have thick brows (lucky you!), then getting them professionally shaped – at least to start off with – can be very helpful, and makes for easier home maintenance. Even if your brows have become sparse, a professional can often improve the shape. (Sarah's were mostly blown off in a gas oven explosion years ago, not helped by over-plucking before that, and they used to skyrocket up at the arch, giving her a rather shocked look. Manhattan expert Eliza Petrescu overcame the problem by carefully plucking hairs above the brows to 'flatten' the arch somewhat, which also worked to create the illusion of widening her thinnish face.)

There's tweezing, waxing, threading, depilatories – a bunch of professional ways of shaping and tidying your brows. Whichever you choose, do talk through what's going to happen and the results you can expect with the practitioner first: it's a bit like a haircut – you can sit like a rabbit in the headlights while your brows are exterminated, which happened to Sarah with threading… (Though Jo swears by it.)

At home, we think plucking – with good slanted tweezers – is by far the easiest way to tend brow shape. We have these tips (right) from Jenny Jordan, whose Eyebrow and Make-up Clinic in London is a mecca for those in search of perfect brows. 'If you want to see the difference that brows make to a face, try putting plasters across your brows. Without them, your face has no shape,' says Jenny. 'As you get older, your brows can literally hitch up and hold your face in place. In the past few years, a new, straighter, upwards-slanting shape has emerged which is as good as a facelift.'

A word of warning: avoid over-plucking. If your brows are scanty, neglect them for a bit; applying olive oil or Vaseline every night may encourage them to grow (OK, that's a folk tale but a lot of people swear by it).

HERE ARE JENNY'S TIPS…

Generally

● Always tweeze in bright daylight, with a hand-held magnifying mirror, facing a window.
● Make sure the brow area is clean and grease-free.
● Use sharp, slant-edged tweezers which grip each hair from the root. Pointy tweezers are difficult to use on yourself.

Plot your brow line

● The line slants gently up, starting at a point above the inner corner of your eyes, but with brows never more than an inch apart over your nose.
● It goes out to a wide-angled bend (rather than the old-fashioned extreme arch), above the point where the white begins at the outer rim of your eyeball.
● Then let the line straighten up, winging towards your temples. To find the outer edge, lay a slim pencil (or a slender-handled make-up brush) up from your nostril, past the outer corner of your eye – where it crosses your brow is the natural finishing point.
● The line should be neither fat nor slim, gently tapering to the outer edge – but do avoid the dated 'tadpole' shape.
● Swipe your tweezed brows with a cotton bud dipped in pure tea tree oil, which is a natural antiseptic.
● To fill in the line, Jenny likes to brush on taupe powder so it smudges into the line, and then fixes it with brow gel.

$\mathcal{E}$ Brow pencils: our award winners

Life isn't fair. Just as hairs start randomly sprouting elsewhere on the face (see page 146 for how to tackle that), brows become finer, lighter – and can fade away drastically. Some go grey. Others just get fairer. Or sparser. But a well-defined brow – even if you have to 'fake' it – is near miraculous for helping to accentuate your features and give the face 'structure'. Very high scores for these award-winning products, with a new entry in fourth place

Although brow powders are now available on the beauty counters, we were interested to find that none of those we dispatched did well enough to be included in our winning line-up. Testers definitely preferred these pencils… NB: Do try different shades, and remember that a lighter, softer shade than your natural brows can often work best.

REVIEWS

New CID i-groom Eyebrow Grooming Pencil & Brush

 A truly stupendous average score for a swivel-up propelling brow pencil which boasts a shaped 'rectangular' lead, facilitating thicker or finer strokes, as you choose. There's a built-in brush at the opposite end; several of the award winners feature these, and they certainly are useful for post-pencil blending, as well as grooming stray hairs. To simplify life it comes in one neutral, suits-all-browtones shade.
Comments: 'Brilliant: the most natural eye pencil I have ever tried; so easy to apply and I felt confident using it as there was control over how dark I wanted to go' • 'having pale blonde brows I've struggled with pencils, yet dyeing looks unnatural – this is the first pencil in 40 years of wearing make-up that's worked for me!' • 'so easy to use – I am really thrilled with it' • 'stayed put all day'.

Benefit Instant Brow Pencil

 This is the third time Benefit has submitted Instant Brow Pencil for our book – and it's nudged yet higher in the rankings for this edition. In three shades (we tried Light), it's a more soft-textured pencil, transforming from a creamier texture to long-wear powder, with a brow-brush built right in to the other end of the pencil itself. Benefit pride themselves on brow expertise with over 500 brow bars in 22 countries and if you're looking to have yours shaped for the first time, these bars aren't a bad place to start.
Comments: 'Amazing; really, really pleased with the results which give a very professional make-up artist feel to my brows' • 'did a great job of making my brows look tidier and more uniform; loved the attached brow brush – overall, a great product!' • 'very natural, good quick-fix' • 'glided on so effortlessly – great to use! Asked my husband and a friend if it looked natural: both said my brows looked great, not fake at all' • 'I'm a convert, I don't usually use a brow pencil but this was so easy to use and gave me an instant lift'.

Suqqu Eyebrow Liquid Pen

We'd heard about this fine felt-tip from make-up artist friend Mary Greenwell – though until we tried it for ourselves, we couldn't imagine how the 01 Green shade

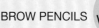

♡ WE LOVE...

Brow pencils are an essential part of our make-up arsenal: without them, Jo says her eyes 'vanish'. She now can't imagine life without Gimme Brow, a Benefit innovation: it's designed like a slightly pointy mini-mascara wand, sweeping on liquid brow colour along with tiny fibres, which bulk up her ultra-blonde, light brows like nothing else she's ever tried. Sarah is another brow pencil devotee – as a victim of over-plucking plus an exploding gas oven! Sarah is another devoted fan of Gimme Brow, and also loves her old favourite, Arch de Triumph Brow Shaper by Soap & Glory, a double-ended pencil with foolproof soft taupe one end and pink highlighter the other. Plus it comes with three pop-out brow stencils, should you feel like playing...

could possibly work. But it does! (To be fair, it's more of a mossy/taupe – and if you're still not convinced, it comes in an actual 02 Brown.) It is great for fine feathery strokes – and we'd recommend it for anyone who may have lost their brows through over-plucking or chemo, as with a little practise the results are super-natural and also totally budge-proof.

Comments: 'Produces absolutely perfect, long-lasting brows with the flick of a brush. My brows looked like they'd been professionally tinted – love this product!' • 'I have never been much of a fan of brow pencils as they do look unnatural and clown-like – but this is a totally different kind of thing and very natural' • 'far from being the lurid green that I'd imagined, the colour is a soft browny-grey which gives a natural appearance; I'm smitten with this little eyebrow marvel and I'll definitely buy another' • 'also tried it as an eyeliner and it works a treat!' • 'no sharpening required and very easy to create a natural shape'.

Shavata Eyebrow Pencil

8.57/10 Clever this: brow expert Shavata Singh's offering is double-ended, giving you a lighter and darker ('dawn and dusk') shade, which you can blend together or use singly to define brows, fill in gaps or bulk up sparse brows. (Blonde testers would have liked a lighter option.) NB The pencil needs regular sharpening for precision: it doesn't come with its own sharpener but testers all had one around the house.

Comments: 'This really helped to give more shape and definition and also made eyebrows look thicker; the colour match was very good' • 'very easy to apply, smooth and creamy, waxy but not smudgy' • 'stayed put all day even when rubbing my eye area; I usually dye my brows but this product matched, stayed put and looked natural' • 'took me a couple of tries to get this right as I have never used one before; well worth the effort as my brows looked more defined and even; didn't budge during the day then came off easily with eye make-up remover'.

Your eyes are changing

…and so should your eye-make-up technique

As with foundation, we can't be as 'prescriptive' in this section as we are elsewhere in this book. (OK. Bossy!) That's because eyes present very different challenges. But here are your options, depending on your particular eye make-up 'challenges'. As make-up artist Terry de Gunzburg explains, 'The eyes become smaller and less "defined" as we age – but you can't just add lots of shadow, because the texture of the skin has changed and too much shadow, or the wrong texture (especially shimmer or pearlised products), can draw attention to wrinkly or saggy areas.'

'Of course, you can draw attention to your eyes,' says make-up guru Barbara Daly, 'but in a different way. Aim for a clean, defined look – smoky if you wish, but never that messy, come-to-bed-look of our youth…'

Try applying an eye base under your eye make-up. Then try again, without an eye base. See which looks better on you. Mary Greenwell believes that eye bases can make your eyes look over-done and over-made-up, but some women feel very self-conscious about the redness of their lids and like an eye base (aka eye primer) to smooth out the skintone before shadow. As an alternative, Mary suggests: 'Try going with the colouration. I love seeing a real eyelid. Apply eye cream and allow it to sink in, so your shadow has something to "cling" to; then put a bit of smudgy brown shadow on the lid – soft, warm, even mossy brown – and leave it at that, with light liner at the base of the lashes, and mascara. That may be enough.'

Eliminate dark circles under eyes with a light-reflecting concealer. Apply the concealer in the hollows under your eyes to brighten the area. (Our recommendations for the best products are on page 56.) A great tip given to us by expert Trish McEvoy for correctors and for brighteners is to stroke the product on as a triangle of lines, one under your eye, then the two sides sloping down to meet at a point on your eye-socket bone: then pat in lightly with a finger to cover the area.

A word on puffiness. If you have puffiness under your eyes, which Sarah does (often due to various ingredients in cosmetics or foods, also hay fever), first stroke an ice cube round your eye area for a few minutes then try a specific product such as Origins No Puffery (which we think is 'genius'!), or one of the other treats for tired and puffy eyes, on page 60. And don't draw too much attention to your under-eyes; a little mascara winged out to your temples, a fine line under the outer third of each eye and a spot of brightener (as above), under your eyes, high on your cheeks and also on the browbone draws attention away from the puffies.

And some secrets for hooded eyes. If your eyelids are actually drooping over your eyes, the only truly corrective option is surgery. But for less pronounced cases, use a highlighter/luminiser under your brow to 'lift' the eye, a very soft wash of taupe on the upper lid to mute it, mascara to define upper and lower lashes, plus fine eyeliner pushed into the lash-line along the lower lashes to draw the attention downwards.

Define the shape of your eyes differently. 'Using a dark shadow to create the "crease" in the socket, as you might have done when you were 20, just won't work,' says Terry de Gunzburg. She advises this approach to open up your eyes: over the lid try a sheer wash of matt eyeshadow, in a neutral shade (eg, mid-taupe – a sort of mushroomy-pink tone, but nothing muddy), then focus on eyeliner and mascara to frame the eyes. Try a sharpened eyeliner pencil or liquid product with an inbuilt fine brush – in grey, deep brown, aubergine or navy – pushed well into the lashes. (If you like, and have time, 'set' liner with a similar shade of powder eyeshadow on top. We often don't bother…)

Top with two coats of mascara. Apply the second coat before the first has dried to avoid clumping. We think soft dark brown can be more flattering for many women – though Trish McEvoy is a firm believer in black 'to enhance definition', for virtually everyone. (Jo goes for black, always.) Waterproof mascara avoids panda eyes, especially during hot flushes. (For more about eyeliners recommended by our testers, see page 68.)

If your 'socket crease' is unlined and droop-free, use a taupe-y grey or even a pale purple shade to accentuate the socket. We rather like a tip from our smooth-lidded singer friend Lulu, who applies powder shadow to the socket of her eye holding the mirror a good two feet (60cm or so) away, so she can gauge the effect from the distance most people see you from. (But then blend so the edges are seamless using a blender brush, holding the mirror up close.)

Add a touch of highlighter on the browbone. This is universally flattering (except possibly for those who have very high eyebrows, in which case it can make them look loftier). Dot on a touch of ivory or bone-coloured shadow, and if (but only if) the skin is smooth, it can be very subtly shimmering.

If you wear stronger shadow and eyeliner, play down your brows. Terry explains that it's all a question of balance. 'If you're wearing quite a bit of eye make-up, and you add a strong brow, you'll look like you've put on way too much make-up. But if you wear a sheer wash of shadow, and fine eyeliner, you can afford to add a bit more brow definition.' (See page 62 for more brow wisdom.)

There is truly no substitute for analysing the different effects yourself, in a mirror. With a discerning friend if available. Eye make-up is an issue where we can't be psychic and make up your mind for you about what looks best: you're going to have to experiment (do give yourself plenty of time for this), based on the advice above. And, of course, you can go and get free make-up consultations in-store from most brands, which might give you valuable tips and info (even if it's to show you what you don't like).

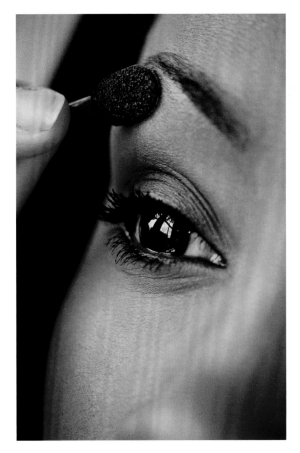

Eyeliners:
our award winners

Mascara is only half the answer for lashes, which invariably become sparser over the years. An eyeliner, applied right into the lash line, also works extremely effectively to create the illusion of thicker, longer lashes. There are many options: pencil, gel, liquid, cream – and they all make a big difference to 'eye-oomph'. We recommend you experiment with different textures till you find the formulation that works best for you – and if you've never trialled a gel or cream liner, do give them a go. Testers loved these – with two new high-scoring entries for this edition

AT A GLANCE

Bourjois Effet Smoky Pencil

Wild About Beauty Line & Define Liner Pen

DHC Liquid Eyeliner

New CID Cosmetics i-gel

Estée Lauder Double Wear Stay-in-Place Eye Pencil

Guerlain Eyeliner

REVIEWS

Bourjois Effet Smoky Pencil

8.61/10 An excellent score for this very affordable pencil, which comes in a range of smokily dark shades; we sent out a selection including Dark Purple, Deep Green and Smoked Brown. (We try always to send out identical products but sometimes brands don't play ball!) A creamier pencil for someone who wants a sultry, maybe even smudged effect from their eye definer.
Comments: 'Top marks: pencil goes on perfectly, very easy to apply precisely; smooth texture without being too soft, smudges easily but controllably' • 'comes with a brush on the other end which is ideal for softening and smudging' • 'cheaper than my usual Clinique pencil and just as good for my very sensitive eyes' • 'didn't drag at all • 'I *love* the pointy brush, so you can soften the line precisely as you want it; product wore well all day'.

Wild About Beauty Line & Define Liner Pen

8.5/10 Already an award winner in *The Ultimate Natural Beauty Bible*, this densely pigmented formula in glossy 01 black-max, with soothing chamomile flower water, gathered up rave reviews from another group of testers. The paraben-free, botanical-rich range launched by Louise Redknapp with make-up artist Kim Jacobs has proved a consistent success in our trials.
Comments: 'Extremely easy and precise to apply, just need the lightest of touches; amount dispensed was perfect. Not too runny and didn't clog but smudges easily if you want. I love this product – probably the best liquid eye liner I have used' • 'soooooo easy to use, goes on really smoothly, doesn't drag and you don't have to press hard; I would definitely buy' • 'loved this fantastic eyeliner, took seconds to apply and stayed put all day' • 'my eyes are quite sensitive but I had no problems'.

DHC Liquid Eyeliner

8.25/10 Another great product from this Japanese company, which reflects that country's demanding standards. We rather love that the founder was involved in educational translation until he discovered the positive effects of olive oil on skin and overall health and set about 'making the world a more beautiful place'. DHC products are only available online. We tested this liquid eyeliner in black: no olive oil in it though…
Comments: 'The first liquid eyeliner that actually works for me! The very fine tip – more like a felt pen - makes it much easier to be precise. You can smudge if you want and also good for getting a glam cats-eye look' • 'will definitely persevere as the fine line is very flattering for an older eye; great staying power too' • 'I loved this and so did my 18 year old daughter, best she has ever used!' • 'fantastic product: even being kind to myself I am not the best at applying eye make up but even I

could create a subtle line as well as other effects; my must-buy'.

New CID Cosmetics i-gel

The subtitle of this tells you pretty much all you need to know – Long Wear Gel Eye Liner Trio with Brush – and our testers had the Bronze, Copper and Stone version. There's a built-in mirror in the lid, while the brush is flat.

Comments: 'Very long-lasting: stayed put from first thing in the morning till I got home from the office' • 'I've tried many liners but have never been able to achieve the clean-lined look before – this takes away all the hard work' • 'a dream to apply and love the colours (great for green eyes)' • 'haven't used liner in years but am converted: so easy to apply, with no dragging.'

Estée Lauder Double Wear Stay-in-Place Eye Pencil

As the name implies, this double-ended pencil (colour one end, blender/smudger the other) comes from a capsule Lauder collection created to deliver specifically long-wear results. It features silicone technology to deliver stay-true colour for up to 12 hours. We normally ask for black or dark neutrals, but on this occasion our testers enjoyed the subtly shimmering Bronze shade, one of seven jewel-rich tones.

Comments: 'Anyone should find it easy to apply precisely, and also very smudgeable – and it stayed like that until I took it off, how refreshing!' • 'very useful and versatile, and lasted well' • 'creamy, easy to apply and sticks to your skin until you remove it' • 'what a dream, perfect consistency for an eye pencil, went on smoothly and evenly, and precisely, as long as I kept it sharp'.

Guerlain Eyeliner

Steady of hand? Fond of a kitten flick? Love a touch of Marilyn…? This is your best eye-lining bet: the only liquid-style option to have impressed testers, it offers a long, pen-like lid for calligraphy-style application. Testers had Noir Ebène 01, a black-brown and one of three sultry long-wear shades.

Comments: 'Love it, love it, love it! Compared with other liners performed well, lasted all day (and some nights!) • 'gorgeous, stylish product which adds a touch of old-fashioned glamour to my dressing table' • 'like the way it can be used for a thin line or a dramatic, thicker line – all effects easy-to-achieve' • 'fine line against lashes makes them look thicker; lasted all day but easily removed at night'.

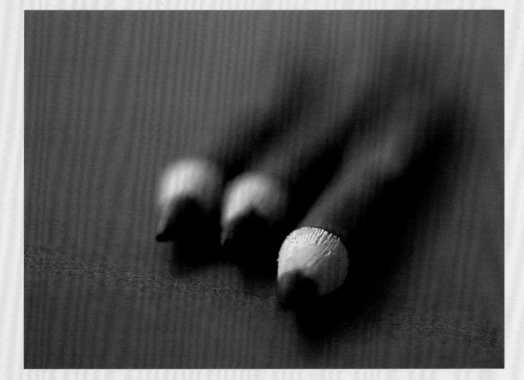

♡ WE LOVE…

Jo is a sucker for a smoky eye pencil, in particular the new Bobbi Brown Long-Wear Eye Pencil, with its richly-pigmented formula. But to enhance the staying power, she often layers a gel or cake eyeliner over the top – favourites are the 'matching' Bobbi Brown Long Wear Gel Eyeliner or Laura Mercier Tightline Cake Eye Liner (you need the 'matching' Eye Liner Brush). Sarah has found her all-time favourite eyeliner with Laura Mercier's soft, smudgy Caviar Stick Eye Colour in Sand Glow, which she accentuates with Aerin's Cool Gel Eyeliner in Effortless Brown for evenings.

Cream eyeshadows: our award winners

Cream shadows are easiest to blend on more 'mature' eyelids – and in a pale neutral can also become a fabulous base for other shades. They're also a lazy, 'everyday' option for a fast make-up effect if you swipe on a taupe-y neutral shade. The right formulation is a must, though – because you want to avoid 'creasing'. With that in mind, we dispatched another batch of cream shadow options to our testers, asking for feedback on smoothness, ease of application and endurance. (As always, we asked for neutral shades that would suit all of you…)

AT A GLANCE

Bobbi Brown Long-Wear Cream Shadow

Benefit Creaseless Cream Shadow/Liner

bareMinerals 5-in-1 Cream Eyeshadow SPF15

Shu Uemura Cream Eye Shadow

REVIEWS

Bobbi Brown Long-Wear Cream Shadow

8.55/10 'At last, a cream eyeshadow that stays on and doesn't crease', promises the Bobbi Brown blurb – and as our testers' comments go to show, this pretty much lives up to that. In a cute small pot (you dip with fingers or use a synthetic brush), it offers a 'breathable polymer technology' (which delivers the long wear and makes it crease resistant), and it's also recommended 'for oily eyelids'. Bobbi is of course known for her super-wearable shades – and there are 20 to choose from, mostly matt but some with a slight shimmer. Our testers trialled Cement, which they found good for daytime on its own, or as a base for evening colours. NB: As some testers pointed out, the little pot is not the most portable.
Comments: '10/10 for the easiest to apply eyeshadow I've ever used, either with brush or finger; the smoothest most velvety texture, matt finish but not flat; have binned all my other eyeshadows and bought several more of these' • 'made the slightly crêpey skin on my eyelids look as smooth as a teenager's again' • 'long, long, long, long-lasting! Stayed put with great finish and same colour – work means my make-up can be on for 16 hours, this was still fresh at the end' • 'seemed to fill all imperfections; made eyeliner easier to apply and last longer on top of it; wish I'd discovered this before' • 'loved the creamy texture which was easy to apply, and the colour, and it lasted! But found the opening of the pot too small for fingers once the contents went down a bit, so you need a brush' • 'gave soft wash of colour that you could build up, didn't cake at all, just a smooth veil of colour'.

Benefit Creaseless Cream Shadow/Liner

 8.25/10 Crease-proof, smudge-proof, offering 'buildable' colour with a choice of 12 shades. Our testers tried Flatter Me, a creamy metallic rose gold colour, with quite a lot of shimmer (some felt too much) but a smooth, flattering finish, they commented. No applicator is provided, so you may need a brush. Benefit may sometimes seem like a young range but pros love their make-up 'Fix-Its' (and so do we).
Comments: 'Can I give this 11 out of ten? Easy peasy to apply, and so simple to layer up if you want to, use both fingers and brush; shimmery but subtle finish, a sheen rather than shadow – yes, oh yes, I would buy, I loved this and so did the other women in my family (had to lock it away) – it gave me so much pleasure!' • 'very easy to use with a brush, spread easily to give a wash of colour and could be built up into stronger coverage; so you could have it subtle or dramatic' • 'lasted about four hours' • 'felt like a creamy powder, if that makes sense! Quite smooth to use, and easy to blend in and didn't cake' • 'packaging is adorable

♡ WE LOVE...

Oooh, lots in Jo's case, most particularly her Ellis Faas Creamy Eyes pen-style shadow in neutral brown E105 (a taupe-y brown) which can be used very subtly or (unlike some) reapplied for a much more intense smokiness. She also likes the award-winning Bobbi Brown Long-Wear Cream Shadow you can read about, left, in Ash – a medium brown – and Bone (as an eyelid base/brow highlighter) but adds: 'The jar opening's a little fiddly, so this is best used with a synthetic shadow brush, not fingers. It lives up to its long-wear promise, though.' Sarah's new rave product is Bobbi Brown's fantastic Long-Wear Cream Shadow Stick, which is exactly what it says – a lasts-all-day cream shadow in a small pencil. From 18 shades, she loves Smokey Topaz, a soft shimmery mushroom, which looks gorgeous smudged round eyes.

– glass container, with a large lid in a pretty little box, makes applying it feel like a ritual'.

bareMinerals 5-in-1 Cream Eyeshadow SPF15 ❋

7.83/10 Like our tester panel, we are fans of this popular mineral-based brand's new set of 'Advanced Performance' eyeshadows in ten soft shades. The five benefits are a super-charged primer, long-wear colour, an eye-brightening formula, lid-smoothing formula and an SPF15 (useful, but of course it won't last all day, even though the colour will, according to our testers who all commented on how long-lasting it was). As they proclaim, one stroke, a quick smudge with a finger and you're good to go out the door. Wear alone for a subtle daytime sheen or top up with a stronger colour for evenings. NB: Wearing one of these neutral shades is particularly good for older eyelids which can tend to be less than even-toned, and sometimes veer to redness.

Comments: 'Fantastic primer, which did brighten up my eye area and reduce the look of redness in my eyes, as well as evening out lid colour and reducing creases' • 'lasted at least 12 hours' • 'top marks – very easy to apply from wand, then smooth on with finger; made my eyes look more open on its own, also a good base for stronger colour – now one of my make-up bag staples' • 'I use it on its own: the subtle shimmer effect is very flattering on my Asian skin' • 'really lightened and brightened my eyes! Stayed on a looooooong time too'.

Shu Uemura Cream Eye Shadow

7.6/10 Loved by make-up artists the world over, Shu Uemura – the range founded by the legendary Japanese make-up artist of the same name – are known for their bold shades – but search hard, and you'll find some wonderful, more neutral (and flattering) tones within the Shu range. Again, the shadow's creators promise that it won't fade, crease – and that this comfortable 'stretch' formula is even waterproof.

Comments: 'Great product; never used cream before but I really liked it for a natural daytime look; lovely and kind to small lines and creases' • 'silky finish that glided on, really smooth and crease-resistant, blended beautifully and stayed put all day and into the night' • 'finish improved when I set it with a little powder, which prolonged it too' • 'best applied with a brush and once I'd achieved an even colour it looked great; slight shimmer which looked best in the evening for me, lasted a lot longer than my usual powder shadow, and the overall finished effect was more dramatic' • 'stayed put brilliantly, lasted all night without any signs of disappearing'.

&Mascaras: our award winners

Lashes get thinner and sparser over time, so mascara is even more essential to help define the eyes and structure the face. However, there's no such thing as a one-type-fits-all mascara – so here are the top recommendations with details of what they do. On this page, the non-waterproof versions – see opposite for mascaras to get you through rain and weepy films!

AT A GLANCE

Non-waterproof

Benefit They're Real

Clinique High Impact Mascara

Origins GinZing Brightening Mascara

Noir G de Guerlain Exceptional Complete Mascara

Waterproof

Paul & Joe Waterproof Mascara

Clinique Lash Power Mascara Long Wearing Formula

Chanel Inimitable Waterproof Mascara

Estée Lauder Sumptuous Waterproof Mascara

TIP

Do replace your mascara every three months for best results and to avoid 'bug' build-up.

NON-WATERPROOF MASCARAS

Benefit They're Real

 8.9/10

We're not really surprised that Benefit's mascara has stormed to the top of the charts: it's been scooping awards right, left and centre, and is now the UK's No. 1 bestselling mascara. Benefit's jokey names belie the fact that their products are incredibly high performing; their own testers saw 94 per cent dramatic increase in lash-length and volume, 'visible lift' to lashes – and 100 per cent experienced long-wear results. Those were pretty much mirrored by our own Beauty Blble testers' lash-enhanced experiences.

Comments: 'Mascara goes on very easily, no clumping; very good lash-lengthening and slight thickening and curl, fairly lustrous looking – quite natural but defined and I only needed one coat' • 'outstanding long lasting results and visible lift – as they say on the packaging' • 'brilliant, brilliant brush – got right into the corners where lashes are small and gave great coverage without clogging up' • 'can I give it 11? It deserves it: great at lash-lengthening, lashes looked thicker but not clumpy, glossy and lustrous. As a mascara junkie, I was super impressed'.

Clinique High Impact Mascara

8.75/10

We love Clinique's precision: this, they say, gives 'up to a 26-degree curl'. We know from experience there's plenty of 'playtime' while you're applying, but the high-impact brush delivers results with just a few sweeps. This too has lash-conditioning waxes in the blend. (Particularly good for extra length and curl.)

Comments: 'Fantastic staying power with a dramatic effect on eyelashes, yet felt natural not heavy' • 'five *****! The best mascara I've ever tried: leaves lashes luscious all day, yet easy to remove' • 'I suffer from blepharitis, a condition which makes my eyes water – yet this really coped well without smudging or running, or irritating my eyes' • 'this was still going strong at 10pm at night' • 'I'm the world's worst for mascara flaking but this one definitely held its own' • 'I'm so happy with the glossy, dark-pigmented results from just one coat'.

Origins GinZing Brightening Mascara ❋

 8.25/10

This lightweight, naturally conditioning formula contains plant extracts including a blend of ginseng, caffeine and other active botanicals plus waxes, Carnauba Palm and Acacia Senegal. Clinically proven, it promises to instantly lift, boost volume and lengthen lashes and impart a deep hue that helps make the eye area look lighter and brighter. Testers were divided about the chunky brush.

Comments: 'Went on easily with no clumping, good lash thickening but not lengthening; lashes looked glossy, lustrous and a bit curlier' • 'no flaking, crumbling or smudging' • 'made my eyelashes look glossy and very glamourous, really opened up my eyes: I'm really impressed' • 'I have tiny lashes and this made them look enormous, brighter and healthy: I thought it was a great product' • 'amazing! A colleague stopped me to say she'd never noticed what lovely eyes I have (I don't), my boss asked what mascara it was, the paper seller even told me I looked much younger and happier…'

Noir G De Guerlain Exceptional Complete Mascara

8.19/10 This is a small revolution in design, offering the first refillable mascara with an integrated mirror, designed by jeweller Lorenz Bäumer. So clever, so sophisticated … so Guerlain. With new generation Ultra-Black pigments, Noir G de Guerlain promises to give you intensely deep colour from daybreak to nightfall, with extra volume, length and curl.)

Comments: 'My eyelashes have never looked better, definitely glossy and lustrous, longer, thicker and curlier' • 'the wand design was pure genius, easy to use and could access lashes absolutely easily' • 'a great formula but does need a specialist remover I found (no one else said this)' • 'fantastic lash lengthening particularly if you wiggled the wand from the root of the lashes through to the end, also gave some curl; didn't clump or flake' • 'my short sparse lashes looked really thick and black; no problems with my sensitive eyes'.

WATERPROOF MASCARAS

As we age, eyes become more sensitive to light, and often to allergens. The result? Eye-wateriness. Our panellists have now put more than three dozen waterproof mascaras through their paces in daily life (as well as the shower and pool). Here are their enduring (!) favourites, with three high-scoring entries. Those promising curl and length did better than volumising ones. Be warned: you need specialist waterproof eye-make-up remover!

Paul & Joe Waterproof Mascara

8.6/10 From a 'cult' brand better known for fashion-forward shades and gorgeous boudoir-esque packaging, a seriously high-scoring mascara that really stayed the distance! Testers universally loved the wand, the finish, the curling effect and the endurance of this mascara.

Comments: 'Wow – this stuff doesn't budge! I didn't have any trace of a smear after a long, hot shower; gave great length, curl and thickness' • 'truly waterproof – the mascara I've been looking for for over 40 years!' • 'no clumping, even after a few weeks of use; stayed put all day' • 'I'm not really a fan of waterproof mascaras but this is a cut above the rest: fluttery, coal-black lashes, a perfectly-shaped wand that coats every lash, and a mascara that stays put through hell and high water'.

Clinique Lash Power Mascara Long Wearing Formula

8.22/10 Ideal for the sensitive-eyed, originally created for the ultra-humid conditions in Asia but wowing us in the West, now. Removes with warm water, not make-up remover! (Several testers failed to grasp this essential fact.)

Comments: 'Didn't budge through a five-mile run and only smudged in the shower because I washed my face with foaming cleanser' • 'incredibly easy to apply, and easy to get to corner lashes; now most definitely top of my mascara list' • 'very natural result, no clumps' • 'stayed on surprisingly well yet it was really easy to remove; a great mascara – oh, and it survived a Body Jam class! (Still not a good look with a bright red face, though...!) • 'the brush was particularly good for defining shorter lashes; it flaked a bit but does have incredible staying power'.

Chanel Inimitable Waterproof Mascara

8.12/10 The revolutionary rubber wand (technical-speak: 'soft elastomer') grips lashes beautifully, enabling a real curling action, plus definition and separation. (Great for sparser lashes, we've observed.) As testers observed, you need a really effective remover to get it off.

Comments: 'Fab product, really great performing mascara, which made lashes longer, thicker, more curly and separated, with glossy lustrous finish – and no mascara to be seen on my face after a weepy movie or shower' • 'didn't budge through rain and weepy movie, though smudged slightly in shower and swimming pool; didn't flake or crumble; lengthening effect very good' • 'especially good on bottom lashes, made them significantly thicker without glooping together, very pretty: my eyes really stand out – cut onions with no problem'.

Estée Lauder Sumptuous Waterproof Mascara

7.8/10 Lauder promise this 'gives you all the thickening of a brush with the definition of a comb', sweeping 'Micro "Y" Lock Fibres' and 'fumed silica' on to lashes, with mica and kaolin clay to boost volume. There's a 'soft-flex' polymer to prevent brittleness.

Comments: 'Unlike many, this mascara really is waterproof – and not clumpy at all' • 'didn't flake, crumble, smudge – amazing!' • 'I was amazed: this was fantastic at lash-lengthening, swept on and lashes just grew and grew' • 'we should all have this tucked away for holidays, weepy movies etc. – the best I've ever used' • 'glossy and luxuriant'.

♡ WE LOVE...

We have both kissed many frogs en route to discovering our perfect mascara. Jo likes a defining mascara for her somewhat sparse and pale lashes; 'volumising' mascaras skate off her lashes without depositing a molecule of colour. A favourite for everyday is MAC False Lashes Mascara, but for any special event she's been blown away by Santhilea Magnetic Lashes, a three-step mascara: sweep on base coat, then use a second small wand to coat the lashes in fibres that give the appearance of false lashes, and 'seal' with the same product used as the base coat. Sarah was in denial for years about thinner 'eye fringe' but can look overdone with volumising mascaras. Her make-up bag staple is Bobbi Brown Intensifying Long-Wear Mascara for day/night, town/country, 24/7. Jo's long-term favourite waterproof mascara is Chanel Inimitable Waterproof Mascara (see left), which survives her summer dips in the Channel without a smudge. Sarah warns, 'do invest in specialist remover for waterproof mascaras or you risk waking with unattractive panda-eyes'.

Eye lash enhancers: *our award winners*

Over the past few years, lash-boosting treatments have developed into a whole new beauty category. However, there is significant concern about the health impact of some formulations (see panel right). For this new edition, our testers trialled a mixture of products including growth-enhancing mascaras, two of which did well. But it is worth noting that neither are waterproof, which our testers flagged up as a problem in some cases. (NB Clarins suggest using their fixing gel, Double Fix' Mascara, over the top.)

AT A GLANCE

Gosh Growth Mascara

Clarins Be Long Mascara

REVIEWS

Gosh Growth Mascara

 8.45/10 This new product from a Danish budget brand, found at Superdrug, performed very well in a difficult category. It works brilliantly as a normal mascara and also contains a 'growth active' ingredient called SymPeptide XLash, based on a hair-restoring complex, which is proven to have a visible effect on the length and thickness of lashes. Plus it offers a rubber brush with teeny 'hairs' to separate and volumise lashes. Our testers were impressed.

Comments: 'Went on smoothly, cleanly and very easily, and even my lower lashes looked much longer; the more days I used it the longer my lashes looked, with a clear difference between day one and 14: I love this mascara, just wish they made it waterproof' • 'definitely made my lashes look thicker, longer and glossy; very good wand design, thin so you can get to the inner and outer corners with fixed short spikes (not brush-like) so no clumping and you can be delicate: you've completely converted me to this product and I was previously a Dior girl!' • 'quality product that gives the same if not better results than mascaras three times the price'.

Clarins Be Long Mascara

8.21/10 Tests conducted on 33 women for four weeks showed that bare lashes increased in length by an average of 1.1mm. It features Be Long Lash Complex, an instant strengthening formula to fortify lashes and boost growth, which contains panthenol (a form of vitamin B5), which is much used in hair care to moisturise and boost, and a matrikine peptide (biotinoyl tripeptide-1), originally used in hair-restorers.

Comments: 'I could really see the lash lengthening effects of this mascara – very impressive product' • 'I loved this mascara which left lashes looking long and healthy but natural. The small flexible brush allows you to get right to the root of the lash and is great for separating lashes, which did not clump at all' • 'brilliant at lash lengthening, left my stumpy bottom lashes looking much longer' • 'definitely worth the money, I would recommend this mascara to anyone – love the classy packaging too' • 'leaves a shiny glossy finish to eyelashes but seemed to take a long time to dry, which I can't get round as I am always in a rush' • 'the wand suits my short fine lashes perfectly, the head bends easily and gives perfect coverage for all my lashes'.

UPDATE

Since this book was first published, problems have emerged with some lash-boosting treatments. One leading brand gave half our Beauty Bible testers sensitivity reactions, eg red, sore, irritated eyes. Similar emails came to www.beautybible.com, and we discontinued the trial. It emerged that the key ingredient is a molecule used in a glaucoma drug to reduce pressure in the eye. This prostaglandin analogue is also known to increase eyelash growth (but only while you use it). The potential side effects are listed on the drug label and, of course, patients are monitored. But even in lesser doses in cosmetic products, which carry no warnings, uncomfortable or even potentially sight-impairing side effects can occur. The FDA in America has recalled over the counter eyelash growth enhancers with similar ingredients, and the only one available is on prescription. In the UK, the MHRA (Medicines and Healthcare products Regulatory Agency) is now investigating products on sale here.

♡ WE LOVE...

Jo tried quite a few and had to give up because they made her eyes itch, but has finally had good results from Rimmel London Lash Accelerator Mascara, which really does seem to have had a slight lash-thickening effect. Sarah has quite thick lashes and the only product that tempts her is Phylia Connect, a 100% natural leave-in treatment for scalp and hair that can also be used on lashes. And don't forget that Joan Collins swears Vaseline is the best lash conditioner ever!

'Wrinkles don't
scare me;
they are a part
of LIFE and I
will and do
EMBRACE them.
But I look at
surgery and that
scares me'

Christy Turlington

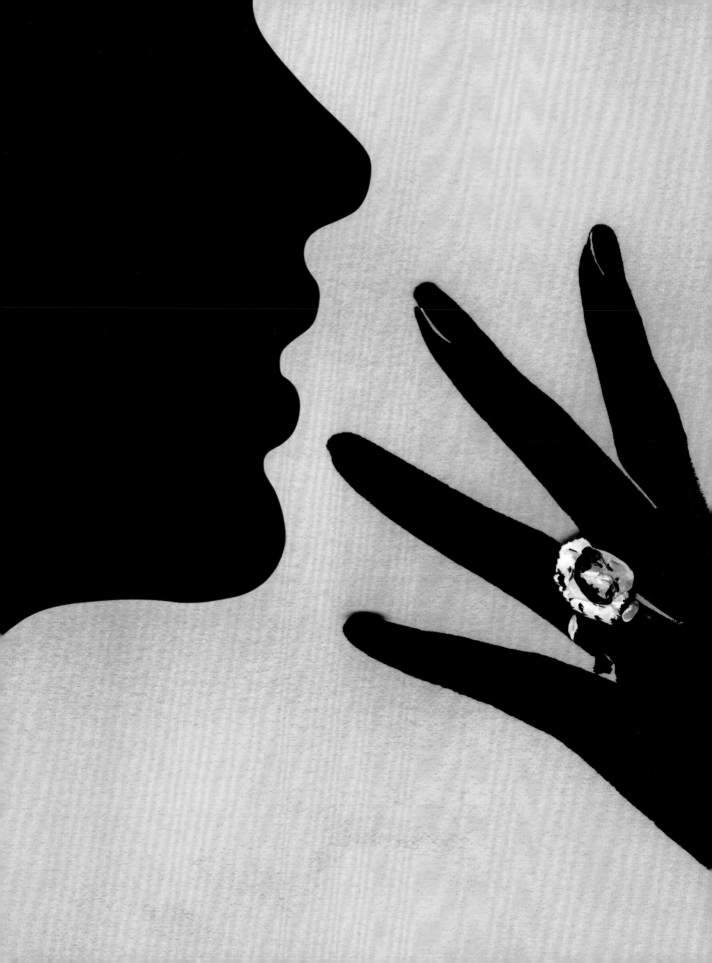

Get glowing – by recharging your skin

A visit to a facialist for a skin-reviving treatment is a rare indulgence for most of us – but in this book we show you the amazing masks, scrubs, creams, oils and transforming techniques that you can use at home to give your skin a real boost…plus insider tips from the experts

There are several ways to wake up your face fast. You can go the professional route: trek to a salon, have your face massaged (or needled as in acupuncture – see page 155), be slathered with creams (and lie there hoping you're not getting a parking ticket). Or you can go the D-I-Y route, which is infinitely cheaper and more accessible. Now, that's not to say we don't love a facial – see a list below for some of our favourite facialists. But realistically, who has the money or, just as importantly, the time to indulge more than once in a blue moon…?

Your daily regime is one thing. But it's easy to be lulled – out of sheer inertia and/or laziness – into doing the same routine for your skin, day in, night out. So we really, really can't encourage you too strongly to try some of the products and the face-transforming techniques in this book.

You can achieve a huge amount – near-miraculous, actually – with a simple, at-home, two-step blitz: a gentle-but-effective exfoliation, followed by a mask. On the next pages, you'll find our diligent testers' top facial scrubs and masks – the skincare wonders that, over the space of 18 months' research for this book, they identified as being the most effective on the market. And on page 212 you'll also find our rundown of the best 'instant face-revivers', packed with glow-getting ingredients that boost skin circulation, and are absolutely fantastic for emergencies (hangovers, jet-lag, or after a cold or flu, when skin can look positively grey). They're as close to eight hours' sleep-in-a-jar as you're going to get.

Throughout this mini-section of the book, we've also included some 'trade secrets': insider tips to try at home, from facialists who we rate and revere – and who, if we had a lunching-lady sort of life, we might see more often ourselves. But even though we're beauty editors, we can't justify that sort of indulgence as frequently as we might like.

But try the products, too, and prepare to be amazed.

5-MINUTE FIX FOR TIRED FACES!

Facialist Suzie Mitchell (who's local to Jo in Hastings) is something of a miracle-worker for tired faces. She has this tip for temporarily 'ironing' away lines from the face and boosting glow.

● Put a little facial oil in one palm and rub hands together, then smooth over face, neck and bosom.
● Rather than fingertips, use the big muscle in the cushion at the base of your thumb, always working upwards.
● Start by fanning out over and round your neck, then work round and up your jaw and cheekbones to the temples, then across and up your forehead to your hairline.
● Repeat, covering the whole face for five minutes. The oil will be absorbed, skin velvety, and your face look rosy and 'lifted'.

> 'You only perceive the *real* beauty in a person as they get OLDER'
>
> Anouk Aimée

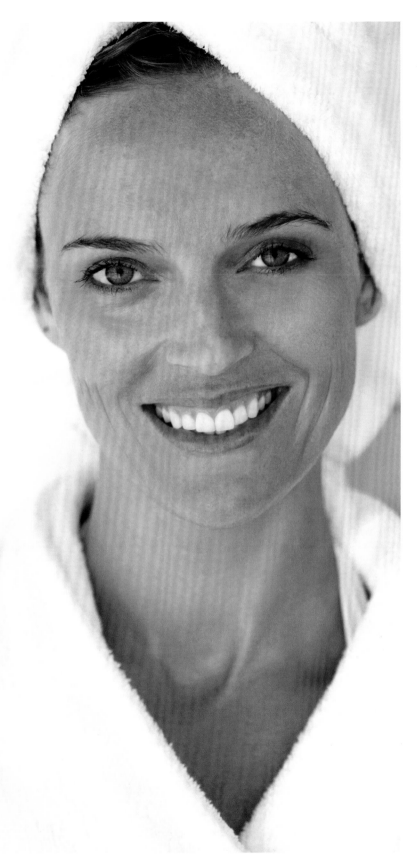

IF YOU HAVE 15 MINUTES OR MORE, TRY THIS!

We adore acupuncturist Annee de Mamiel's facial acupuncture treatment, which she combines with massage. If you can't get to see her (or anyone else), just try this…. Then look in the mirror and go, 'Wow!'.

● Smooth your favourite facial oil over your entire face and neck.
● Cup your hands over the nose and mouth, breathe in and out deeply.
● Tug your earlobes with thumb and index finger. Then with fingertips, use firm, circular movements to massage from behind ears to base of neck.
● From the point of your chin, work up and outwards along the jaw to your ear; then from the corners of your mouth over the cheeks to the ear; then from the base of the nose to the top of the ear. Repeat the whole sequence three times.
● Sweep your fingertips firmly over your eyebrows, then under, then gently pinch along them. Repeat twice.
● Pressing firmly with your middle fingers, circle the eyes beginning above the inner corners and working outwards. Repeat three times.
● From the centre of your forehead, just above the nose, zigzag middle fingers in small, firm motions out to the temples; repeat working up the forehead.
● With the side of your index finger (held vertically), smooth skin from centre of face outwards, beginning with your forehead, then sides of nose, middle of mouth and centre of chin.
● Finish by breathing deeply, hands cupped over your mouth and nose.

OUR FAVOURITE AGE-DEFYING FACIALISTS…

Sarah Chapman
Emma Hardie
Ole Henriksen (LA)
Su-Man Hsu
Abigail James
Amanda Lacey
Sharon McGlinchey (Sydney-based but also London and LA)
Vaishaly Patel

Facial scrubs: our award winners

Dry, dull surface skin cells are the key issue lying between many a woman's complexion and a youthful radiance. When cell turnover slows, the dead surface skin cells don't reflect the light in the same way as a twentysomething's naturally fresh, dewy skin – but the good news is that a gentle exfoliator can go a long, long way towards restoring a healthy glow

AT A GLANCE

Darphin Age-Defying Dermabrasion

Liz Earle Naturally Active Gentle Face Exfoliator

Dermalogica Daily Microfoliant

UrbanVeda Purifying Exfoliating Facial Polish

TIP

To avoid overdoing the use of a scrub on the face, use your ring fingers to massage in, using circular movements. The touch of this finger is naturally more delicate than with the index or second finger, all but eliminating the risk of over-zealous application.

G-E-N-T-L-E is our watchword, though – it's important to avoid anything that scratches or over-buffs the skin – so in our quest to discover the most effective facial scrubs, we dispatched several dozen to our panels of testers (ten for each product, as normal). They had truly glowing praise for some. PS Try using a facial scrub before applying a mask for maximum effectiveness.

REVIEWS

Darphin Age-Defying Dermabrasion

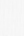

Darphin (originally a French brand, now owned by Estée Lauder) promise this very high-scoring product is kind enough even for sensitive skins, with buffing particles of jojoba, silica, pearl and lava to refine skin texture, plus a corn-derived ingredient to target age spots. Gentian and bisabolol have been added for a soothing action, and Darphin say this can be used as often as every other day. (Though we advise: try it once a week first, and assess results. That may be enough to keep you radiant.) Luxuriously-textured and luxuriously-priced.
Comments: 'Love this, the rich, creamy, lush texture and my glowing, cleaner, brighter skin after; you can use it without water but if it dries out a little, just add a touch then you can really massage it in; a small amount goes a long way' • 'skin never felt taut or dry after' • 'very fine grains exfoliate skin gently, lovely fresh smell, skin looks polished and fresh, clearer and brighter after; people say how good my skin looks' • 'super product that does brilliant job of exfoliating in the most gentle way – really lovely' • 'skin felt so soft and smooth and moisturised, it was wonderful, looks brighter'.

Liz Earle Naturally Active Gentle Face Exfoliator

Featured as one of Jo's 'loves' (see right), this is a softly-softly introduction to exfoliants, if you haven't tried one before. As with the whole Liz Earle range, botanicals feature generously (purifying eucalyptus, which also delivers a 'clean' scent, and lashings of cocoa butter), and – crucially – the skin-buffing action is down to rounded particles of jojoba. Gentle by name and gentle by nature – but effective, too, testers reveal.
Comments: 'Skin felt immediately smoother and really moisturised – and I liked the refreshing, uplifting eucalyptus scent' • 'my husband tells me my skin looks smooth and glowing and I think it's because of this' • 'loved this from the first time I used it' • 'just the right consistency to massage around my face without feeling I was stressing my skin' • 'leaves skin feeling moisturised, unlike most scrubs' • 'no redness or irritation – the best scrub I've ever used' • 'zingy scent helps to wake you up in the morning – even helped with blocked nose from a cold!' • 'a real "wake-up effect": thinking of using this as part of a hangover cure!'.

WE LOVE...

Personally, thanks to diligent use of a muslin cloth at night-time, we go easy on facial scrubs – reserving them for an occasional blitz. For Jo, favourites include Aurelia Probiotic Skincare Refine & Polish Miracle Balm (which smells glorious and can be left on as a mask), or Liz Earle Gentle Face Exfoliator (yes, it truly IS gentle). Sarah uses a flannel at night and in the morning to remove cleanser and virtually never exfoliates. NB Dermatologists are now warning against overuse of exfoliators on sensitive skin.

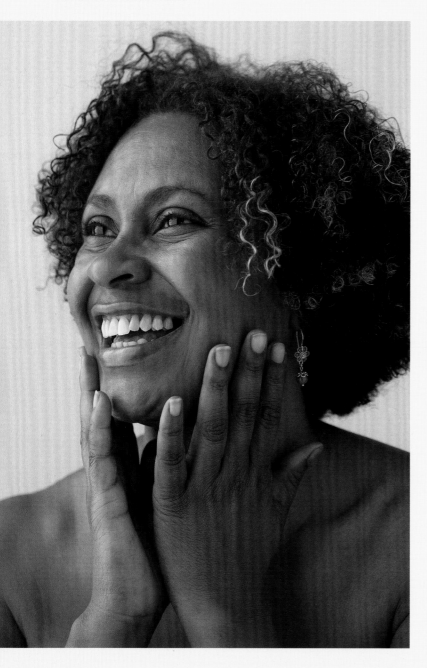

Dermalogica Daily Microfoliant

8.75/10 As the name suggests, Dermalogica tell us this rice-based enzyme powder can be used every day – but please read the comments we make for Darphin about frequent use, (see opposite), before you do that. The powder formula – which shakes out of the container into the hand – activates when you mix it with water, releasing papain (a skin-brightening enzyme), salicylic acid and rice to smooth and boost cellular renewal. To add to its brightening power, bearberry, liquorice and grapefruit are incorporated, along with a skin-calming blend of green tea, ginkgo and oatmeal.

Comments: 'Not grainy at all, felt really soft and gentle, very easy to apply; skin looked really fresh and glowing, and felt unbelievably soft and smooth; people say I look very well; after a month skin looks glowing and refreshed' • 'I use it twice weekly, which is enough, but you could use it daily – a lovely comforting treatment without any harsh abrasiveness' • 'using this regularly has reduced my fine wrinkles and enlarged pores, made skin smoother and my skin feels so much nicer – a very lovely product, and moisturiser goes on much better' • 'husband says my skin looks brighter and fresher, and he's been trying it too and is very impressed!' • 'after a month, skin looks a lot smoother, brighter and more toned'.

UrbanVeda Purifying Exfoliating Facial Polish ❀

8.71/10 This brand relies on the 5,000 year wisdom of the Ayurvedic medical system of India to balance skin naturally. The Purifying range combines cold pressed pure neem, from the ancient evergreen tree much used in traditional medicine, and refreshing essential oils to help remove impurities and prevent congestion, so is particularly suited to more oily skin although we trialled it on a range of skin types. The facial polish helps to reduce excess sebum and improve open pores while gently exfoliating and also hydrating.

Comments: '10/10, great for my oily/spot-prone skin; I usually avoid scrubs but I really like this: skin felt tingly and fresh, I definitely have fewer blackheads and it seems to calm my hormone-related spots' • 'lovely creamy scrub with very fine grains; love the minty fresh smell and my skin feels alive vibrant and ready for anything' • 'skin looked clearer and brighter, make-up glided on better after using this' • 'skin looks very good, young and glowing – was told I look "really well"'.

Anti-ageing face masks: our award winners

We love, love, love face masks. The ritual of slapping on a mask once a week can be a rare moment of pampering in a hectic life. But more than this, we like the results that many masks swiftly deliver: brightening, smoothing, plumping and delivering a surge of dewy moisture to thirsty skins. Plus, some products now feature specific 'anti-ageing' ingredients, such as skin-brightening enzymes. Our diligent panellists lay back and relaxed while trialling an incredibly wide selection of masks – and their top choices, featured here, with two new entries for this latest edition (including an immensely high-scorer)

AT A GLANCE

Filorga Meso-Mask Anti-Wrinkle Brightening Mask

Elemis Fruit Active Rejuvenating Mask

Super Facialist by Una Brennan Rose Hydrate Intense Moisture Mask

Elemis Pro-Collagen Quartz Lift Mask

REVIEWS

Filorga Meso-Mask Anti-Wrinkle Brightening Mask

 9.14/10 Packed to the gills with hyaluronic acid (which has a super-gentle, super skin-plumping effect), this lightweight mask is to be smoothed onto the face once a week for up to 30 minutes to deliver best results. Filorga is a high-tech French clinic which offers treatments like mesotherapy (a 'needling' technique') and peels to chi-chi Parisian women: this, they promise, is like 'mesotherapy' in a mask. Not strictly possible, of course, but testers were wowed.
Comments: 'Top marks: my skin felt like velvet and also looked uplifted; it made skin tone more even and I think I looked younger... Make-up went on more evenly as my skin was so smooth' • 'exquisite, fresh-smelling product that felt great, more like a moisturising cream than a typical taut-making mask' • 'improved my dehydrated skin's appearance and quality every time I used it' • 'my skin looked very good for a few days, younger and very healthy' • 'I didn't like using face masks as I hate removing them after, but this was as easy as taking off my normal cleanser; I haven't found anything as good among the many I have tried' • 'absolutely gorgeous to use with instant stunning results: skin looked younger, plumper and glowing'.

Elemis Fruit Active Rejuvenating Mask

8.86/10 The first of two award winners from Elemis in this category, this mask contains strawberry and kiwi for radiance-boosting, macadamia nut oil, shea butter – and kaolin clay, which is deep-cleansing, helping to refine the skin and banish dullness. (Interestingly, they recommend it for smokers – which we don't recommend! – because of the circulation-boosting effect.) It's not tight, but it does 'set' more than the other winning masks.
Comments: 'Top score for a perfect mask! My skin looked fresher, less puffy, more "perky", dreamy texture, smells like a fruit smoothie, my face was rejuvenated' • 'skin looked fresh and smooth, definitely brighter, which improved with regular use' • 'loved this creamy, light mask which felt a little tingly but not uncomfy, skintone improved, definitely healthier, and could actually see the difference' • 'skin softer to the touch and dewier-looking, gives a clearer-looking complexion than my usual mask' •

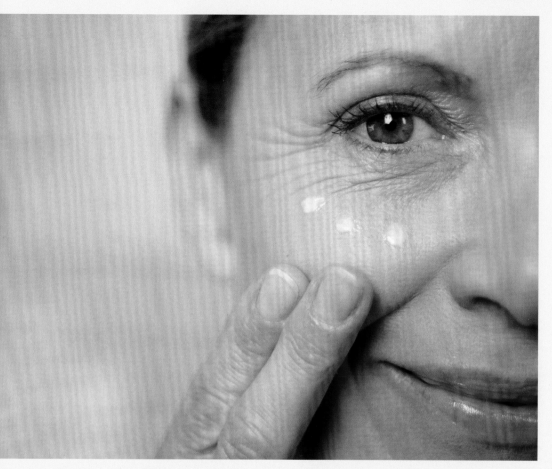

♡ WE LOVE...

Jo's bathroom shelf is always rather crowded with face masks. When skin's feeling ultra-dry, she reaches for super-rich Aurelia Probiotic Skincare Cell Revitalise Rose Mask, or the equally lavish and nourishing L'Occitane Immortelle Cream Mask. Sarah Chapman Skinesis Instant Miracle Mask leaves her skin, she swears with a 12 year old's complexion (albeit only for a few hours…). She's also a big fan of Bliss Triple Oxygen Energizing Mask, which fizzes and foams on the face to deliver a booster of brightening vitamin C – and is a truly fast fix (just three minutes is all it takes to wake up her face brilliantly). Sarah's two top miracle-workers are Dr Bragi Intensive Treatment Mask – a fabric mask that has an instant youthifying radiant effect – and Darphin's Youthful Radiance Camellia Mask, which plumps up skin and makes it more even-toned.

'make-up went on like a dream and stayed put so I felt far more confident after just one treatment'.

Super Facialist by Una Brennan Rose Hydrate Intense Moisture Mask

8.81 / 10 One of the UK's leading facialists put together this range exclusively for Boots, offering three masks – including this super-nourishing, soothing, calming option. Gently scented with Damask rosewater and geranium (testers did love the smell), it features skin-caring ingredients of white willow extract and vitamin E with marshmallow for re-plumping. It's a fast fix: just five minutes to a renewed complexion.

Comments: 'Skin looked clear and healthy with an even skin tone, if you like the scent of roses, this is a great product and good value' • 'it definitely smooths, plumps and brightens skin, reduces fine lines slightly, and is very reasonably priced' • 'the quality and softness of the product and the delightful rose smell gave this a real pleasure factor' • 'skin felt clean and soft, looked perkier and more hydrated; make-up glided on – I loved this'.

Elemis Pro-Collagen Quartz Lift Mask

8.78 / 10 Much richer and creamier than the first Elemis entry, left (and pricier, too), this is from the spa brand's state-of-the-art Quartz Lift collection. Quartz, they tell us, enhances cell communication, while argan offers a 'facelifting effect' – and two other botanicals (padina pavonica and noni) relax and smooth the skin. There's also an 'anti-pollution complex', and Elemis call this 'the take-home facial'. As for our testers…?

Comments: 'Top marks! Instantly lifted and toned my skin, revealing a more radiant complexion, felt glorious and beautiful smell; left with such a soft, glowing skin and fine lines smoothed out, really hydrated and plumped out skin' • 'usually have salon treatments but this could persuade me to do it at home; skin very much rejuvenated, glowing, smooth, soft and tight – seemed to contour it' • 'skin did feel as if I'd had a salon facial – glowing and not taut at all' • 'pleasingly moisturising, left skin very soft and more toned without feeling tight'.

Facial oils: *our award winners*

The best facial oils sink softly into skin, plumping and nourishing without ever feeling tacky or greasy. Specific ingredients are often chosen for their age-defying properties, helping to brighten skin or lessen wrinkles. We asked our beauty sleuths to help narrow down the choices for you – and here are their top choices, all natural, from over 150 that we've now put through their paces

We love oils for mature skins. The right blend of essential oils can work to balance oilier complexions and they're also ideal for touchy skins, which may react to synthetic preservatives: oils are naturally self-preserving, so don't need anything extra to extend their life. As Geraldine Howard, of Aromatherapy Associates, observes: 'Think of facial oils as "food" for the skin; moisturisers as the water. Skin needs both to keep it soft and supple.'

A few drops is all it takes. While they're sometimes expensive (because of the cost of the concentrated botanicals in the blends), a bottle of facial oil typically lasts for much longer than a jar of cream. Only use as much as your skin needs: usually three or four small drops (literally) is enough. It should sink in quickly, so if skin looks greasy ten minutes later or the next day, you've used too much.

We like to apply facial oil under night cream for a double-whammy of effectiveness. Great for skins prone to dryness at any time – or in winter, when central heating wicks the moisture out of skin. Alternatively, put a little cream into your hands and blend it with facial oil using your fingers then apply. We're great believers in 'customising' our treatments to deliver what our skin needs, and this is a great way to make a not-quite-moisturising-enough night cream a bit richer.

You can custom-make your own blends and you will find several simple recipes in *The Ultimate Natural Beauty Bible*. Or you can opt for one of the many pre-blended oils that are now widely available. Once the exclusive preserve of French women, who learned early on how powerfully skin-caring facial oils can be, there are now dozens and dozens of options on the market – which is why we've put them through their paces.

REVIEWS

ESPA Replenishing Face Treatment Oil ❀ ❀

Our testers were overwhelmed by the effect of this intensely nourishing product designed to rehydrate and smooth fine lines. On a base blend led by coconut, sweet almond and jojoba oils, this aromatic product contains neroli and sandalwood essential oils to help revitalise skin and stimulate cell renewal with vitamin E-rich avocado and patchouli extracts to soften even the driest skin. (NB: Most testers asked for a different container with a pipette to deliver drops rather than teaspoons: ESPA please note).
Comments: 'this product rapidly become one of the best things I've ever used. My skin looks radiant and feels moisturised and nourished but not greasy at all' • 'this made my skin feel plumper and slightly firmer, pores seemed smaller, jawline slightly firmer and overall condition of skin improved' • 'hubby said skin looked great – and he never notices! So effective it was worth the higher price' • 'does my skin look better? YES YES YES! It has really, really

AT A GLANCE

ESPA Replenishing Face Treatment Oil

Aurelia Cell Repair Night Oil

Liz Earle Superskin Concentrate

AD Skin Synergy Night Treatment Facial Oil

MV Organics Rose Plus Booster

improved my skin far beyond my expectations' • 'fine lines around eyes and lines on my forehead less visible'.

Aurelia Cell Repair Night Oil ❀❀

9.15/10

From the all-girl British company that won our first Best New Brand award in 2014, this BioOrganic 100 per cent pure boosting treatment works in tandem with your skin's nightly repair mechanism. The bevy of botanicals includes Kalahari, and mongongo oil, kigelia and baobab plus hibiscus to provide a formula that works on all fronts, to nourish, repair, firm and tone, fight free radicals and reduce cell-damaging oxidative stress. Plus a relaxing blend of lavender, rose, mandarin and neroli essential oils to waft you off to sleep.

Comments: 'Loved this: skin looked brighter, fresher, smoother and plumper in the morning: have definitely noticed an improvement in my skin. When I didn't use it, I really noticed the difference' • 'smells absolutely divine, really relaxing; sinks into the skin quickly, no greasiness, the recommended two to three drops is plenty and my skin was so lovely and smooth I felt quite radiant' • 'amazed by the instant result: softer skin, pores less noticeable, complexion looked more radiant, rested and refreshed – oh my word, how much do I love this! Simply the best find for me – my skin has never looked so good' • 'skin looks glowier and softer: my husband and mother both commented'.

Liz Earle Superskin Concentrate ❀❀

9.15/10

This previously came top of the facial oils category in *The Green Beauty Bible*, but when we sent it out to our mature testers, they awarded it a micro-mark higher than its previous score (which was 9.1/10, in that case). Which, to us, just goes to confirm what we know: that our trials are incredibly consistent! This is one of Jo's favourites (see We Love…).

Comments: 'Skin was immediately much smoother and after four weeks the difference was quite dramatic, my skin was more toned and firm' • 'my combination/dry skin looks youthful and I think the aromatherapy oils help me unwind and sleep better' • 'I'm 45 with slight wrinkles, dry skin, tightness, sun damage – and this product makes me look younger! Definitely plumped my skin, made jaw line more toned and helped my lines on my forehead' • 'my sensitive skin is smooth and soft; particularly liked the instruction to inhale the fragrance, which seemed to calm my mind before bed'.

AD Skin Synergy Night Treatment Facial Oil ❀❀

9.12/10

Therapist and former PR Amanda de Ayala poured years of insider knowledge into her small signature (AD) range, which includes this super-nourishing oil. It's based on £8,000-a-kilo cold-pressed rosehip oil from Chile – an ingredient renowned for its age-defying benefits – together with jojoba, sweet almond, evening primrose and vitamin E. Sarah is a big fan. The delectable scent's down to a skilful active blend of essential oils of rose, lavender, palmarosa, ylang-ylang, neroli, frankincense and jasmine.

Comments: 'I've had several people ask if I have been on holiday because of the healthy look to my skin' • 'seemed to replace the plumpness skin loses over time, making it look younger' • 'the inclusion of lavender makes it relaxing to wear while going to sleep, and I've noticed a reduction in fine lines' • 'I was surprised how well this sinks in, and after a few days I received comments on how well I was looking' • 'my beauty therapist commented on how well-hydrated my skin is' • 'my wrinkles were less noticeable and my skin more nourished' • 'I loved this and it lasts for AGES!' • 'skin glowing, but less redness'.

MV Organics Rose Plus Booster ❀❀❀

9.07/10

This brand originated in Sydney, Australia from facialist Sharon McGlinchey, who oversees every detail, and is one of Sarah's all-time favourites (as well as A-listers including Emma Watson). Suitable for all skin types, Rose Plus Booster (the rose comes from super-previous Bulgarian rose oil and rosehip oil) is particularly good for dry, delicate and hormonal complexions and calms redness from damaged blood vessels and rosacea.

Comments: 'Wow! I am quite devoted to how my skin feels now – less dry and flaky, less red, more even, really good. This is a hero product – the tiniest amount of this magic oil has made an amazing improvement to my sensitive dry skin in a few weeks' • 'far and away my favourite product: sinks into skin quickly and I love the rose fragrance. My skin looks brighter and fresher. I will save up to buy more because it is so economical' • 'there's nothing I didn't love about this product: smelt amazing, a pleasure to massage into skin, my skin glowed after using it, I had compliments and there are only seven ingredients, all organic – I rest my case'.

♡ WE LOVE…

As well as long-term favourite Liz Earle Superskin Concentrate - 'I absolutely adore the smell: neroli, lavender and chamomile', Jo has embraced L'Occitane Divine Youth Oil, another gloriously-scented face treat, featuring the same wonderfully aromatic immortelle oil as the Divine Cream which has so wowed our Beauty Bible testers in the past few years. Sarah loves AD Skin Synergy Night Treatment Facial Oil, which also won favour with testers, and also OV Naturals Triple Rose Nourishing Organic Facial Oil, a handmade treat from a tiny business in Somerset. A new favourite is Kiss The Moon After Dark face oils, in Calm, with jasmine, Roman chamomile, ylang-ylang and sandalwood – bliss in a bottle.

Learn the new foundation rules

As your face changes, so should your approach to creating a flawless canvas…

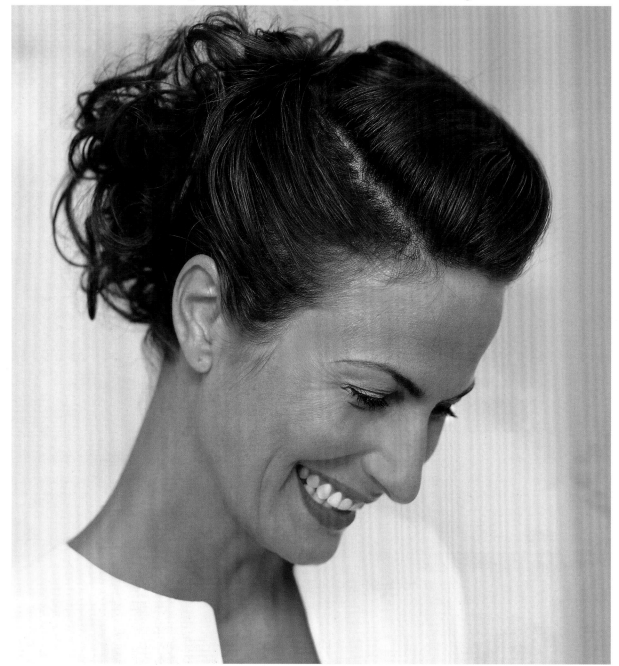

Throughout this book, we're very prescriptive about what works and what doesn't – because we know what really works, and we're giving you the inside info. (That's what we're about.)

However, there are two areas of make-up – foundation (aka base) and eyeshadow – where we can't be totally prescriptive, and where you'll need to experiment to see which of our various proposed options work for you. Some will, some won't.

We suggest setting aside a little playtime to experiment with the different techniques (and maybe even products), to see which give you the best results. We don't have a webcam on your computer so we can't look and tell you which works, which looks best – but if you use two mirrors (one hand mirror, to get a side view), you should be able to judge for yourself. If you're not certain, ask a friend who you trust.

What we know for certain, though, is that the products you've been using through your twenties and thirties are pretty unlikely to make you look fabulous once you hit forty – let alone beyond…

As Trish McEvoy says: 'As we get older, we lose evenness (principally due to cumulative sun damage), clarity, colour and definition. That's the difference between a young face and an older one. Your aim should be to recreate these as naturally as possible.'

HOW TO APPLY YOUR BASE

The better your skin, the lighter the foundation. That's the rule – according to Mary Greenwell and other make-up pros we respect. But she adds: 'Every woman over forty has to wear foundation. Ironically, up until that point it can sometimes be ageing.'

Echoes Terry de Gunzburg: 'I could get away without foundation until my forties, but no longer. Skin doesn't look neat – or even clean, in some cases – because the skintone is no longer uniform (which also makes you look tired). Your complexion may be a bit red, or look a little shadowy and grey or sallow. But this doesn't mean just applying more of the foundation you've always worn (if you have). Layers of heavy foundation make all lines look worse. If you have always worn quite a lot of base, you probably need to use less and with a lighter touch. You want uniformity – but you don't want a mask-like effect.' Never use your base as an all-over corrector/concealer. If you have flaws, use a corrector/concealer sparingly, just where it's needed. For the best effect, you need to learn to 'layer' products (as we explain here).

● **So: start your 'layers' with a primer.** (See page 89 for more information, and which ones our testers liked best.) Applied after your moisturiser (and don't forget to let this sink in for at least five minutes) and/or serum, a primer adds softness and luminosity, can go some way towards evening skintone, and helps turbo-charge the staying power of your make-up.

● **Rethink your foundation.** 'Nothing too matt, nothing too heavy,' is Mary's wisdom (she likes cream bases best). Our recommendations for Anti-Ageing Foundations, see page 90, are another good place to start. The 'finish' should not be too matt; a little dewiness or 'light' is flattering, but not so much that you look shiny. If you have oily skin, go for oil-free; dry skin, choose one labelled 'moisturising'. The big new option is mineral powder foundations, which many experts including Trish McEvoy and Jane Iredale (the pioneer of mineral make-up) recommend, particularly for conditions such as acne and rosacea. See page 92 for more.

● **Test the foundation shade on your neck.** 'Just below the jaw is the right place,' says Mary Greenwell. 'Your base should match your neck, not your face or even the jawline itself, and should "disappear" to avoid that tell-tale join line.' Be brave, and check it out in bright daylight, adds Barbara Daly.

● **Try a foundation brush.** We're big fans of these, and so is Terry de Gunzburg. 'I don't like sponges but I do like brushes,' she says. 'You can control the quantity that you apply and you can "layer" the foundation on a little at a time, using the brush to make tiny feathery strokes that tap it into the skin and pores. Apply a little foundation to the back of your (clean) hand, and pick the foundation up from there with the brush, a little at a time. You can always add, but it's harder to take away. Then use the warmth of your fingers to "press" the foundation into the skin, which makes it look natural.' (NB: We're big fans of all the products in Terry's By Terry make-up range: after all, she is the woman who created the legendary Touche Eclat/Radiant Touch for YSL, and there is probably nobody who understands light-reflecting particles and how to introduce radiance into make-up products better than her. She's very funny about her line, insisting: 'I created it for women who want to look as good as their daughters. Or their husband's mistress.' A very French approach…!)

Alternatively, use your fingers to smooth in your foundation, from the word 'go'. Fingers are Mary Greenwell's preferred 'tools', also Barbara Daly's. 'They

Can you fix an open pore? We know these bug you from the number of emails to www.beautybible.com, over the years. Pores tend to 'stretch' as we age, especially for those who've had oily skin in the past. Conversely, they can be very obvious on dry skin. The old advice was to avoid moisturising the affected area – but first, that's not practical and also we'd rather you protected your face with an SPF. And actually we suggest reading the comments made about award winners in our Miracle Treatments, Serums and Night Creams section as many testers observed improvements in tightness of pores as a result of using certain products featured there; ditto, the clay-based mask in our Face Masks section. But do avoid toners which can over-stimulate sebaceous glands. For a quick fix, try patting on a primer or line-filler – they can make pores vanish in a flash (albeit temporarily) and are your fast track to pore perfection.

are warm, and so help "meld" foundation into skin,' Mary says. (We say: try a brush, try your fingers, and see which gives you the best effect. Sarah favours fingers most mornings – with brushwork for dress-up days – but Jo finds fingers take off as much as she's putting on so uses a brush. So the mantra is 'experiment'!) Don't feel you have to apply it all over your face, says Barbara Daly. 'Start from the centre and blend out, so by the time you get to the fine hairs at the side (don't worry – everyone has them), there's nothing there.'

Remember, your base is not a corrector or concealer. So, once you've applied your foundation, stand back and take a look. If you still have flaws you want to hide, such as brown spots, red cheeks, scars or dark circles under your eyes, read on.

COVERING REDNESS, AGE SPOTS AND OTHER FLAWS

While Trish McEvoy believes every woman of a certain age should own a corrector, concealer (see below for the difference) and luminiser, they are certainly essential for camouflaging hyperpigmentation (brown spots), redness and other blemishes. Her advice: 'After you've primed skin, take your corrector (always matt, yellow- or peach-based, with deeper peach for women of colour), and dot it on with a little brush, then press it in. Very important to dot and press, do not sweep it on. If it needs more blending use a little make-up sponge.' You can then apply cream/liquid foundation, or brush on mineral powder base if you need it. Setting with translucent powder over liquid foundation is optional. 'Technology has advanced so tremendously that many formulas today are long wear and don't need powder,' says Trish.

'My grandmothers lived long into old age and they were always BEAUTIFUL to me. They *loved life* and it showed in their faces'

Penélope Cruz

And what's the difference between a corrector and concealer? Sometimes very little: though generally correctors are lighter and aim to correct colour and tone on very red cheeks or rosacea – rather than a concealer which sits on a blemish such as under-eye dark circles or a scar to conceal it. For more pronounced flaws, you might want to use a corrector followed by a concealer. (For more camouflage advice on covering rosacea and acne scarring, see page 168.)

For frown lines, try patting on a silicone-based filler, which will soften the edges (more on page 94).

Brighten up with a luminiser. Aka a light-reflecting pen (see page 56). These magic wands add luminosity to your high planes: cheekbones, upper brow, forehead – and you can dab a tad on your bosom and shoulders. As well as accentuating the positive, they draw attention away from the negative areas.

Set your make-up with face powder. This will definitely make it stay in place longer. (Disappearing make-up is a perennial problem for thirsty skins, and also anyone who's experiencing hot flushes.) But it has to be the right powder – feather-light and barely-there – and it must be used judiciously on the areas that need it rather than all over the face. A finely-milled, translucent loose powder will reduce pore appearance too, says Barbara Daly.

Apply face powder with a fat eyeshadow brush. (Yes, really.) Mary Greenwell advises using an eyeshadow brush (albeit the largest of these you can find) to target powder on the areas of the face that tend to shine: nose, chin, centre of forehead. Also try putting it on very lightly over your eyelids before you apply make-up. Leave the rest of your face naked of powder: you want to see the radiance, and powder may dull that.

One exception to the rule: By Terry Voile Poudre Eclat. This whisper-light, transparent face powder has the subtlest light-reflecting pigments which correct and even out skintone, mattifying while still leaving skin luminous. It also seems to add a veil of 'softness' to the skin. (Like all of the By Terry products it is far from cheap but a pot will last you just about for ever.) Rose Lumière is a colour that works on all skintones except black and Asian. To set your make-up for a long evening out, an all-over dusting of Terry's powder is the key. But this time, use a large round-headed brush, please.

ANTI-AGEING
AWARD
WINNERS
BEAUTY BIBLE

Make-up primers:
our award winners

We challenge you to discover the difference that a cosmetic primer can make to how well your make-up lasts and how much smoother your complexion appears

REVIEWS

Smashbox Photo Finish Foundation Primer

9.14/10 Bounding into new first place comes Photo Finish Foundation Primer launched by the cosmetic brand born from making-up stars for shoots at the legendary Smashbox photo studios in LA. This very light liquid was formulated for normal to dry skin but there are five other options: for oily or blemish-prone, dry, dull, sensitive or lined skins.

Comments: 'Blended in perfectly: the overall finish is brilliant – non-greasy and fresh – and foundation lasts a lot longer, also fills in lines' • 'a friend I hadn't seen for a while said I looked great' • 'visibly reduced my pores, like no other primer, wrinkles less noticeable, foundation lasted longer and my face was flawless!' • 'fantastic base, left skin smooth and velvety, BB cream sat perfectly on top'.

Guerlain Météorites Perles Light Diffusing Perfecting Primer

8.57/10 Delicate petal pink pearls are suspended in this gel primer, and diffuse when massaged into the skin to give a radiant glow without – miraculously – adding shininess. (In fact, there are absorbing powders to neutralise sebum.) It has the usual signature Guerlain violet-y fragrance (which we love, love, LOVE...).

Comments: 'Really loved this product, easy to use, fantastic packaging, sank in quickly and made my skin feel like silk; enhanced radiance and an excellent base for make-up, which lasted longer – my skin glowed through the day' • 'gives a gentle, pretty glow which lasts all day' • 'make-up looks satin-smooth on top of this smooth, light serum, which left a sheen on my skin, and my friend said how good it looked; I like the ingenious pearls' • 'gave a much more smooth and professional look, fabulous fragrance, foundation glided on'.

AT A GLANCE

Smashbox Photo Finish Foundation Primer

Guerlain Météorites Perles Light Diffusing Perfecting Primer

Clarins Instant Smooth Perfecting Touch

DHC Velvet Skin Coat

 WE LOVE...

Somewhat to her shame, Jo often does her make-up on the train and, like Sarah, she has recently switched to Charlotte Tilbury Wonderglow, which creates a (yes) wonderfully glowing, line-blurring, radiant base for make-up. You can also dot it on top of foundation to perk up your face at any point. Clever.

Clarins Instant Smooth Perfecting Touch

8.39/10 Clarins do tell us that this little pot of silky-smooth skin perfector CAN be used all over the skin – over day cream and under foundation/powder – but the dinky size of the jar means you might get through it quite quickly, even though you need very little actual product.(It can also be used on specifically lined areas, as an instant smoother.) It contains a 'Line Minimiser Pigment' for soft-focus effect, plus 'Acacia Micro-Pearls' which plump up to fill any lines.

Comments: 'The rich, silky texture is very easy to apply and sank in immediately; definitely enhanced radiance and is an excellent base for foundation – the glow lasted throughout the day; this little pot can work wonders' • 'you need to apply just a little then let it sit for a few minutes before applying foundation or else it gets mixed in; made skin look brighter and smoother and has encouraged me to use a primer more regularly'.

DHC Velvet Skin Coat

8.33/10 Japanese beauty brand DHC is becoming a bit of a 'cult' – thanks to products like this. Just two or three drops of this primer, smoothed into skin, are all it takes to create the promised velvety matte canvas – and DHC also trumpet this product as a shadow and eyeliner primer, too.

Comments: 'I absolutely loved this primer. It glides on like velvet and provides a fantastic base and left skin silky smooth all day. I didn't have to reapply make-up at all during my long working day' • 'friends commented on how good my skin looked, it's now a make-up bag essential' • 'brilliant for smoothing out fine lines in the under eye area, under my concealer' • 'great product in a handy tube, definitely a must' • 'helped smooth out lines and wrinkles'.

Anti-ageing foundations: our award winners

There are now foundations designed specifically for older skin that give good coverage to hide imperfections and create a more radiant, even tone

AT A GLANCE

Clarins Skin Illusion Natural Radiance Foundation SPF10

Lancôme Teint Miracle

Bobbi Brown Skin Foundation SPF15

Benefit Hello Flawless Oxygen Wow Brightening Makeup SPF25

TIP

The most important thing with foundation is still the right colour: but don't try it on the back of your hand – the skintone is invariably dramatically different. Use a Q-tip to try it just below your jawline. If it disappears, it's the right shade.

In the past few years, a whole new category of bases has emerged to cater to the wannabe-fabulous-at-forty-plus market. Anti-ageing foundations mostly do double-duty: instantly evening out skintone (one of the most instantly de-ageing tricks) plus moisturising, and some contain ingredients to help perfect skin over the longer term (firming/plumping/damage-limiting, etc). The snag is that foundation should only be applied where you need it – definitely not as an all-over 'mask' – so there's a limit to what can be achieved in terms of serious ongoing improvements. Here are the high-scoring bases which seriously impressed testers, including new award-winners appearing for the first time in this latest update. Ace bases, indeed.

REVIEWS

Clarins Skin Illusion Natural Radiance Foundation SPF10

8.89/10

The secret moisturising 'weapon' for older skins in this antioxidiant, anti-pollution foundation is a 'time-released micro-patch', so Clarins tell us, to reduce dehydration. The medium-coverage formula enhances radiance thanks to pink algae extract and (cosmetically) a 'pink opal powder' for an opalescent glow, alongside light-optimising pigments for a soft focus effect. It offers light sun protection (NB: Only where applied) – SPF10 – and there are also ten shades available. (Our lot were dispatched 107 Beige.)
Comments: 'Brilliant! Amazing a foundation so light can cover so well' • 'my partner asked me what on earth I'd done as I looked so much better after putting my make-up on; he said he wished he could get away with wearing make-up!' • 'just amazing: covered so well, looked so radiant and un-made-up – love, love, love…' • 'helped to cover the dark circles under my eyes well' • 'skin felt softer and looked plumper – the best foundation I've ever used,

smelt divine and a little went a very long way' • 'I have already recommended to lots of my friends following their compliments on how good my skin looks. I absolutely love this product – I am converted for life!'.

Lancôme Teint Miracle

8.81/10

One of Sarah's own favourites (see We Love…), this is the product of 10 years of research (with 770 women involved in Lancôme's studies). The aim? Quite simply to improve the way skin absorbs light. The result is this luminous foundation featuring a new generation of optical pigments and incorporating 40 per cent water – so it's amazingly light, yet gives great coverage, with the bonus of a UVB-protecting SPF15 (but only where you've applied it).
Comments: 'The best foundation I have ever had and I am totally converted: it is light but seems to conceal flaws; someone complimented me about my complexion in a photo' • 'radiance was definitely enhanced, but no shine on skin for a change, so easy to apply and stayed in place all day – no retouching required' • 'made my skin look glowing and soft all day, a couple of friends commented how well I looked' • 'made me look far more polished, an excellent product: I felt it did enhance radiance and lifted my complexion'.

Bobbi Brown Skin Foundation SPF15

If it's a supremely weightless formula you're after, look no further. (We'd almost categorise this as 'foundation for foundation-phobes'.) Though it's super-lightweight in texture, coverage is good and impressively long-lasting, with an SPF15 to help against UVB. We appreciate Bobbi's acknowledgment that skin comes in all tones: our testers received Beige, but there are 16 other shades.
Comments: 'The best foundation I've ever used! Felt weightless and comfortable as if it wasn't there' •

ANTI-AGEING
AWARD WINNERS
BEAUTY BIBLE

'stayed put all day, without the usual oily patches on my forehead, and the colour was true to my own skintone; no tell-tale lines' • 'more dewy than powdery: it evens skin, blurs light blemishes – loved it' • 'easy and quick to apply for a natural look' • 'over the last ten years I have tried many types of foundation and all have ended up unused and in the bin. They have always felt heavy (even light formulas) and I could feel them on my skin. This has completely converted me'.

Benefit Hello Flawless Oxygen Wow Brightening Makeup SPF25

8.21/10

This new award winner from the hugely successful San Francisco-based cosmetic company boasts Oxygen Wow Hydrating Complex to give a plumping effect as well as brightening, plus a useful SPF25 (but do remember it won't last all day – and it's not intended for serious sun-bathing just batting round city streets or strolling in the park). You can build up the oil-free (but not drying) formulation easily for light to medium coverage. In nine shades from Ivory (two options – for yellow or pink undertones) to Nutmeg. Beauty Bible testers were indeed 'Wow-ed'…

Comments: 'I have tried lots of different foundations and this was one of the best. Covered without looking heavy, my skin looked great, even, fresh, much brighter and healthy-looking' • 'I loved this brilliant product, which made my skin look a million times better than it does normally' • 'easy to blend and smooth, and I could leave it more sheer in places, which I liked a lot' • 'makes my skin look as if it's under a soft focus lens, very flattering; loved the light-as-air formula, which covered the redness on my cheeks and small blemishes' • 'I actually was complimented on how well I was looking'.

♡ WE LOVE…

At the launch of By Terry Terrybly Densiliss (terrible name for a truly stupendous product), Jo was just one of the many beauty editors who refused to leave the building without this new foundation in her paws, and has since recommended this luxe-priced base to countless friends. Sarah's new revelation is Suqqu, a Japanese brand that offers liquid and compact foundations, which are feather-light but cover well. They last and last without caking, breaking up (due to UV light) or settling into lines.

Concealers: *our award winners*

Many cream concealers (usually a little thicker than cream foundation) we've tried are not suitable for under-eyes, as they can look cake-y – but the top scoring products here (with two new entries) do claim to work well for dark circles. So, depending on your needs, you may only have to invest in one double-duty concealer for your make-up bag.

Benefit Erase Paste

8.62/10

A seriously spectacular score for a product from a pretty light-hearted brand – which actually does serious products. This concentrated creamy formula principally targets discolourations and flaws but can also be used on dark circles, as the three shades are specifically 'brightening'.

Comments: '10/10 for thread veins, small blemishes and pigmentation, also made wrinkles look less obvious – but not enough for scars; blends in very well and looked natural' • 'I used it on moles, blemishes, scars, wrinkles, pigmentation and it covered them. I also used it on my daughter who has acne – it was incredible to see the difference'.

Wild about Beauty Smooth Cover Concealer Kit ✿✿

8.33/10

The kit contains two shades of concealer plus setting powder in a neat little compact with applicator. The creamy formula is enriched with skin nourishing and calming ingredients, and works as a primer too, they say.

Comments: 'Love this great product – very easy to apply and blends easily; fantastic for dark circles and covers blemishes beautifully' • 'covers redness but still looks natural' • 'excellent coverage – a must-have' • 'left skin feeling like silk and didn't gather in fine lines round my eye area'.

Crème de la Mer The Radiant Concealer SPF25

8.13/10

A ritzy silver palette with a mirror in the lid accompanied by the perfect synthetic brush for application. Don't rely on the SPF, though, as it's applied so sparingly (but useful for age spots, we'd say).

Comments: 'Very easy to apply and blend, it sort of melts into the skin; brilliant for dark circles' • 'great on pigmentation' • 'covered thread veins and age spots completely, and blended into wrinkles: I was very pleased overall'.

♡ WE LOVE…
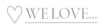

To erase redness, Jo dips her finger in the product that collects around the neck of her foundation tube (By Terry Terrybly Densiliss) – which makes for a perfectly matched shade, in a slightly thicker and more covering format. Sarah now uses Liz Earle Light Reflecting Concealer daily around eyes (see page 57) and also in forehead furrows. Charlotte Tilbury The Retoucher (in nine shades) is brilliant for camouflaging pigmentation.

Try a mineral foundation

Mineral make-up has been a huge beauty buzz over the past few years, and many women around our age are converts. But it does require a new set of make-up skills, so if you're going to try a mineral foundation, we want to ensure you optimise your chances of great results

Two things we'd say: the first is that provided you use a good product and follow this advice, you will get great coverage – one friend used Susan Posnick's ColorFlo to camouflage the flaming redness after she had her face lasered (and went out dancing, she was so confident). Second, mineral make-up need not look dry or caked if you start here…

Moisturise your face first. The mineral powder will adhere to the natural oils of your skin, but as there's no natural moisture in a mineral foundation you need to add some extra. If skin's too dry, the powder will end up looking just like that – powder. (As usual, wait ten minutes for moisturiser to sink in before applying make-up.)

Use a specific mineral foundation brush. Some of these are 'kabuki-style': stubby and short-handled. Because they're almost circular, they work for the 'swirl and buff' movement that's best for applying this type of make-up (see below for details). Some brands – such as Susan Posnick – have the powder in the handle of the brush, so of course you use that.

Tip a little of the powder into the lid of the jar. If the powder is loose (rather than contained in the brush handle), never, never dip your brush directly into the mineral make-up – you'll pick up way too much. A little is all you need. If you require more, gently tip a tad more into the lid, and swirl your brush in that. But all you'll need is a pinch or so.

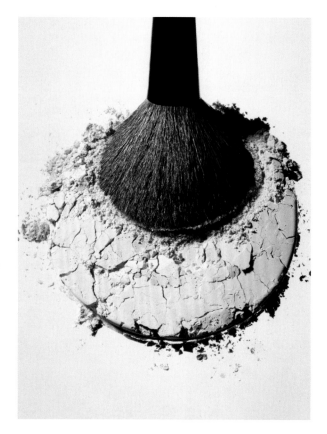

Then tap the brush. This dusts off any excess powder.

Swirl and buff. You apply mineral foundation by holding the brush at right angles to your skin, not at a sloping angle. Then rub the brush on to your skin using circular movements, particularly focusing on areas you want to conceal. You can gradually build coverage this way, until it's the level you want. This isn't like normal face powder where you want to skim it over the surface: you're really aiming to buff and push the powder into the skin. As with all foundation techniques, it takes a little practice, but is worth persevering.

Spot-target any veins, etc, with a fingertip dipped in

powder. This is a great tip we picked up: rather than continuing to layer on mineral powder, you can put a dab on the end of your finger and press it on to something you want to conceal (a broken vein, an age spot). The heat of your finger helps the powder to meld into skin.

Try a setting powder if you find your mineral make-up disappears. In general, women report to us that mineral make-up lasts for longer than regular foundation. But if that's not the case with you, try a specific mineral setting powder (such as BareMinerals Mineral Veil). Do not, however, try setting mineral make-up with your regular face powder: the textures don't work well together.

Mineral make-up: *our award winners*

Mineral make-up appeals to women for two reasons: in powder form, it's easy to swirl on to the face (though you may need a bit of practice, see our how-to, opposite), and many users like the fact it's 'natural'. All mineral foundations aren't created equal, though. If you are looking for a truly 100 per cent natural product, check out the daisy rating of the award winners listed here (for more see page 7). NB: We list other excellent mineral make-up products in our book *The Ultimate Natural Beauty Bible*, but not all those were tested on mature skins – unlike these winners.

Antipodes Performance Plus Mineral Foundation with SPF15
❀ ❀

With a base of finely milled Australian earth minerals including kaolin, zinc and titanium, this offers Vinanza Performance Plus, which promises to decrease water loss from the skin so it stays soft and hydrated. Also to decrease the excessive melanin production that causes freckling and pigmentation, and reduce redness and flushing. In four 'hues', you are recommended to reapply regularly and top up with Mineral Finishing Powder.

Comments: 'Loved this product: the coverage was fantastic and very buildable, from very light then enough to cover small blemishes: I recommend to everyone' • 'balanced my skintone marvellously, toned down my shiny skin so for once it looked dewy without looking greasy and lasted for several hours; didn't look at all cakey' • 'very natural lovely coverage: I am converted to mineral foundation now' • 'felt fantastic on my skin, even in the scorching heat' • 'makes my skin look so much better than other foundations, love it'.

Inika Mineral Foundation SPF15 ❀ ❀

This product from another leading Australian brand offers concealer, foundation and powder in one natural product. In eight shades from porcelain pale to much darker, this promises to be ideal for skin conditions such as acne and rosacea, as well as effectively covering scarring and pigmentation.

Comments: 'Fantastic. I have tried a lot of mineral foundations but this was by far the best, gave my skin a glow usually only associated with youth' • 'dewy, non-powdery finish, and covered redness on

AT A GLANCE

Antipodes Performance Plus Mineral Foundation with SPF15

Inika Mineral Foundation SPF15

Bobbi Brown Skin Foundation Mineral Make Up SPF15 (Light)

Youngblood Mineral Cosmetics Natural Mineral Foundation

♡ WE LOVE...

Jo's never been a fan of the mess mineral powder make-up can cause, so now uses the excellent bareMinerals Ready SPF20 Mineral Foundation. Sarah often recommends bareMinerals Complexion Rescue Tinted Hydrating Gel Cream to anyone with problem skin.

cheek area very very well' • 'my new favourite foundation, gives very natural finish with healthy glow, covers and unifies, improves skin' • 'fab product, so weightless yet great coverage, including (disguising) open pores, invisible on skin and not dry feeling'.

Bobbi Brown Skin Foundation Mineral Make Up SPF15 (Light)

Bobbi promises this is 'mineral makeup reinvented': a blend of mineral powders triple coated with vitamins, moisturiser and conditioners, plus film formers, which is then triple-milled into the finest particles for a light sheer finish that looks like skin and can be built up to cover blemishes and imperfections. In eight shades.

Comments: 'I used my own make-up sponge to apply, which was very easy, gave good sheer coverage, very natural and dewy but just enough' • 'not at all messy to apply, very fine finish: covered small blemishes and open pores and evened out skin tone, especially good for summer' • 'you can build up coverage gently to cover imperfections, balanced skin tone and made it look flawless' • 'a beautifully professional mineral foundation, which gave flawless results. I love it'.

Youngblood Mineral Cosmetics Natural Mineral Foundation ❀ ❀

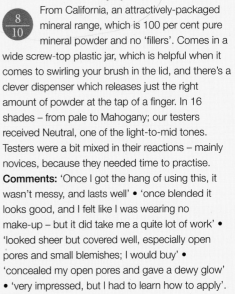

From California, an attractively-packaged mineral range, which is 100 per cent pure mineral powder and no 'fillers'. Comes in a wide screw-top plastic jar, which is helpful when it comes to swirling your brush in the lid, and there's a clever dispenser which releases just the right amount of powder at the tap of a finger. In 16 shades – from pale to Mahogany; our testers received Neutral, one of the light-to-mid tones. Testers were a bit mixed in their reactions – mainly novices, because they needed time to practise.

Comments: 'Once I got the hang of using this, it wasn't messy, and lasts well' • 'once blended it looks good, and I felt like I was wearing no make-up – but it did take me a quite lot of work' • 'looked sheer but covered well, especially open pores and small blemishes; I would buy' • 'concealed my open pores and gave a dewy glow' • 'very impressed, but I had to learn how to apply'.

Wave a magic wand over your lines

Fact: most of us are cowards when it comes to physical invasion of our one and only face with a syringe. (And we say: that's no bad thing.) But as an alternative to Botox and line-filling injections, there is a new generation of cosmetic wonder products which make lines vanish in a flash

You may have decided, like us, that doctor-administered fillers aren't for you. But after a certain stage can there be a woman among us who hasn't glanced in the mirror and wondered what we'd look like if a magic wand was waved over this furrow, or that laugh line, or the annoying little groove – or 'marionette' line – that's just started to run from mouth to chin? Yes, we've all been there…

Which is why we are very, very, VERY excited about the latest trend to hit the beauty scene. Call them 'faux fillers', if you like – but what they really amount to is Polyfilla for faces: products that you apply to your lines and hey, presto! They're gone. Of course, it's all an illusion. But who really cares? Because isn't that what make-up is actually all about? (And personally we love them!)

Bear in mind, of course, that topical fillers will never be as effective as those applied with a syringe by a cosmetic doctor. True volume can only be created when the 'volumiser' is applied deep in the skin's fat layer, and that's not going to happen when you merely pat something on. (If you really want to go down that route, see page 46 to arm yourself with all the right questions to ask before anyone comes waving a syringe in your direction…)

Choose your product. There are two categories of these products (known to insiders as 'optics'). The first is purely cosmetic: the Polyfilla-types – called 'line-smoothers' or 'line-fillers', which have a temporary effect only. As well as delivering those blink-of-an-eye results, the second category of these line-diffusing fillers also offers anti-ageing benefits, which claim to work with regular continuous use to fight those pesky grooves.

Essentially, how do they work? According to Steven Hasher, Vice-President of Research and Development for GoodSkin Labs (an exciting and somewhat hush-hush new division of Estée Lauder Worldwide), 'Imagine a cloaking device – similar to the technology used to make planes invisible to radar.' He goes on to explain in more detail that by taking different sizes of spherical particles – including nylon, talc and silicones – and matching them to the skin's own 'refractive index' (that's the way light naturally bounces off the skin), you can hide and veil the wrinkles… We would add that although this type of line-concealer has anti-ageing benefits, we'd say you also need a 'miracle' cream, or an eye treatment product – rather than relying on a faux filler alone to treat lines and wrinkles.

Remember: practice makes perfect. Unlike a face cream, there's a little bit of extra work involved in applying these fillers – and just maybe, a bit of experimentation, while you establish which technique works best for you. (Persevere. It's worth it.) Here's our advice:

● Most of these products have tiny nozzles or pen-style applicators which dispense just a little product – and with those, we've found that squeezing the product along the length of the line, then patting it in lightly with the ring finger, delivers the best turn-back-the-clock results.
● Try this over make-up, but also underneath: some fillers won't shift if you apply foundation over the top, although we recommend leaving the 'filler' for a minute or two before applying base. There's really no way round it: you need to experiment.
● Carry the product round in your kit for on-the-go touch-ups since our experience is that none of them – yet – endure from breakfast to dinner without a little repair work.

So which to choose – 'Polyfilla' (for instant results only), or with the addition of precision-targeted anti-ageing ingredients…? We can't make up your mind for you. So we suggest you read our testers' comments on both types of line-filler, opposite.

Line-fillers: *our award winners*

AT A GLANCE

L'Oreal Wrinkle Decrease Collagen Filler Double Filler Intensive Wrinkle Reducing Care

Benefit The Porefessional

Cosmetics à la Carte Skin Veil

 WE LOVE...

Jo originally went into something of a decline upon discovering that TRI-AKTILINE Instant Deep Wrinkle Filler is no longer available in the UK (although it is still on sales in the States, so she brings it home from travels to visit family). But she's also a convert to Benefit The Porefessional, which rocketed to the top of the line-smoothing charts in our last update of this book. Jo likes the fact it's skin-toned, so it really does look natural when patted into lines, blurring them quite astonishingly. Sarah is a total convert to B. Flawless Targeted Wrinkle Filler, a real beauty steal from B., which is exclusive to Superdrug.

For anyone troubled by lines, wrinkles and grooves, these are utter magic. We've even managed to dissuade women from opting into Botox treatments by demo-ing the instantly line-blurring power of some of these 'line-fillers', which work by depositing optical pigments, silicones and synthetic ingredients like nylon into lines to minimise (and in some cases, even eliminate) their appearance. As a bonus, some of these also contain anti-ageing ingredients which target the lines themselves, over time. There are now dozens of options, of which our testers rated these highest (including a new entry). Most others, they observed, performed far less well, with plenty languishing in the line-filling doldrums...

L'Oreal Wrinkle Decrease Collagen Filler Double Filler Intensive Wrinkle Reducing Care

8.29/10 A convincing new winner for this new edition with a silicon-enriched formula that also contains collagen biospheres, which apparently inflate up to nine times in volume to help fill in wrinkle furrows. The small tube has a slanted nozzle to make it easy to apply. Promises immediate results plus a longer term, targeted anti-wrinkle action. You can also use it as an all-over moisturiser come smoothing product.

Comments: 'I absolutely loved this gel/cream which definitely made my complexion smoother, with no caking or patchiness when I applied foundation' • 'you only need a small amount for each line and it didn't shift or rub away when I put tinted moisturiser on top' • 'I'm a fair old cynic about these products but there is definitely a difference both immediately and long term' • 'It does what it says, lessens the lines and wrinkles around my eyes and on my forehead. Hydration and blurring lasted the whole day and wrinkles less prominent in the longer term. Am buying more products in the range' • 'gave me extra confidence as my skin looked a little younger, which made me feel good'.

Benefit The Porefessional

8.11/10 Don't be misled by the name of this product Although The Porefessional does a fab job of minimising the appearance of open pores (something we know bothers many of our mature readers, since the pores stretch over time), the other well-kept secret action of this lightly skin-tinted silicone-rich product is to blur lines.

Comments: 'Went over make-up really well; made face look softer and dare I say it... younger – and husband said I looked "fresh"' • 'goes onto skin effortlessly and leaves you with a completely flawless complexion; I am amazed something so easy to use produces such dramatic effects that last such a long time' • 'perfect product to put on my pores and fine wrinkles, knowing they'd be smoothed/neutralised in close-up situations' • 'skin looked even and fine lines dramatically reduced; lasted all day without the need for touching up' • 'other fillers I've used have looked white and chalky, but the tint gets rid of this – Benefit should definitely do more to market this as a line-smoother as it truly does the job well'.

Cosmetics à la Carte Skin Veil

7.87/10 A product that Jo, too, rates highly: a sleek silver mirrored compact, this is super-easy to use: it features a velvety sponge which you can swipe over lines and wrinkles, under or over make-up (most testers preferred the latter). The optical pigments also work to minimise the appearance of open pores (great around the nose), and it can also be used all over the face as an under make-up primer. Skin Veil comes in three shades: Original (untinted for any skintone, which our lot received); Vanilla (for paler complexions) or Honey (for medium-to-dark skintones) – although none deliver actual coverage. Very easy to use.

Comments: 'The texture is like a creamy/satiny foundation which goes on invisibly and gives a fabulously smooth, luminous quality, with the illusion of flawlessness; I am totally addicted!' • 'I applied with fingers, and my foundation went on easily over it; all seemed to blend together to cover and plump' • 'fine lines seemed to disappear, worked best under mineral powder foundation, made my skin look air-brushed! Loved it as a primer' • 'this really gave a very natural look that lasted all day'.

Be very, very nice to your feet

...every single day. We put more stress on our feet than any other part of the body. And, as leading podiatrist Margaret Dabbs says, 'Foot pain shows on your face.' (Like any pain actually)

Feet are the foundations of the body: when they go wrong, it impacts on our whole being. Plus we want our tootsies in the best possible shape, not just to look good but to take us walking, which is nature's greatest medicine – good for our heart and lungs, and for improving bone density (of our lower half), doesn't strain the joints – and gets us from A to B absolutely free. Walking can also work as a weight-loss technique, if you put in the miles regularly and vigorously.

All of which means that after about 35, we need to think of our feet in terms of much more than ways to show off fabulous shoes and glam nail polishes. Foot problems before that aren't unknown, of course – though they're usually shoe-related (corns and bunions, in particular). But as we age, feet become more problematic. And our experience is that whenever we stop walking regularly – because of illness, injury or simply painful feet (Jo was once almost crippled by an allergic reaction to MSG, Sarah by an ingrowing toenail) – then it's not long before everything feels like it's falling apart.

Remember: foot 'wellbeing' is vital. Overleaf, you'll find answers from one of the most respected 'foot pros' that we know, to help you tackle specific foot problems. Because unless feet are happy, the rest of you is going to be miserable – and that's going to add ten years to how you look. Give them some daily 'foot love' and you'll float along, looking like a spring chick!

Treat yourself to some sexy, comfy shoes. Once upon a time, comfy shoes equalled 'old lady' shoes. Well, baby, look at the comfortable shoe selection NOW! The reason's simple: as the population ages, we're just not giving up on fabulous shoes. We're both absolutely fetishistic about shoe/foot comfort because we walk wherever we can, and we now have a wider-than-ever choice of shoes which look great – but, very importantly, cushion our feet. (This is crucial because the collagen in the sole of the foot dwindles, along with the collagen in our faces.)

Look for these brands we love: Taryn Rose, Clarks (don't write them off because they've been seriously jazzed up), Ecco (ditto), Terra Plana, ShoeTherapy pumps (with posture-correcting soles), Aerosoles, FitFlops and Chie Mihara, a fantastically funky but wearable Spanish brand Jo recently discovered, which is increasingly widely available. And Sarah adores her Ugg boots! All these have extra 'padding' beneath the ball of the foot. (NB: We find those 'party feet' gel insoles squish your toes, putting pressure on the top, so aren't ideal for everyday wear – although fine for the occasional cocktail *soirée*.)

Buff, buff, buff. One of the basic but avoidable ways feet become painful is through the build-up of hard skin – on the balls of the feet, the big toes, and/or heels. A minute of daily exfoliation is literally all it takes to prevent this. (See below for our thoughts on medi-pedis, to get you started.) Lightly whisk a foot file (see page 101 for recommendations) across areas of hard skin. Do not use pressure because this 'compacts' the layers of skin, making the problem worse, according to medi-pedi guru Bastien Gonzalez. NB: We like to buff dry or slightly damp feet, rather than wet ones – on a towel to avoid unalluring 'foot dandruff'.

Massage, massage, massage. Bastien's other critical piece of advice is to use a moisturiser every single night to keep feet soft and comfy. And really, really work that balm or butter into hard skin areas with your fingers like a deep-tissue massage so it breaks down any 'compacted' skin.

Treat yourself to a medi-pedi. This isn't about polish and paint (though you can sometimes tag those on to the end): it's about ultra-efficient removal of hard skin, correct trimming of toenails (to avoid ingrown nails), nail-buffing, cuticle TLC and diagnosis of any problems, which can then be professionally addressed. Once you've had a medi-pedi (we have them every couple of months), it is much, much easier to do the maintenance at home. In fact, given the choice between having our face and our feet attended to, we'd choose feet every time.

Go mad with a nail polish. This is one area where you don't have to worry at all about being 'age-appropriate'. So go a little wild: crazy metallic jade; pillar box red; Chanel's classic vampy burgundy/black Rouge Noir. It'll make people smile. Especially you. (And that takes ten years off.)

'Give them some daily *foot love* and you'll FLOAT along, looking like a *spring chick!*'

TIP

If you have purply bruised toenails, as Sarah often does from horses lovingly stamping on her toes with metal shoes, Hollywood nail legend Jessica Vartoughian advises putting a pale polish over the base coat, before you apply a colour, to camouflage the bruising. Neat.

Put your best foot forward

... and treat any foot woes. Podiatrist Margaret Dabbs's London clinic is where beauty editors (and many other foot-aware folk) head, when feet need not just a treat but actual treatment. So we turned to Margaret for some sole-searching advice on how to stop common foot problems in their tracks

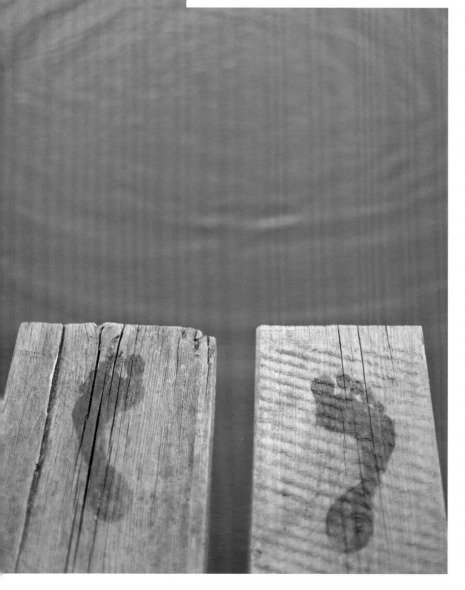

Actually, the biggest problem that Margaret sees in older feet, she says, is dehydration. As we age, the skin thins, we lose subcutaneous (just-under-the-surface) fat, and our tootsies become as dry as the desert. Fascinatingly, that's partly a side effect of the circulatory system preferentially looking after the female organs, and directing blood there. 'Your feet are the end of the road,' explains Margaret. The rest, though, is down to us not looking after them – so, if we may repeat earlier advice, it's vital to moisturise every night.

What's more, it's important not to wear closed-in shoes without socks or tights: 'The moisture from your feet drains into the shoes, drying out the skin – and your feet and shoes are liable to get a tad whiffy, too,' says Margaret. (Open sandals with bare feet are fine because they let your feet breathe.) Now deal with…

Calluses and corns. A callus is a thickening of the surface layer of the skin – hard skin, in other words – which usually forms in response to pressure, often on the ball of the foot, the heel and/or the underside of the big toe. Well-fitting shoes, plenty of moisturising and regular buffing should keep calluses in check, while seeing a podiatrist for regular treatments is also a boon. For corns, professional attention is vital – ideally, as soon as you get one.

A corn is a tiny, cone-shaped mass of

hard skin with a visible centre; it can be excruciatingly painful. The key is to consult a podiatrist who's experienced in biomechanics (the action of how you walk) to find the cause – which could be tight shoes, toe deformities, sticking-out bony bits or an unbalanced gait. As well as treating the corn, you should get advice in order to prevent a recurrence; they may suggest supportive inserts called orthotics, which can be individually made (expensive) or, increasingly, off-the-shelf (much cheaper).

Warts. These small, rough lumps on the skin, caused by a virus, occur mostly on feet (where they're called verrucas) and hands. Most clear up spontaneously in time (could be a long process though). But since they're contagious and unsightly, treatment is worth exploring. Margaret Dabbs uses a 'holistic' combination of cryosurgery (freezing) and acupuncture: 'It's really successful over about three sessions,' she reports. Pharmacist Shabir Daya, who specialises in natural remedies, recommends this regime: twice daily, apply Manuka Paint, which contains a powerful antifungal and antiviral herb called horopito plus antibacterial manuka (tea tree). Cover with a plaster. Also take L-Lysine 1000 mg, one tablet twice daily on an empty stomach, to help prevent the virus multiplying, plus the herb astragalus (an effective immune enhancer).

Thick toenails. This is a perennial problem for Sarah, again due to horses stamping affectionately on her toes! Medically called 'onychogryphosis', it's also known as Ram's Horn Nail. It's safe to file thick toenails down with a sturdy emery board or foot file, advises Margaret, adding that podiatrists can reduce them speedily with a diamond file. But the damage to the nail bed is likely to be long-term, so don't expect nails to grow back quite normally.

Morton's neuroma. Women over forty sometimes get a shooting pain in one foot when they get up in the morning. This

may be down to a condition called Morton's neuroma, where a nerve is compressed, usually in the space between the third and fourth toes. Acupuncture can help, but in some cases surgery may be necessary.

Plantar fasciitis (PF). Inflammation of the plantar fascia, a band of tissue that stretches from your heel to your middle foot bones, causing intense pain. One thing we know: FitFlop sandals help this foot condition (and many others). Among fans is Olympic long-jumper Jade Johnson who had PF; she was given foot exercises to do in sand by her physiotherapist but found she got 'the same effect from wearing FitFlops for 20 minutes daily. They were really helpful in getting my feet working and pain-free quickly.'

Bunions. These inflamed and painful bumps on the side of your big toe joint afflict about one woman in three in the West. The moment you notice a problem, consult a qualified podiatrist specialising in biomechanics and human movement. The underlying cause is usually the foot shape you inherit, but looking after your feet – and in particular wearing roomy, softer, foot-shaped shoes (eg, trainers) – may help. Wearing toe separators round the house may also be helpful (check out Beech Sandals, which are a specific type of footwear that separates the toes). Avoid high heels and pointed toes except briefly for glam occasions, and don't wear

flip-flops continuously. If you need surgery, make sure the surgeon is really experienced: we've heard horror stories of general orthopaedic surgeons (who do just a few bunions a year at most) taking out too much bone. Sometimes, says Margaret, the problem is actually arthritis on the joint: this can be cleaned out via keyhole surgery, but may need repeating.

THE BEST EXCUSE WE KNOW TO BUY NEW SHOES

It's not just the pointy-toed and heeled Jimmy Choos that may be putting pressure on your feet. (Actually, we're rather keen on wearing flimsy, pretty shoes because it means you have to keep your feet looking good.) Supportive footwear – from Birkenstocks to trainers, via FitFlops and MBTs – may all cause problems if you don't replace them annually. 'They definitely benefit your feet, building to an optimum in about six weeks,' says Margaret Dabbs. 'Then you need to wear them to maintain the improvements. But be aware that the footwear itself will wear down over time – so you'll begin to notice hard skin building up. The bottom line is: don't over-wear supportive footwear – and buy a fresh pair regularly.' Experts also recommend not wearing the same shoes two days running – both for your feet's sake and because leather needs a rest.

TIP

'Always cut toenails straight across: don't curve and dig down into the outer corners,' advises Margaret. A poor pedicure resulted in a sore toe for Sarah when the therapist dug down one side of the nail, causing a small but very painful build-up of hard skin. It was only diagnosed when she had a pedicure at the fantastic Beverly Hills salon of the 'Hollywood queen of nails', Jessica Vartoughian. We think it pays to invest in your feet: good shoes, good pedicurists and podiatrists, top-notch salons.

Foot treats: our award winners

First you buff (see opposite for foot files), then you slather. That's our mantra for soft, supportive, supple feet. After a certain age, feet cry out for richer emollients to deal with cracked heels and hard skin, which can ultimately have a wider impact on health, affecting how we walk. At the same time, we want products to put the spring back into our step – that's where reviving botanicals (think camphor, rosemary, mint) can work mini-miracles. So, good news: the foot treats listed here had our valiant testers skipping with delight

AT A GLANCE

Dr Organic Virgin Olive Oil Foot & Heel Cream

Liz Earle Foot Scrub

Aveda Foot Relief

CCS Foot Care Cream

Margaret Dabbs Intensive Care Hydrating Foot Lotion

REVIEWS

Dr Organic Virgin Olive Oil Foot & Heel Cream

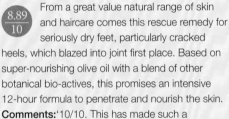 From a great value natural range of skin and haircare comes this rescue remedy for seriously dry feet, particularly cracked heels, which blazed into joint first place. Based on super-nourishing olive oil with a blend of other botanical bio-actives, this promises an intensive 12-hour formula to penetrate and nourish the skin.
Comments: '10/10. This has made such a difference; I have poor circulation, diabetes and had damaged skin on my feet. It is now lovely and soft' • 'I loved the light refreshing fragrance and thick creamy texture, which left my feet soft and silky, feeling cool and refreshed. Please, please recommend it to people' • 'helped swollen ankles and so moisturising and cooling, real pleasure to use – I love it' • 'immediately moisturised my dry feet and heels. Result!'.

Liz Earle Foot Scrub

8.89/10 As you can see, this is not an emollient to slather on but a rinse-off scrub. However, our testers found it to be a real treat for feet so here it is. Already an award winner in *The Ultimate Natural Beauty Bible*, it scored again for this book. With natural pumice to whisk away hard skin, the softening, stimulating elements include avocado and wheatgerm oils, plus essential oils of peppermint and rosemary.
Comments: 'My feet felt like a newborn baby's – soft and tingly clean, all soreness and tenderness gone' • 'adored the clean, fresh-smelling peppermint fragrance and my feet felt great after using this' • 'feet were refreshed, smoothed and moisturised – I was very impressed with this product's effectiveness' • 'easy to apply this creamy foot scrub as it is thick and doesn't drip or make a mess; after a few uses the rough hard skin on my feet felt much smoother' • 'my feet felt very pampered after using this product'.

Aveda Foot Relief

8.72/10 Already a seriously high-scorer in our books, we dispatched this to a panel of ten mature testers. The lavender and rosemary oils deliver instant welcome refreshment, there's a moisture surge from castor and jojoba oils, and all the while, salicylic acid (from willow bark) and lactic acid help gently soften calluses and rough patches.
Comments: '10/10! I've used this product on my very dry feet twice daily; it's creamy and I love the fragrance; worked exceptionally well, feet feel refreshed, cool and silky soft' • 'I get a lot of hard skin on my feet, leaves them soft and smooth, as well as cooling and refreshing; it's expensive but you only need a little dab' • 'a really refreshing effect – lovely cooling sensation that lasted a long time'.

CCS Foot Care Cream

 8.71/10

To be honest, foot products don't come more – well, pedestrian than this… Used by professionals, it's richly-textured – packed with glycerine and urea (though lanolin-free) – and has a somewhat clinical eucalyptus aroma. Though this cream may never get your beauty-hound's heart beating overtime, testers nevertheless gave it a really high score!

Comments: 'The most effective foot cream I've ever used: deeply hydrating and the effects are cumulative and long-lasting' • 'this thick lotion works really well on hard skin: my tootsies are going to be in tip-top condition in sandals this summer!' • 'skin on feet has lost its scaliness'.

Margaret Dabbs Intensive Care Hydrating Foot Lotion

 8.5/10

Personally, with the amount of walking we do, our feet would probably look like rhino hooves without monthly or so medi-pedis from Margaret Dabbs's team. (Can't recommend too highly.) But that's not what secured this a Beauty Bible Award: our completely independent testers really liked this rich, creamy, lemon myrtle-scented lotion, packed with healing organic emu oil (which is anti-inflammatory and anti-fungal, too).

Comments: '10/10 for this lovely creamy smooth foot cream. I have very, very dry skin on my feet and this made them smooth, soft and great smelling. So enjoyable to use and so effective' • 'rich cream that sank in well and really softened hard skin' • 'very good moisturiser indeed, instantly absorbed and kept hard skin patches very much under control' • 'a friend commented my feet were looking good' • 'Wow! Left my feet feeling as if I was walking on air – soft, silky, moisturised, expensive but worth every penny'.

♡ **WE LOVE…**

Jo has been using the very rich Kashmir by In Fiore, a San Francisco brand (find it here via Victoria Health). 'The very grounding blend of essential oils – including a ton of patchouli – is great, last thing at night.' Sarah is a foot cream fetishist because of the huge difference it makes to toe to top wellbeing (not to mention pedi-prettiness). As well as the Margaret Dabbs product (yes, it's an investment but it really lasts), she finds Soapsmith Body Butter Melt, a rich balm, works a treat on feet.

Foot files: *our award winners*

Hard skin is Public Enemy Number One when it comes to happy feet. Rather than an occasional blitz, we prescribe a nightly buffing session when that day's skin build-up can be lightly scuffed away. (For serious hard-skin removal after a long period of neglect, there's nothing to beat a professional pedicure, or a visit to the chiropodist – or a medi-pedicurist, those brilliant hybrids of the two.) The key with a foot file is to find one that is hand-friendly, so it's comfortable to hold and allows for the perfect 'angle' when you access your soles and heels. These award winners were several steps ahead of the competition, and read on for a top-scoring entry. NB: If you have diabetes it's always best to consult your health professional before using anything like this.

Diamancel #20 the conqueror

 9.25/10

A wowzer score for this classic, top-of-the-range foot buffer. Like a giant, raspy metal nail file, it's thin and quite flexible (washable, too), making it easy to buff feet with almost no pressure.

Comments: 'Most effective on the balls of my feet where I tend to get hard skin; definite improvement in condition and smoothness' • 'love it, love it, love it! • 'just a couple of swipes leaves you with baby-soft skin'.

Tweezerman Pedro Callus Stone

 8.87/10

Tweezerman recommend using this wet for best results; first the rough side (for removing calluses), then the fine side (for smoothing).

Comments: '10/10 for this double-sided rough pad, which whisked away rough skin so it was soft and smooth with no irritating bits left!' • 'resounding yes to this: the smoother side was also excellent for rough elbows'.

Margaret Dabbs Professional Foot File

8.56/10

Designed to use once a week on dry skin, this file uses compressed Crystal Technology and partners Margaret's Foot Lotion (left).

Comments: Hard dry skin came away very easily and after three days I had none: very impressed' • 'really easy to hold and manoeuvre into position; helps absorption of cream too' • 'the most marvellous foot file I've ever used'.

♡ **WE LOVE…**

Since the launch of the MICRO Pedi – a battery-operated foot-buffing tool – Jo has abandoned manual foot-buffers, and spends a minute or two three times a week removing all traces of hard skin. (Put a towel on the floor to catch the 'foot dandruff', though!) Sarah returns time and again to an old-fashioned foot file (the sort you get in high street chemists), which works perfectly for her.

Maybe, just maybe, switch your fragrance

Most of us by now have acquired a 'perfume wardrobe' (as a couple of scent-o-philes, ours are more walk-in closets, actually). Or maybe you're one of those women who've worn a 'signature scent' all these years. Well: don't be surprised if gradually your favourite fragrance smells different on your skin. Or, which is also very common, fades faster...

You are not hallucinating. There's a reason. As Roja Dove (the oft-quoted *professeur de parfums*, **who is an old and valued friend of ours) points out, 'Skin tends to become drier from perimenopause onwards and that affects fragrance – because it interacts with the oils in your skin. Less oil means there's nothing for the fragrance to "grip" on to.'**

As a result, evaporation is speeded up, which also fast-forwards the process of the fragrance's development. So the base notes swoop in much sooner, and you'll get a more fleeting encounter with the top and heart notes.

But you should also be aware that there's another reason why fragrance may not smell on you as it once did: the formulation may have changed. New laws and guidelines governing fragrance ingredients have led to many ingredients being withdrawn – either for reasons of potential irritancy or for environmental conservation reasons – which has forced fragrance brands to tweak some legendary confections.

We do suggest trying Roja's tips, right. Then you may well find that your favourite fragrances smell 'right' on you again. Or if not, then he's come up with a shortlist of scents (which we echo) to explore now you are *d'un certain âge*. (You can feel a little bit smug that on younger women, most of them smell way too grown-up and elegant – a bit like a little girl trying on mummy's shoes.)

ROJA DOVE'S TIPS FOR HELPING FRAGRANCE

Use a pH-neutral body wash. This won't strip away your skin's natural oils, which are already in shorter supply than they were. (Many body washes trumpet their pH-neutrality on the label, but as a short cut, you'll find them in ranges including Dr. Hauschka and Garnier.)

Apply moisturiser before you apply your scent. This gives the scent something to 'cling' to. On your body, use either a totally unscented lotion (or oil), or the 'matching' body lotion to your usual fragrance. (Most neck creams aren't so scented that they'll interfere with your fragrance choice, but they will help by counterbalancing dryness.) 'Layering' the body lotion or oil that matches your scent, in our experience, actually 'time-releases' the scent during the day as you warm up (which you may well do quite a lot!) and cool down.

Try something new. If the advice above doesn't help with your current scent, look for something different – it could be a wonderful discovery! Don't rely on scent-strips in stores (except for eliminating things you really aren't ever going to like); it's crucial to know how something's going to smell on your skin. Apply to your well-moisturised pulse-points, allow a few hours to develop – and don't be rushed. Which means that duty free is not the place to find your new 'signature scent'; go to a department store, an independent perfumery or a specialist fragrance store – there are more and more of these, showcasing fabulous 'niche' brands in which there are some truly sublime creations.

N°5

CHANEL

PARIS

10 *FABULOUS* FRAGRANCES FOR *FABULOUS* OLDER WOMEN

This list – compiled by Roja Dove – features some of the most divine fragrances, which, if you don't already know them, are worthy of at least a brief encounter, but we suspect might have you falling in love…

GUERLAIN *Shalimar*

GUERLAIN *Mitsouko*

JEAN-CHARLES BROSSEAU *Ombre Rose*

LANVIN *Arpège*

CHANEL *No. 5*

HOUBIGANT *Quelques Fleurs*

YSL *Rive Gauche*

ESTÉE LAUDER *Private Collection*

CHRISTIAN DIOR *Diorella*

NINA RICCI *L'Air du Temps*

SEM

'ATTITUDE
is *everything*'

Diane Von Furstenberg

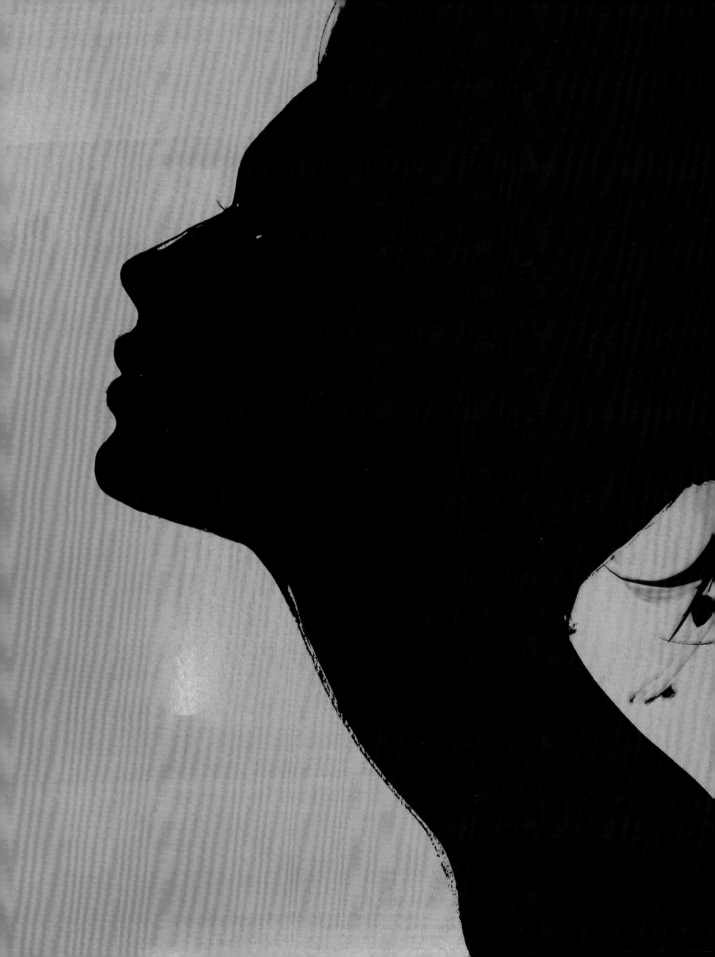

Get a great hairstyle

(And if you like, tear up the rule book into a million pieces)

We may be bossy about how to clean your face or apply foundation so that it takes years off you, but we don't feel that anyone should be prescriptive about what hairstyle suits who at what age. That's because – as legendary Manhattan stylist John Barrett says – today, almost anything goes for older women. Pixie short-cuts. A bob. A funky-chunky textured cut. Long hair. Think: is Julianne Moore cutting her hair short and getting a perm? Is Daryl Hannah or Joanna Lumley? No way. And nor do you have to. But there is *one* absolute rule: you've got to keep it in fantastic nick.

What we've done is to create a montage of some fabulous-looking hairstyles. Use it as your inspiration if you don't feel your current style is working for you and you need ideas. You might also want to keep your own cuttings folder of women whose hair you think looks fabulous. Tearsheets aren't just for teens: they're a great communication tool at any age. Don't be shy to take this into your present stylist – or to a new one: please don't be afraid to divorce your current hair beau if they can't give you a good hair year – and workshop the ideas with them. (Actually, at this age, you really don't need to be shy about anything, any more…)

Personally, we recommend opting for the very best cut you can afford (also colour, see overleaf). We prioritise hair over clothes, because unlike even the most favourite jacket or pair of shoes, your hair is something you wear every single day of your life. Going around with good hair makes you feel amazing, whatever else is iffy. And it can make such an impression on other people.

If you've had the same hairstyle for years, think about this: is this your 'signature' style? In which case that's absolutely fine. We know plenty of women who've had the same style for-flipping-ever, and we can't imagine them any other way – think Goldie Hawn, for instance. With those visual markers in place, your actual age can be almost unnoticed. What may need to change, however, is your colour.

If you spot someone with a great haircut, ask them who looks after their hair. We do it. Our friend Lulu does it. Honestly, that person will just be flattered.

Don't decide on a new cut while you're wearing a salon robe. The style should suit the type of clothes you wear, and your stylist should

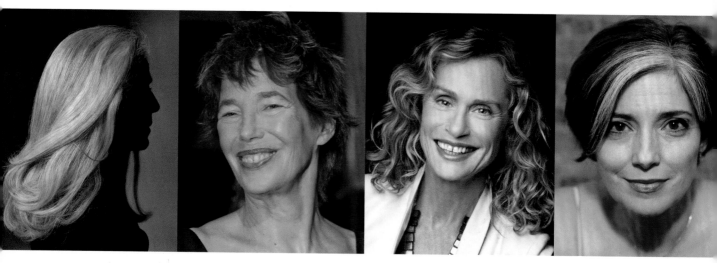

always, always see you in your 'everyday' clothes before cutting your hair for the first time. They should also take into account the texture of your hair, which is the ultimate deciding factor for any style. Never trust a stylist who decides on how to cut your hair having only ever seen you after a shampoo; Jo once walked out of a New York salon – with dripping hair – when this happened to her.

Which means: ideally, schedule a consultation before you get your hair cut. Use this face-to-face (which you should never be charged for) to give your stylist a potted history of styles you've loved – and hated – so they can get an idea of your favourite looks. Let them run their fingers through your hair, and feel its weight and texture.

Be truthful with your hairdresser about the amount of time you have for upkeep. Can you wash and blow-dry it every day? If you opt for a short, precise cut, have you got time and funds to have it trimmed every three to four weeks? If you want to dedicate your life to your hair, that's your call, but if you want low-maintenance hair so that you can get on with everything else you want/have to do, you're going to need a style that can be tousled dry with some styling product, or tied back, or pinned up simply. Honesty pays. What do we do? Jo takes her shortish layered style to the hairdresser once a week, and has a blow-dry, then goes again a week later. Sarah mostly does her own hair with the amazing John Frieda Volume Airstyler, a round heated brush, which styles, volumises and makes hair shiny smooth. She

actually finds long hair's easier (except for the time it takes to condition and dry) because she can tie it back for riding, etc – and it only needs trimming every six weeks.

Avoid razor cuts like the plague. Sarah spent months in recovery after an attack! Always, always talk through with your hairdresser how they're going to 'texturise' the ends, if that's part of the look you're going for, or thin out very thick hair. Razors can roughen the cuticle and the tips; the hair appears more dull because you've disturbed the reflective surface, and it can go as flat as a crêpe Suzette. That's our experience (and that of others) – and if anyone comes within 20 paces brandishing a razor in the direction of our hair, we're outta there.

If you have very curly hair, go very short – or go very long. Anything in-between is unbelievably high-maintenance and can have a massive 'broom' effect. (Or you could consider a Brazilian keratin hair-straightening treatment, though be aware that in tandem with banishing the frizz, it can flatten your previously fulsome hair. The results can be temporary – but one friend nearly had a nervous breakdown; nothing gave her back the volume she'd taken for granted.)

And for more on which cut suits which face shape... Visit www.beautybible.com/faceshapes. We have archived on our website some drawings from our previous book, *Feel Fab Forever*, which offer guidance about cuts and styles that suit particular face shapes. You might find it useful.

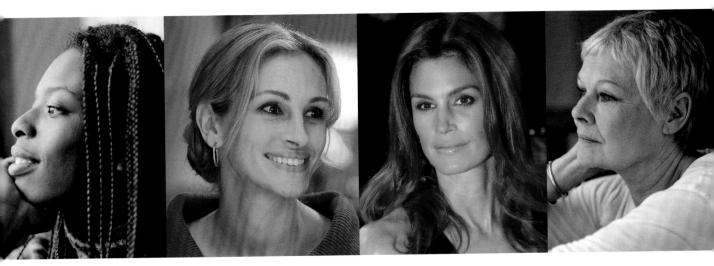

Learn to speak the language of hair colour

If it sometimes seems as if your colourist is speaking another language – well, he (or she) is. So here are all the key terms translated into real-life words – which should help you achieve the look you want, whether you're having your hair coloured in a salon or doing it yourself

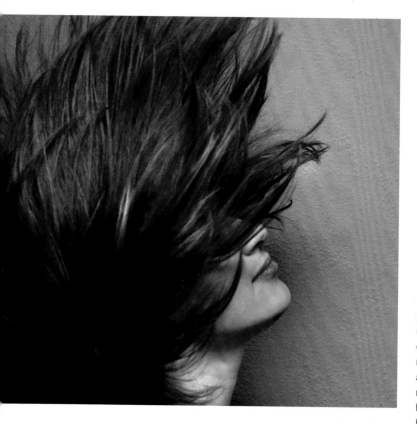

TIP

After colouring, never shampoo before 24 hours. This will help the colour to 'set', so it takes perfectly.

We truly, truly recommend, though – if at all possible – that as you start to develop grey, you have your hair coloured professionally at least once, and then at least occasionally. We know that hair colouring can be pricey and can carve huge chunks out of your diary to maintain. A sympathetic colourist, however, will be able to advise you on the best shade for your skintone. If they're really generous-spirited, they may be able to point you in the direction of a particular shade in a drugstore/chemist brand that might work for you, or at least tell you where on the Hair Colour Level Charts you are (see right), and what level of shade would work best with your (undyed) colour.

HAIR COLOUR GLOSSARY

Baliage (aka balayage) The technique of painting highlights directly on to the hair without using foils (see Highlights, right); this can enable a colourist to get closer to the parting/roots with the bleach. Can give a 'beachy' look and lessens the occurrence of unwanted regrowth lines sometimes associated with foil highlights or those pulled through a cap – but best left to true hair colour artists.

Demi-permanent colour Lasts up to 28 shampoos. Contains lower levels of peroxide (which means it's less harsh and drying) than permanent colour. It's great for creating natural-looking tone changes (such as taking brown hair to a rich auburn shade) and will cover grey. Gradually fades back to the underlying shade.

Double process A technical term for having single process colour (all-over colouring of the hair, see single process, below), at the same hair colouring session as having your highlights done.

Glaze (aka Gloss) A pigment-laden or clear liquid used to enhance a hair colour temporarily.

Highlights Streaks or chunks of lighter colour (created through the use of ammonia/hydrogen peroxide), applied through the hair – usually using foils or pulled through a cap.

Permanent colour This doesn't wash out, and requires the roots touching up every four to six weeks. It contains both ammonia and peroxide, so it can lighten, darken and/or completely change your hair colour; it can also cover grey.

Peroxide Otherwise known as hydrogen peroxide, extensively used in hair colouring as a 'developer' or 'activator'. Its role is to open up the cuticle and allow bleach or colour into the cortex of the hair.

Rinse See temporary colour, below.

Semi-permanent colour Washes out after six to 12 shampoos. This enhances natural hair colour but won't lighten it and won't cover grey, although it can soften its appearance. (NB: The reason hair colouring companies cite the number of washes rather than a time-frame is that some of us wash our hair every day, others as occasionally as once a week.)

Semi-temporary Not to be confused with semi-permanent: this colour lasts from four to six washes, contains no ammonia and isn't mixed with a 'developer' such as hydrogen peroxide.

Single process All-over colouring of the hair, from the roots at the scalp right through to the ends, in one step.

Temporary colour Simply coats the hair shaft and rinses out after one shampoo. These cannot lighten hair, but only temporarily brighten or darken.

Tint May sound subtle, but this is an alternative phrase used by hairdressers to describe permanent colour.

Tone-on-tone colour Another phrase for demi-permanent, see left.

HAIR COLOUR LEVEL CHARTS

Now you've mastered this, get your head around Hair Colour Level Charts. This is why so many women head for the salon to have colour done (and that includes us). There is an absolutely fiendish system for numbering hair colour: there are 12 levels, with one representing black and

TIP

Home hair colouring can be incredibly messy. We are very, very impressed by some new innovations – including Precision Foam Colour from the John Frieda brand – which are 'mousse-like' once they have been mixed, rather than liquid. This means they are drip-free, don't wreck all your towels and there is no need to cover every surface in the bathroom before applying – because unlike most, they don't splatter all over the place. A truly welcome haircare revolution.

12 representing ultra-light blonde. As a general rule, the first number on the label of a box of hair colour will tell you the colour level of that product. However, your own base colour – and where it falls in that spectrum from one to 12 – will affect the final shade on you personally. This is why colourists advise that you don't stray more than one or two shades lighter or darker than your current natural hair colour, for optimum results.

But remember: no matter what the language of hair colour, one picture speaks a thousand words. It's all very well being able to speaka da lingo when it comes to knowing your semi-permanents from your demi-permanents – but in our experience, the biggest challenge can be successfully communicating actual shades and colours to a salon colourist. So: you say 'brown'. Your colourist could be thinking: anything from milk chocolate to dark chocolate. At the same time, what's 'red' to you might be pillarbox to a colouring professional. (Yikes.) This, we think, is where photographs truly come into their own: brandishing a cutting torn from a glossy of the colour that you are hoping for, in front of your hairdresser, can save an awful lot of confusion. (And, potentially, tears.) We recommend keeping tearsheets of anyone whose hair colour you'd love to emulate. You can then talk through what's actually achievable and – crucially – what the upkeep would be.

HAIR COLOUR LORE

The golden rule of hair colour is this: don't stray more than one or two shades from your natural colour. It won't suit your skintone, and will be a nightmare of upkeep. Now read on! When it comes to covering a whole head of grey, don't go darker. Not only does it showcase greys and regrowth, but it can look opaque, like you painted your head with shoe polish. Generally, you should request a single process (see our GLOSSARY) and highlights that bring your natural hair colour one shade lighter, because it will add dimension and disguise the greys, and flatter your complexion. If you're thinking of going blonder, a shade or two lighter can be very flattering – especially because skin gets sallower with age, and a few fine streaks can wake it up. But going too light can be just as ageing as going too dark. Here's a quick way to tell, from Manhattan colour maestro Louis Licari: 'If you have to put on more make-up to make your new colour work, you've picked the wrong shade. The one colour you should absolutely avoid when you're over 40 is raven black. It will sap life and colour from your face.'

HColoured haircare: our award winners

Statistically, most women colour their hair from mid-life onwards (and many of us, of course, start much earlier). But we know that many of you don't take advantage of the growing number of products specifically created to put back some of the shine and life that colouring can take out, as well as preventing colour fade

AT A GLANCE

Shampoo

Aveda Camomile Shampoo

Aveda Clove Shampoo

Korres Shampoo for Coloured Hair with Sunflower and Mountain Tea

Pureology Hydrate Shampoo

Conditioner

Aveda Camomile Conditioner

Korres Conditioner for Coloured Hair with Sunflower and Mountain Tea

Pureology Pure Hydrate Conditioner

Lee Stafford Beach Blonde Conditioner

Liz Earle Botanical Shine Conditioner for Dry/Damaged Hair

It's a fast-growing section of the haircare market, and our testers trialled shampoos and conditioners for different shades of coloured hair, including many new options, which resulted in a new entry for blondes. You may like to choose a product that targets your specific haircolour – or go for one of the other, suits-all-hairtones products.

SHAMPOO REVIEWS

Aveda Camomile Shampoo

8.78/10 Aveda's high-scoring colour care products feature deeply conditioning babassu oil, which leaves hair silky and helps to revive colour. The formulas are infused with plant-derived ingredients to refresh colour naturally – in this instance, chamomile and calendula, enriched with beta-carotene to enhance golden tones. It was trialled by blonde testers, who loved both this and the 'matching' conditioner (see opposite).
Comments: 'Great product, left hair feeling light and clean, helped brighten and freshen up my blonde highlights' • 'good gloss on my ashy-blonde hair, and made it more manageable and a bit more golden' • 'made my dry blonde hair blonder, softer and more shiny: I would buy' • 'great shine – best for golden blondes rather than grey blonde'.

Aveda Clove Shampoo

8.71/10 Well, well, well: when Aveda put forward a brunette shampoo, it scored a few micro-points behind the blonde Camomile option! Definitely a go-to brand for coloured hair, then – and with that signature Aveda scent to revel in, throughout. Here, find detoxing clove, brown-

enriching coffee plus antioxidants, to shield from environmental challenges.
Comments: 'Really enhanced my colour – delighted' • 'gave colour a new lease of life and fantastic shine' • 'after three weeks my grey is usually starting to show through but with this it lasts another week' • 'hair has so much more shine and looks incredibly healthy; colour richer' • 'couldn't see re-growth and emerging grey as much after using this' • 'improvements in manageability I'd never have thought possible'.

Korres Shampoo for Coloured Hair with Sunflower and Mountain Tea

8.67/10 A new entry from this much-loved Greek range, which has spent ten years developing hair care that avoids using the usual synthetic chemicals, particularly silicone. Korres products are stuffed with active botanicals – in this case from the island of Crete – and promise colour protection with deep moisturisation. Our testers agreed that it delivered.
Comments: 'Lathered well without needing to use masses and felt clean but not dried out. Looked healthy, was fresh-smelling and definitely easier to style, looked lighter and bouncier' • 'made my hair more manageable, shinier, glossier also smoother so I didn't need to use straighteners as much' • 'I loved this – it made my hair look like I had visited a salon, newly highlighted and beautiful shine. I got lots of compliments'.

Pureology Hydrate Shampoo

8.19/10 Pureology – a new-ish botanically-rich vegan colour-care range under the L'Oréal umbrella – has done well in our anti-ageing

ANTI-AGEING AWARD WINNERS BEAUTY BIBLE

hair categories, here with a highly concentrated shampoo (each bottle is said to last 80 washes), which is zero-sulphate and delivers their 'anti-fade' complex, to optimise colour protection for any shade of coloured hair.

Comments: 'Prolongs the brightness of my colour, delivered a beautiful gloss and shine, improved manageability and the overall look of hair, so yes, it's anti-ageing!' • 'no problems with scalp irritation which is important because I occasionally get psoriasis on my scalp; helped to keep colour "truer" for longer and hair is in much better condition' • 'very impressed, this nourished my hair so colour became brighter and lasted longer'.

CONDITIONER REVIEWS

Aveda Camomile Conditioner

8.78 10 The 'matching' conditioner to the winning shampoo (for blondes and lighter shades of hair). By popular demand, Aveda's colour-care range also comes in one litre bottles.

Comments: 'Works best if used as instructed! Leaving in for five minutes or longer gave great shine to my grey-blonde hair' • 'excellent for brightening and freshening blonde highlights/colour but probably not rich enough for people with very dry ends' • 'gave good gloss and manageability to my ashy-blonde hair' • 'easier to get a brush through, and made my dry hair softer, more shiny, easier to straighten'.

Korres Conditioner for Coloured Hair with Sunflower and Mountain Tea ❀

8.44 10 A very high score for the botanical-stuffed conditioner that matches the award-winning shampoo. Sunflower and mountain tea are, they tell us, natural sources of polyphenols, a type of antioxidant that help protect hair colour and sheen from the rigours of frequent shampooing, styling agents and UV exposure. This range also contains organic extracts of dittany and marjoram from the island of Crete (like armchair travel really, except in the bathroom).

Comments: 'Love this conditioner, very easy to apply and gave silky soft healthy-looking hair, blonde colour more radiant and light reflective' • 'styling much easier and detangling quicker' • 'I started using this the day after a full head of highlights; weeks later the hairdresser commented how bright my colour still was' • 'amazing! Hair less

frizzy, shinier, healthier looking, smelled great and looked fantastic'.

Pureology Pure Hydrate Conditioner

8.19 10 For more about the range, see the shampoo write-up opposite; meanwhile, here's the feedback from testers.

Comments: 'Hair looked really shiny and healthy after first use, definitely brightened hair, easy to comb through and didn't dry frizzy before blow-drying; hair felt great, not heavy, and in far better condition despite using hair striagheners etc' • 'I used this just after having my hair coloured and I do think they have improved the colour for longer, very impressed by gloss, shine, manageability' • 'I have dreadfully frizzy hair and while using this I could omit my usual leave-in conditioner'.

Lee Stafford Beach Blonde Conditioner

7.93 10 A great performance from this new entry against dozens of others. Perhaps unsurprisingly, there's a 'Pro-Blonde Complex', in this fade-proofing conditioner.

Comments: 'My dry, not very glossy, short hair became shiny, lightened, brightened and easy to style: I have been complimented on several occasions' • 'really seemed to "lift" my tired looking, curly/frizzy hair, making it look very healthy: it was lovely to blow-dry after' • 'my very fine hair now feels silky, with a little bit of shine, not weighed down and is very easy to style; it was very easy to use and I really liked it' • 'liked the fragrance and it was very easy to comb this through my highlighted hair; this made hair silky and less flyaway'.

Liz Earle Botanical Shine Conditioner for Dry/Damaged Hair ❀

7.6 10 Although there's only one shampoo in Liz's range, conditioners are matched to hair type. So our tinted testers trialled the Dry/Damaged version, which features blue seakale (for colour protection) and lashings of yangu oil, sustainably harvested by a Kenyan forest community.

Comments: 'Amazing! I have long, thick wavy hair and this not only moisturised my highlights beautifully but there's a huge improvement in manageability' • 'without doubt the best conditioner I've ever used on my hair, which looks smoother, healthier and in lovely condition • 'only need a small amount as it's very rich; took good care of fresh highlights' • 'lovely fresh, natural and clean smell'.

♡WE LOVE...

WE LOVE...

Of the haircare out there that's specifically targeted at coloured hair, Jo has always liked the John Frieda Sheer Blonde range and is particularly keen on the Sheer Blonde Colour Renew Shampoo and Conditioner, which rise to the challenge of keeping her very, very highlighted hair shiny and soft. But we're both converts to the Liz Earle range – the conditioner did well with our coloured-hair testers here – to the point where (ssssh, don't tell!) we've been known to sneak tubes into the aforementioned West End salon, having found its moisturising, glossing action brightens our highlights and prolongs colour.

TIP

To camouflage grey roots on dark hair, or dark regrowth in blonde highlights, – any combi really! – invest in Color Wow Root Cover Up, the brush-on powder now available in seven shades from platinum light blonde to black, via red.

*H*Moisturising haircare: *our award winners*

We get so many emails from readers concerned about dull, dry hair. The dryness can be linked to hair colouring, diet, or simply be a manifestation of the fact that as we get older, everything seems to desiccate a bit. A mini-revolution in the haircare market has seen a raft of haircare products calling themselves 'moisturising' – so we wanted to know: how hair quenching are they, really…?

AT A GLANCE

Shampoo

Kevin.Murphy Hydrate-Me.Wash

Alterna Caviar Replenishing Moisture Shampoo

Sebastian Professional Strengthening and Repair Shampoo

Aveda Dry Remedy Moisturizing Shampoo

Conditioner

Alterna Caviar Replenishing Moisture Conditioner

L'Occitane Repairing Conditioner for Dry and Damaged Hair

Kevin.Murphy Born. Again Essential Treatment

Aveda Dry Remedy Moisturizing Conditioner

Sebastian Professional Strengthening and Repair Conditioner

Here's the low-down on both shampoos and conditioners, with two new entries, one shampoo and one conditioner. (NB: Normally we're sceptical about the need to use 'matching' products, but it does seem to have paid dividends for some testers, as with coloured and volumising haircare.)

SHAMPOO REVIEWS

Kevin.Murphy Hydrate-Me.Wash

9/10

Packaged rather like a wine box, this super smoothing hydrating wash is formulated for normal to dry hair, or even the very dry type that 'just cannot be repaired'. It contains lots of antioxidants such as kakadu plum, vitamins A and C, plus hydrolysed silk extracts, to give hair a healthy glow, they say, and stop it losing more moisture. No sulphates or parabens.
Comments: '10/10. I LOVE this rich and creamy shampoo; works like a dream, leaving hair soft and silky, and scalp feeling fresh and clean – and I just adore the fragrance. A little bit of affordable luxury' • 'very practical sturdy packaging with outlet at the bottom, lefty my slightly oily hair squeaky clean with excellent gloss' • 'the most moisturising shampoo I have used, my hair loves it' • 'after drying, both with a drier and naturally, my hair felt very soft and silky, easy to manage and looked healthier and shiner'.

Alterna Caviar Replenishing Moisture Shampoo

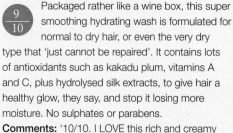
8.69/10

This boasts 'a transformational blend of hydrating marine botanicals' plus an Age Control Complex, a proprietary enzyme delivery system so the keratin-nourishing ingredients are better absorbed, plus colour protection. Oh and protection from UVA and B – and, interestingly, from artificial light sources too. Not cheap but lasts a long time, testers remarked.
Comments: 'Thick shampoo but very easy to work through hair; hair felt soft and smooth, healthy and shiny, less frizzy and not weighed down' • 'made my hair feel clean and fresh, and more manageable' • 'best shampoo I have ever used, hair felt soft and detangled, definite improvement in texture, much glossier, detangled much easier and ends improved' • 'fantastic shampoo for my long hair, worked really well at cleansing and felt nourished, lovely and soft, and much glossier after'.

Sebastian Professional Strengthening and Repair Shampoo

8.39/10

Sexy, sleek packaging – but that's not what swayed our testers, who highly rated this shampoo, designed to repair, strengthen and protect hair. It's also 'colour safe', Sebastian tells us, so could have been trialled in that category – but was primarily judged by our ten-strong panel for its moisturising qualities.
Comments: 'Hair looks better than it has in years; I thought I would always have greasy hair and scalp but not any more' • 'very easy to apply, delicate fragrance and user-friendly packaging; left hair really shiny and manageable, tangle-free and easier to style; I could leave it for a day or two longer than usual' • 'left hair clean but not stripped of natural oils' • 'fab rich product which made hair a bit shinier, lighter and softer'.

Aveda Dry Remedy Moisturizing Shampoo

8.21 / 10 Aveda have risen fabulously to our anti-ageing haircare challenges, with several new entries in this edition. This mega-moisturising shampoo offers meadowfoam oil, jojoba, sunflower, buriti and soybean oils, which all work to lock in hydration without weighing hair down – and Aveda groupies will love the signature scent. Testers loved the 'matching' conditioner, too (opposite).

Comments: 'Smoother, healthier hair – didn't always need conditioner if I was in a rush' • 'my normally dry, coarse hair felt lustrous and silky, with a subtle sheen; I washed hair every other day instead of every day but it didn't lose its bounce' • 'my hair's been manageable and in great condition ever since I've used this' • 'on bad days my hair can resemble a Brillo pad, but this has really helped with the dryness'.

CONDITIONER REVIEWS

Alterna Caviar Replenishing Moisture Conditioner

8.94 / 10 Designed to be used with the shampoo that did so well with our testers, this was a clear new winner outperforming previous products. It features a similar cocktail of ingredients plus lipids (oils) such as linseed and sunflower oils, shea butter and also algae extract.

Comments: 'my dry, frizz-prone hair felt well moisturised and was smooth, healthy and shiny' • 'definitely helped with tangles in my hair, which can be dry and look dull; delivered good gloss and left hair beautifully soft' • 'made my hair much silkier and glossier' • 'almost smelt like a moisturiser, made my hair softer and fuller'.

L'Occitane Repairing Conditioner for Dry and Damaged Hair ✤

8.5 / 10 Formulated with a natural vegetable complex of five essential oils (angelica, lavender, geranium, ylang ylang and sweet orange), this new entry is designed to help repair dry, damaged, colour- or chemically-treated hair. It promises to strengthen and nourish, detangle, soften and add lustre – our testers say it does.

Comments: 'I have seen a definite improvement in my dry coloured hair, which immediately felt silky smooth and manageable, it styled very well

with blow drying' • 'smoothed my hair and gave it a really good gloss which lasted 'til the next wash' • 'I was surprised that it really did condition my very dry ends, my hair felt fabulous, and looked smooth and moisturised'.

Kevin.Murphy Born.Again Essential Treatment ✤

8.3 / 10 The ingredients in this Australian offering are so small that they can pass instantly into the cortex of the hair, according to the blurb. Essential oils are the key ingredient, which help to moisturise, repair and regenerate, and improve colour retention. Paraben free with a significant amount of natural ingredients, like its partner shampoo opposite.

Comments: 'I loved this treatment. Totally wowed by it. I was expecting huge frizzy disasters but my hair is so soft, shiny and seems to hold its style for longer' • 'very easy to comb through and my hair looks much healthier, easier to manage, with lots of shine' • 'made my hair look volumised and shiny, very smooth with fewer split ends; loved the results, the aroma and the rich creamy texture of the product'.

Aveda Dry Remedy Moisturizing Conditioner

8.29 / 10 Here, the 'sister' product to the Dry Remedy Shampoo opposite: a rich, penetrating hair treat we've used ourselves over the years, to glossy effect. Aveda groupies will love the signature scent.

Comments: 'My hair really needed some TLC and I was surprised to see the difference after just one wash' • 'hair felt thicker and lustrous' • 'gave hair much-needed body/condition and helped to tame very dry "tufty" short sections'.

Sebastian Professional Strengthening and Repair Conditioner

8.14 / 10 The conditioner which 'matches' the top-scoring shampoo in this moisturising category (see that review for more info). Again this attracted several top marks and made for very happy, glossy testers.

Comments: 'Getting a glossy result outside the hairdressers is a challenge on my thick, coarse, coloured hair but this worked!' • 'creamy and easy to apply, this transformed my hair; also bouncy, full and manageable' • 'I needed a minimal amount to get my hair glossy, shiny, frizz-free and manageable'.

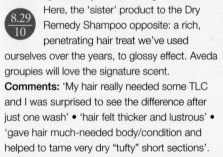

♡ **WE LOVE...**

We're both enraptured by the stupendous and natural Phylia de M. range, from California, which restores a child-like softness even to our very thirsty hair. Sarah also rates the Ogario range of semi-natural hair care by a north London hair stylist, Norris Ogario. Meanwhile, Jo recommends the light, swingy shine delivered by the Sebastian Hydrate range – 'plenty of reflective gloss, but it doesn't weigh hair down at all'.

TIP

When your hair looks really dry and thirsty, add a dab of moisturiser to the palms of your hands, distribute over your palms and fingers and run your fingers through your hair. It will do just a little to quench hair's thirst until you can wash and re-moisturise with one of the conditioners here, or apply a mask.

Give yourself more hair

– by pumping up the volume. Hair 'oomph' is a real issue. In general, it becomes a little thinner as we age – and with less of it, volume's even more important if you don't want your locks to look skimpy...

Thinning hair is a very common beauty woe shared by women from forty-something-plus. We're not necessarily talking full-blown, hormone-related/stress-related hair loss: simply the fact that over time, there seems to be less to play with – and most of us could do with a little extra oomph in the hair department.

So we asked stylist Andreas Wild (from the John Frieda salon in Mayfair, London) – who looks after both our mops quite wonderfully! – for his advice on dealing with fine and/or thinning hair.

Have your blood checked to see if you're missing any nutrients. If thinning is associated with the menopause, it could be that you're missing some nutrients – in particular, iron. Women often lose hair around the hairline in pregnancy but it grows back – whereas menopause-related hair loss seldom does.

Work with what you've got. Talk to your stylist about the best cut for your face and shape – and the amount of hair you have. Take pictures with you of styles you like (as with any haircut, frankly), but in particular talk to your stylist about how practical that style might be for you, with your individual volume of hair (or lack of…).

● Shorter hair is almost always easier to manage – and looks younger and fresher; in addition, length weighs the hair down, so shorter may equal bouncier. Shorter-than-chin-length bobs or more gamine cuts may suit heart-shaped faces with a 'right-angled' jaw-line (think Judi Dench), but won't suit anyone with a longer face.

● Actually, there is a simple equation to see if short hair will work for you (see illustration, left). If the measurement from your ear lobe straight down to the level of your chin is more than 5.5cm/2in, you probably won't suit shorter hair. Truly!

● A chin-length bob often works well for women with finer hair (but do remember hair will 'lift' when it's dry, so it should be a good centimetre below your chin when wet).

● If you are tall, broad-shouldered and anything less than slender, bear in mind that you need enough hair on your head to balance your body shape.
(PS Look on our website – www.beautybible.com/hairstyles – to find drawings of which styles work best for which face shapes.)

Camouflage any hair loss at the hairline. The hairline is the first thing people notice about you, so if your hairline is receding, try a soft, graduated fringe – side-swept if you like. Damp hair down in the morning and pop a couple of big rollers in it to keep the oomph up (or use heated rollers).

Don't try to put too much volume in. On some heads, all that extra va-va-voom will just go flat after a couple of hours; better to choose a sleeker, lower-maintenance style requiring less wrist action.

Prep hair for styling with a volumising shampoo and conditioner. We trialled some of these (see overleaf), to help you identify those which work best. Then use a specific thickening lotion or volumising mousse.

Apply a regular strengthening treatment. Kérastase has a dedicated 'Extreme Strengthening' range which many stylists (including Andreas) recommend.

Never overuse heated hair appliances. Dryers, straighteners, curling tongs, etc will damage and weaken hair. When drying, towel hair to damp then lift the roots with a smallish brush or your fingers. Put medium-sized Velcro rollers on and around the top, let hair dry while you do your make-up. Remove rollers and finger-comb or brush smooth.

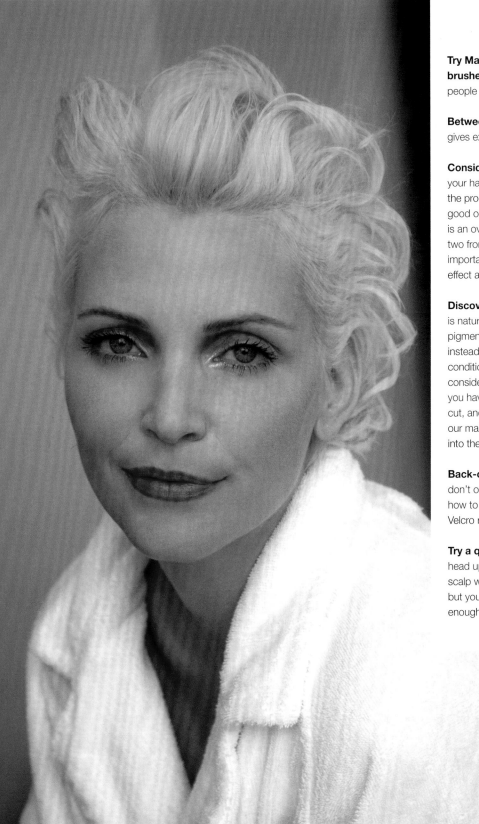

Try Mason Pearson Sensitive Pure Bristle brushes. These were specially developed for people with thinning or very fine hair.

Between washes, use a dry shampoo. It gives extra volume.

Consider colouring your hair. Colouring your hair tends to make it thicker because the processing actually swells the hair. A good option for non-grey or partially grey hair is an overall tint – no more than a shade or two from your natural colour (VERY important), with balayage (highlights) to lift the effect and make it look more natural.

Discover the upside to grey hair. Grey hair is naturally coarser and thicker than pigmented hair – so don't fight the grey, but instead concentrate on keeping it in great condition. Depending on your skintone, consider adding soft blonde highlights. NB: If you have grey hair, never have a 'mumsy' cut, and remember: make-up (applied as per our make-up chapters) helps stop you fading into the background.

Back-combing can be helpful. But again don't overdo it: ask your stylist to show you how to just tease the roots before you put in Velcro rollers, or when you take them out.

Try a quick fix, when hair's flat. Turn your head upside down, and vigorously rub your scalp with your fingertips. It won't last long but you'll get a welcome instant lift. (Long enough for a lunch or a meeting, anyway.)

Volumising haircare: our award winners

For hair that's starting to look thin, limp or flat, there are now formulas to help create greater fullness and oomph...

AT A GLANCE

Shampoo

Alterna Caviar Anti-Aging Bodybuilding Volume Shampoo

Percy & Reed Bountifully Bouncy Volumising Shampoo

Gielly Green Volume Shampoo

Jo Hansford Volumising Shampoo

Conditioner

Phyto Phytobaume Volume Express Conditioner

Jo Hansford Volumising Conditioner

Alterna Caviar Anti-Ageing Volume Conditioner

Happily, the haircare industry, recognising this problem, is lavishing hundreds of millions of research dollars (and euros) into creating products that give hair extra body, bounce and root-lift. Our more flat-haired testers have now trialled more than three dozen shampoos and conditioners in this category, and got pretty pumped up about these products – which include a high-scoring new entry in each section. Previously shampoos tended to score higher than conditioners but this new round of testing reveals some fabulously effective but lightweight products for fine, limp hair.

SHAMPOO REVIEWS

Alterna Caviar Anti-Aging Bodybuilding Volume Shampoo

 8.39/10

With Alterna's hallmark Seasilk blend of hydrating marine botanicals and hi-tech extras (Age Control Complex, Enzymetherapy and Color Hold), this claims to give thicker, more voluminous hair, with weightless moisturisation and added lustre. Our testers agreed.

Comments: 'A small amount lathered and cleaned well, roots were not so flat and hair felt thicker; my hair looks its best all day and style lasts longer because I don't need oily serums to calm frizzy bits: I will recommend to all my friends' • 'a great shampoo: gave me less frizz, more shine and a boost of volume, which is what it promised, so a Big Tick from me' • 'lovely gloss, very impressive, and not static which is brilliant' • 'definitely gave more bounce and body, hair felt terrific! I love this' • 'expensive but a little goes a long way and the results are so worth the price: I am completely converted!'

Percy & Reed Bountifully Bouncy Volumising Shampoo

 8.11/10

A new, high-scoring entry from a London hair duo that is winning awards all over the place (including a Cosmetic Executive Women industry award for Best New Brand). Our testers certainly loved this 'amplifying' formula, which is packed with blueberry extract, grapeseed oil, sweet almond oil, vitamin B3 and aloe vera gel, delivering shine as well as oomph. (In our experience, some volumising shampoos can sometimes be a bit drying.)

Comments: 'Hair was bouncy and fuller, felt healthier and lasted all day and into the next' • 'worked very easily through hair, lathered well and gave the squeaky clean feel when rinsed, was manageable and combed through very easily' • 'my fine hair is noticeably shinier and I did notice a volumising effect, which would have been more if I had used rollers; since using this, my hair is more manageable, smoother and slightly thicker' • 'I could feel the shampoo building the volume immediately; left my hair shiny and thicker, manageable and easy to brush with less breakage than usual: I love this range and have encouraged a friend with similar hair to buy it'.

Gielly Green Volume Shampoo ✤

 8/10

From a small, boutique, eco-minded London hair salon, Gielly Green's signature haircare is more natural than most, without SLS, parabens or synthetic fragrances. Thickening, strengthening (herby-scented) botanicals here include argan, neem and sea buckthorn oils, plus Dead Sea minerals and mud.

Comments: 'I have the limpest hair ever and this really made a huge difference – my hair didn't feel weighed down at all, and if I styled it, it stayed like that without any extra product like hairspray' • 'this shampoo is amazing, made my hair lovely and bouncy, not heavy and limp and definitely not as greasy as before' • 'top marks for squeaky clean, glossy hair with nice volume – although it doesn't last more than a day, it's much, much better than my normal shampoos' • 'really easy to apply, foamed up quickly, washed out perfectly and left hair squeaky clean; didn't sting my eyes – and my hair looked and felt fabulous'.

Jo Hansford Volumising Shampoo

Part of a new range from the 'first lady of colour' Jo Hansford, who looks after the Duchess of Cornwall and Elizabeth Hurley, the volumising products improve structure and boost the roots, as well as encouraging growth while moisturising the hair follicle.

Comments: '10/10. My baby fine hair had lots of volume, felt thicker, dried like a dream and was easier to manage: I want to repurchase!' • 'hair felt very clean and definitely more volume, which delighted me – loved that my hair looked in such good condition and there was more of it. Very noticeable result and a friend commented so it wasn't just me' • 'I absolutely love this shampoo: it smells gorgeous, my hair feels lovely and my scalp doesn't itch: hair looks thicker and glossier, and even the colour seemed brighter' • 'left my hair bouncy and full of life with a lovely shine'.

CONDITIONER REVIEWS

Phyto Phytobaume Volume Express Conditioner ✻

From a leading French brand, this new award winner was specially developed for fine and/or limp hair, and promises to make a flat mop look voluminous with a gorgeous shine. It's enriched with red seaweed, elder and gleditschia extract for body and bounce.

Comments: 'My hair looked in much better condition, bouncy and full, and the volume lasted until the next wash. Loved how sleek and glossy it looked too. So easy to apply and rinse out' • 'great for the summer to add volume to my very fine hair' • 'easier to style when using this product, hair more hydrated and the product has got rid

of any frizz' • 'at first I didn't like the thicker feeling but I'm used to it now and hair stays put better, not limp at the end of the day: I love using this product now' • 'definitely more body after drying/styling, so much healthier looking and shiny: people have been commenting: I'm so chuffed!'

Jo Hansford Volumising Conditioner

Another partner product here, this time to the newcomer shampoo (opposite) from hair expert Jo Hansford. In addition to conditioning panthenol, sweet almond oil plus a unique blend of vitamins A, B1, 2 and 6 smooth, soften and moisturise.

Comments: '10/10: I was hooked from Day One. As well as adding volume, it addressed my fine, heat damaged, over processed hair: it just felt wonderful, so easy to manage and styled beautifully' • 'lovely to apply and orangey scent so pleasant that my husband uses it – good for my itchy dry scalp, and made my hair more bouncy so less styling required: shiny gloss so good that I had lots of comments' • 'I was amazed at added volume over several uses: hair looked and felt very thick and lustrous, in a natural looking way: also easier to blowdry into a style'.

Alterna Caviar Anti-Ageing Volume Conditioner

Like its matching shampoo (opposite), this contains a bevy of nature cum science technologies, and also trumpets its 'freefrom' credentials (no parabens, sodium chloride, phthalates or gluten). It's specifically formulated for fine thin hair, a common problem as we know from Beauty Bible readers.

Comments: 'Win! Win! This has all the benefits of the moisturising conditioner as well as volumising so I was thrilled – I can't recommend it highly enough' • 'my hair had more body, looked lovely and shiny and it gave me lots of good hair days, made me feel so much more confident in myself' • 'texture of product reminded me of Mr Whippy! Made hair feel light and slightly fluffy, so smooth that I liked stroking it after!' • 'hair definitely felt and looked thicker and with added volume, which lasted until the next wash' • 'even without using my usual volume mousse or spray my hair felt nice and thick: I actually went three days without washing, something I haven't dared do for years'.

Hair masks: our award winners

File this under 'essential weekly maintenance', whatever your age. Packed with replenishing oils, nourishing botanicals – and sometimes shine-boosting silicones – we've long believed that hair masks are a must for every woman. More and more women agree with us, and in response the hair industry now offers multiple mask choices. Our testers trialled several dozen, using once a week over a period of time. Alongside their feedback on instant and longer-term benefits, they awarded some pretty stellar scores…

AT A GLANCE

Aveda Damage Remedy Intensive Restructuring Treatment

Gielly Green Repair Mask

Louise Galvin Sacred Locks Treatment Masque for Fine Hair

Kiehl's Olive Fruit Nourishing Conditioner

TIP

Any hair mask will work better if you apply some heat. Wrapping hair in a hot towel is one way. But the heat doesn't last long – so instead, our friend Philip B applies conditioner to hair and then blasts it with a hairdryer for 15 minutes, 'twisting' the hair. This is particularly good with oil treatments, though these are best applied before shampooing.

REVIEWS

Aveda Damage Remedy Intensive Restructuring Treatment ❀❀

9/10 A convincing new winner in this popular category with this treatment mask from Aveda's best-selling Damage Remedy range for hair weakened by chemical processing, heat styling and environmental pollutants. Recommended for an intensive weekly treatment to help repair, seal and smooth even the most damaged hair, this contains strengthening quinoa protein and plant oils for silkiness and shine.

Comments: 'An excellent treatment, which delivers in terms of strength and softness; used regularly on my chemically treated hair I saw a marked improvement in feel and condition' • 'top marks: easy to work through, gave a lovely shine and no candy floss ends!' • 'gorgeous fragrance, gave my very curly hair a lovely silky consistency and more shine, really softened my hair which made it easier to style: quick and effective' • 'I am massively impressed and so delighted with this; gave my fine thin hair volume and texture, with no styling products; economical and easy to use'.

Gielly Green Repair Mask

8.81/10 This eco-minded London hair salon and spa in London's Marylebone have two deeply nourishing masks in their boutique haircare line: this new entry's based on mud, alongside neem oil, sea buckthorn oil and what they describe as 'ancient minerals' from the Dead Sea. Argan oil (used for millennia by Moroccan women) is a buzz ingredient in hair circles – and in this lavish formulation certainly worked its re-glossing magic here.

Comments: 'Thick, creamy product: I used a shower hat after applying and kept it on for 20 minutes, and was delighted with results' • 'my hair has not looked this good since I was a teenager; I kept saying to my family "feel my hair!" because it was so soft – gave bounce, volume, brought out highlights and smells divine' • 'after a few weeks of use am happy with improvement in softness, volume, depth of colour and subtle sheen – definite anti-ageing effect' • 'this product has a real "wow" factor and I could see improvements from the very first use'.

Louise Galvin Sacred Locks Treatment Masque for Fine Hair ❀

8.75/10 This luxurious winning mask targets fine hair, which can so often be weighed down by conditioning treatments. Louise's products have done very well in our previous books, including *The Green Beauty Bible*, as they use naturally-derived ingredients in place of synthetics/ polymers/petrochemicals/silicones, etc. The treatment masque deploys a form of honey combined with wheat proteins, with twice-weekly treatments recommended.

Comments: 'Very easy to work through wet hair; on first use, hair was glistening!' • 'helped keep my colour bright, hair stayed conditioned rather than becoming dry and brittle, definitely helped with smoothing and making it manageable' • 'loved this product, so easy to apply and divine smell; left hair squeaky clean, easy to manage and thicker – the first product I've found that really works well on a consistent basis' • 'hair much more manageable, smoother and nice shine'.

Kiehl's Olive Fruit Oil Nourishing Conditioner

8.75/10

There's an even richer Hair Pak in this range, but our testers actually trialled this lavish conditioner as a hair mask, since it's designed for dehydrated, damaged hair. Replenishing ingredients include avocado oil, olive fruit oil and lemon extract, which gives an uplifting zestiness.

Comments: 'My coloured, rather dry hair was shinier and manageable – usually a wet bird's-nest after washing, really tangled and difficult, but this was one of the best conditioners I've used, it was easier to comb out, and left hair light and smooth' • 'delivered an incredible shine; the first time I used it hair was noticeably greasy but definitely a case of less is more for good results; tangle and static-free hair, light and shiny' • 'simple to use, sensible plastic tube, lovely product and very economical; my once-dry hair was softer and more shiny, easy to comb through and to style, which left me more in control'.

♡ WE LOVE...

How much space have we got…? Coloured hair is thirsty hair. So we follow our own slavish advice to use a hair mask once a week, and in Jo's case, that could be generous lashings of the Liz Earle Botanical Shine Conditioner for Dry/ Damaged Hair, Ogario London Restore and Shine Hair Masque, from a small London hairdresser – and when she's feeling flush, she springs for a massive tub of surely the most gloriously scented hair mask in the world, Léonor Greyl Masque aux Fleurs, 'which is just packed with jasmine. After a bout of over-styling, this rescued my "fried" hair in a month.' Sarah has two favourites: Ojon Restorative Hair Treatment, which is a solid oil that needs warming – a bit messy and takes time but gives great shine – and also for simpler but truly fab results, she uses Jo Hansford Intensive Masque, slathered on to dry hair and left as long as possible before shampooing and conditioning as usual.

Hair shine sprays: *award winners*

We don't necessarily advise using these all the time, but for an instant boost when hair looks less-than-glossy, they're a boon. Long term, however, hair masks, moisturising haircare – plus hair-nourishing foods and supplements (oily fish and omega-3 supplements) – are more effective for improving the shine factor. The challenge is that some of these sprays make hair appear greasy rather than shiny. (Start off by using a little, applied to the ends of your hair from the back, so if it's too heavy for your hair, you'll get through the day without it all going lank.) Although there aren't a gazillion options out there, some did go down reasonably (if not spectacularly) well.

A word of warning: do use these sprays before getting dressed in anything you care about – one tester found three spots of shine spray on her T-shirt, and as she says: 'If it had been a new expensive outfit I would have been heart-broken.'

Moroccanoil Glimmer Shine Spray

7.87/10

A new winner: you physically pump the argan-rich shine spray on to hair (so do make sure to keep your distance, even though it's 'non-greasy'). Moroccanoil have taken the hair world by storm with this range, here with a new entry which guards against frizz and environmental damage, adding 'luminosity' to brunette hair.

Comments: 'Created gloss rather than shine on my medium-length fine hair; very light so didn't weigh down my hair or make it greasy' • 'I sprayed some on my hands too, and applied to ends after blow-drying, which made hair look sleek and reduced dry ends' • 'controlled the short fine new hairs in my parting and gave very effective shimmery shine'.

Aveda Brilliant Spray-On Shine ❁

7.44/10

Aveda have done exceptionally well in the haircare department in our book, here with a shine-boosting finishing mist which also tackles flyaways. For all hair types, there's vitamin E as well as Pro-vitamin B5 (to 'temporarily mend split ends').

Comments: 'Made my long hair – thin but lots of it – look good, nice and shiny with no flyaways; no greasiness and no residue at the end of the day' • 'shine lasted a long time; I would definitely buy. Brilliant' • 'amazing shine on my thick coarse grey/white hair which lasted all day'.

Paul Mitchell Soft Style The Shine Spray-On Polish

6.83/10

As well as instantly delivering gloss, this is recommended for use before straightening irons, with a protective shield offered by jojoba, aloe, henna and rosemary, plus silicones. (You can also apply it to bare skin for 'a touch of glamour', Paul Mitchell tell us.)

Comments: 'Gave my fine, wispy baby-like hair a natural sheen/gloss that I liked and lasted through the day' • 'surprised how light this spray is, hair wasn't damp/limp after use, and did stay in place longer' • 'good for my thick coarse coloured hair, which is dry and not responsive to my usual shampoo/conditioner'.

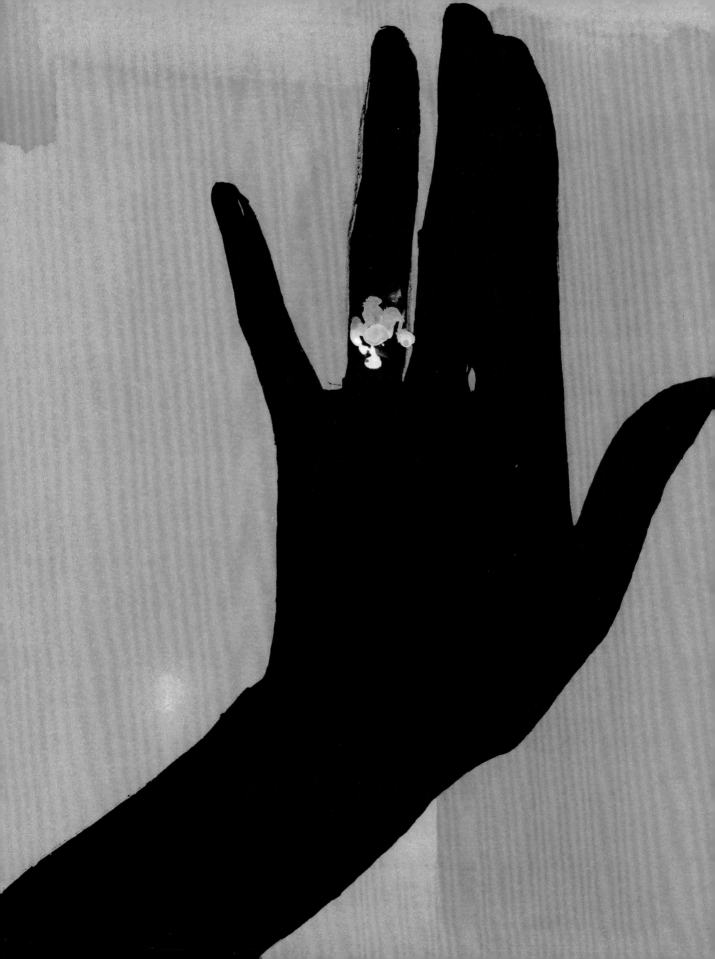

'I've been living
in this EXCELLENT
body for over 60 years.
I *LOVE IT* so much.
As long as it doesn't
get too fat, or too thin,
doesn't break –
I just think,
"Thank goodness!"'

Joanna Lumley

Treat your hands with

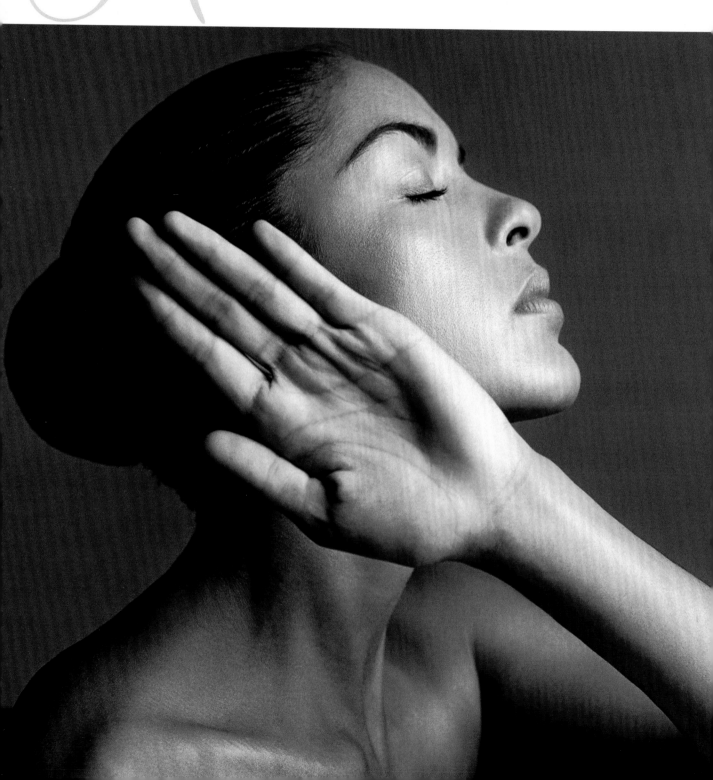

the same care as your face

Every time Madonna's photographed with her hands on view, bitchy tabloids rush to point out that they haven't aged as well as her face. (Good tip: she often covers them up in gloves, long and lacy for evening, soft leather for day.) We don't go in for bitchiness, but if Madonna's hands are a better clue to her real age – fiftysomething-ish – than her very famous *visage*, she's not the first woman that's true for. There's a very, very simple rule to ensure ageing isn't fast-forwarded when it comes to hands. It is this: lavish them with the same attention as your face. (They are equally visible, after all, though that's so easily forgotten.) Which means…

Shield them from sun damage. Either use a body sunscreen on the backs of your hands and forearms, or a hand cream formulated with a built-in SPF. Remember to reapply after washing – so the tube needs to be neat enough to carry in your handbag. Basically, get in the habit of putting an SPF on your hands as part of your morning beauty ritual – post-sleep cleansing, moisturising, SPF-ing, etc. (Apparently it takes 16 to 21 times of performing a task to make it a habit. That's less than a month, for something which is truly going to keep the years at bay.)

Scrub, every week. Just as a once-a-week exfoliation does wonders for facial dinginess, so the same is true for hands. When you're exfoliating your face (and your body), scrub the backs of your hands. It helps treatment products penetrate quicker, while also instantly brightening by buffing away the surface cells. We'd also like to tell you about a product which is frankly a bit of a party trick of ours: Yes to Carrots Feel the C Pampering Hand & Nail Spa. We were turned on to this because it did incredibly well with testers in our book *Beauty Bible Beauty Steals* – and quite rightly so. It's a tub of Dead Sea salts blended into a skin-nurturing oil mixture, which you use as if washing your hands. We have yet to try this out on anyone who isn't blown away by how bright, moisturised and incredibly soft their hands are, in about 15 seconds flat. (One friend said she couldn't stop her beau holding her hand.)

TIP

Please don't forget the obvious: wear gloves whenever you're washing up, gardening, and maybe even handling paper – it makes nails as dry as the Sahara. If you can't bear to wear gloves while you work with papers (we can't), make sure you slosh on really oily hand and cuticle cream before and after. And don't use your nails as staple removers, to tighten Phillips screws, or dig out stones from horses' hooves… they were not designed for those purposes.

Slap on a mask. When you put a mask on your face, put it on the backs of your hands. Couldn't be simpler. (If you're in the bath, that means keeping them above the water-line. Er, obviously…)

Slather on a rich hand cream overnight. Last thing at night before switching off the light, uber-moisturise your hands with lashings of hand cream. For a shortlist of those which our testers found had anti-ageing powers, turn to page 126. Conventional beauty wisdom says that it helps to apply cotton gloves over the top, but we're not convinced: the cotton 'wicks' the cream off the hands, and they feel frankly odd to us. In the same way that night creams and facial oils applied at night harness the body's skin-repairing mechanism, this is true with hand creams. Where the cotton gloves can be useful is if you're slathering on a cream while, say, watching a movie on telly; stops your greasy paws from getting all over everything.

Hand and nail problems – and the fixes...

Dry and ragged cuticles. This is just another manifestation of (not to put too fine a point on it) the gradual dessiccation of the body. A cuticle oil massaged into nails overnight will go a long way towards fixing this problem, while boosting blood flow to help encourage nail growth (yet another thing that slows with age). For specific recommendations of cuticle treatments, see page 128.

Flaking/splitting nails. The oil treatment mentioned above will help prevent flaking – not immediately, but over time. Submerging hands in water isn't helpful – but it's what rubber gloves were invented for (if you really can't bear the feel of them, try surgeons' latex gloves – provided you're not sensitive to latex – which feel like there's nothing there). Avoid acetone-based nail polishes – the only exception to this rule being the slightly-unlikely-at-this-stage-in-life event that you have fallen for a glitter nail polish: a quick blitz with an acetone-based polish remover is preferable to endless, endless rubbing and soaking with a regular polish remover to get the glitter off. And NEVER, EVER buff if your nails are weak. Oh goodness no, no, NO! – and don't let perfectionist manicurists do it either: shriek, jump out of your chair, run, whatever it takes to stop them, or your nails will suffer for months.

Nails that snap. Over-dry, brittle nails will simply break. Again, oil treatments help. Our testers review nail strengtheners on page 128, but the chemical types should be used for short bursts (not more than a month) – otherwise nails become over-strong, and prone to snapping rather than bending flexibly when challenged.

Ridges. Very, very common, these. Length-ways ridges can respond to very, very gentle buffing; your nails need to be naked for this (although again, as above, you can oil them first). Buff lengthways, but never to the point where you create 'heat'. (And note our caution about buffing above…).We recommend the excellent Jessica Flawless nail treatment, also Zoya Get Even Ridge Filler Base Coat; another good option is Essie Ridge Filling Base Coat. Occasionally, a ridge becomes a split, for which the best solution is a 'patch' applied at a nail salon, while it grows out, or a false acrylic nail. Yet again, you need to boost nail health while it's growing out with stimulating oil massage of the nail bed.

For all these, try nutritional supplements. Sarah is a bit of an oracle on weak nails – her weak spot – and sadly notorious with the manicurists at John Frieda, who are practically as relieved as she is when they grow at all. (Think horses, gardening – and, simply, fragile nails…) The thing that really, really works for her is Sun Chlorella (tiny pillules of food state green stuff, see page 176). Pharmacist Shabir Daya also recommends taking a magnesium supplement at night (as important as calcium for bones, nails and

TIP

Taupes, oranges and frosted nail polishes can be desperately unflattering to older hands. (No matter how hard Chanel try to persuade us that they are this season's must-haves, and no matter how long the subsequent waiting-lists…) Ironically, mature women often choose taupes because they think this will distract from hands they feel self-conscious about, but instead pale pinks, soft crimson – and even deep berry/wine varnish, which has become a modern classic – will bring nails (and hands) back to life.

teeth, plus it keeps you calm!) and, if budget permits, silica (aka horsetail), also an important compound for nails.

And eat good food. Try to consume oily fish (salmon, mackerel, sardines, tuna, etc) two to three times weekly for the omega-3 essential fatty acids, which help nails, skin and hair (not to mention brain and pretty well everything else…). If you don't like fish, try a supplement with fish oils, or plant oils if you're veggie. Also make sure you get enough protein for the iron content – iron deficiency is a common cause of flaking nails as well as thinning hair (Sarah finds a steak a week works a treat; veggies should consume lots of wholegrain cereals and flours, leafy green vegetables, blackstrap molasses, pulses such as lentils and kidney beans, dried apricots and figs). And everyone needs lots of multicoloured veg for the vitamin C which is vital for iron to be absorbed.

Camouflage sun spots on the back of hands. Try self-tanner on hands and forearms as this reduces the 'contrast' and thus the visibility of sun spots. Medical peels and lasers are a pricier – and potentially riskier – way to deal with sun spots: we suggest reading the advice on page 186 before you go there.

Veins. Ah, the Madonna problem. Many of us develop large, bulging veins on the backs of the hands, partly to do with the skin relaxing and thinning with age (as well as the gradual loss of fat), so they become more visible. It is, technically, possible to have the veins on the backs of the hands 'stripped out'. The surgery is akin to the way varicose veins are treated, but in general only one hand is operated on at a time as hands can be painful and swollen for the first few weeks after surgery and tender for some time after that. (For more advice which covers all forms of cosmetic surgery, see page 46.) Personally, we'd counsel an attempt at Zen-like acceptance of veins. Gratitude for the miraculous tasks our hands perform on a daily basis – from typing to texting, writing to playing the piano – helps, we find.

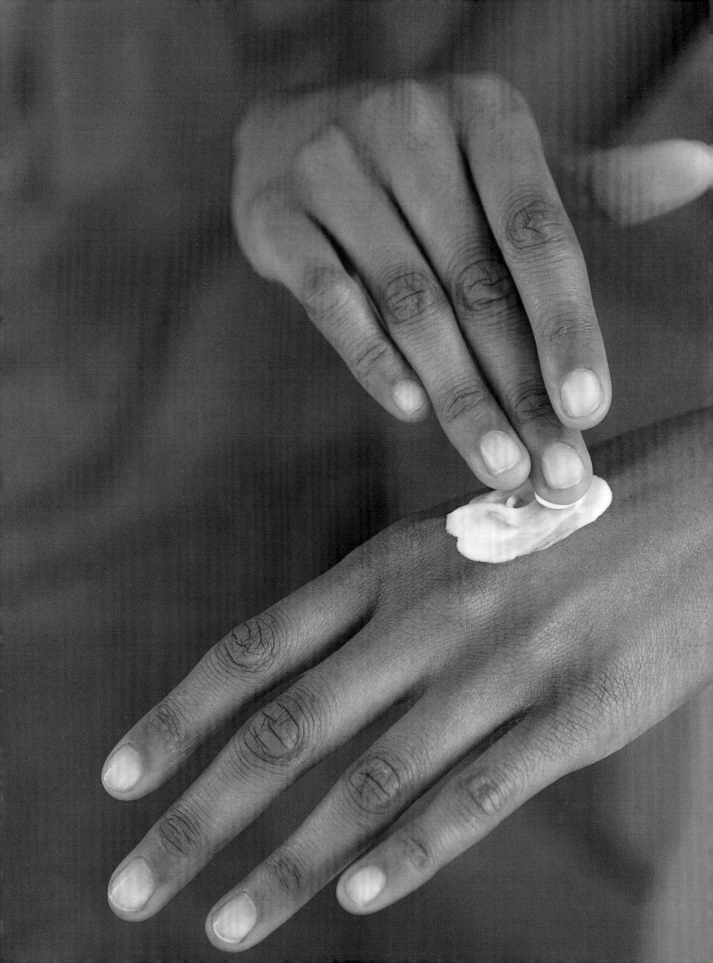

Anti-ageing hand treatments: *our award winners*

Because hands give your age away faster than a glimpse in your passport. Because hand-creaming is one of our favourite (and most frequent) beauty activities. Because there is now a raft of creams that promise not only to soften and moisturise but also to help eliminate signs of ageing, by harnessing many of the same ingredients as facial care. For all those reasons, we assessed dozens of hand creams for specifically age-defying actions, rather than just something to leave hands smooth and velvety. Were our testers wowed…? You bet. Look for a super-scoring new winner at the top of the leader board, among four newbies

AT A GLANCE

Tisserand Intensive Hand and Nail Cream

Jurlique Rose Hand Cream

Barefoot Botanicals SOS Barrier Hand Cream

MV Organic Skincare Hand Rescue

Alpha-H Age Delay Hand & Cuticle Care Cream

Circaroma Replenishing Hand Cream

REVIEWS

Tisserand Intensive Hand and Nail Cream ❀

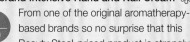

9/10
From one of the original aromatherapy-based brands so no surprise that this Beauty Steal-priced product is strongly aromatic, principally lavender. Our testers mostly loved it but commented that some might not. As well as some synthetic chemicals, it contains jojoba seed oil and lavender oil as top ingredients plus other essential oils and naturals.

Comments: 'If you like lavender, lavender, lavender, you will like this! The texture is very easy to smooth in, absorbed within seconds, nice and moisturising' • 'the perfect consistency, a really nice hand cream that worked very well as overnight treatment too' • 'good old-fashioned tube, a hero product that nourished cuticles like a dream, left hands hydrated with no greasy texture' • 'wonderful – rich, nourishing and easily absorbed: my hands now feel very soft, skin plumped and radiant looking, nails nourished and less brittle'.

Jurlique Rose Hand Cream ❀ ❀

8.94/10
Stuffed with a garden-full of botanicals and deliciously scented with *Rosa gallica* flower extract, this rich protective hand cream promises long-lasting hydration as well as natural antioxidant protection. Soothing too, with camomile and calendula.

Comments: 'Top marks for this product. Perfect consistency, soaked in beautifully, old lady skin definitely more supple and less papery-looking, AMAZING rose smell and it's much less greasy than my existing hand cream: feels totally luxurious, I would buy again and definitely as a gift for friends and family' • 'moisturises wonderfully – immediately transformed my somewhat reptilian hands into baby soft ones; the nicest hand cream I have used in a long time, and a really good moisturiser for the face too!' • 'hydrating not at all greasy; skin looks so much brighter/clearer; already plan on buying this for Christmas and birthday presents as I am so impressed' • 'this lovely cream really made a difference to my unsightly cuticles'.

Barefoot Botanicals SOS Barrier Hand Cream

8.86/10 We were a teensy bit surprised when Barefoot put this forward for our anti-ageing category, as we think of it more as a super-moisturising 'barrier' cream for dry/sensitive/eczema-prone skin. But part of the reason hands look 'old' is that they're dry and papery, because of moisture loss – so the shea butter, macadamia/sunflower/jojoba oils, chickweed and mallow extracts work to trap the skin's own hydration, soothing and smoothing at the same time. Very, very light lavender scent to this cream.

Comments: 'Skin looked smoother, fresher and younger and felt comfortable for hours' • 'lovely hand cream – hands are super-smooth, just wonderful' • 'improved dryness and nails less prone to breaking' • 'lovely hand cream with gorgeous fragrance that worked on my "nurse's" hands; cuticles less ragged' • 'recommended to anyone looking for a "natural" hand cream that works – it does what it says on the box!'.

MV Organic Skincare Hand Rescue

8.83/10 This cult natural Australian brand, developed by passionate beauty therapist Sharon McGlinchey who formulates and oversees every detail, is one of Sarah's favourite desert island must-takes and this rich multi-tasking hand cream lives by her basins. Testers particularly noted the pump dispenser, a feature of all the products, which keeps product bug-free and also dispenses exactly the right amount of product so though expensive, it lasts a really long time.

Comments: 'Much much better than my usual hand cream: love the pump which gave just the right amount, absorbed instantly, and I really noticed a difference in the brown spots on my hands – quite shocking as I have never seen that before' • 'I am not a hand cream fan as I hate the tacky feeling on my hands but this was quickly absorbed and I do love the feeling of my beautifully soft hands. Despite the cost, I will rebuy – it has finally converted me to hand cream' • 'I absolutely love this hand cream, works beautifully, smells great and I will buy for myself' • 'I can't count the number of hand creams I have and this is my favourite: NO CONTEST! A one-stop shop for moisturising hands, nails, skin – softens everything like magic wand. LOVE IT'.

Alpha-H Age Delay Hand & Cuticle Care Cream

8.71/10 Although AHAs (alpha-hydroxy acids) may be problematic for sensitive faces, they can be great for hands and bodies – helping to exfoliate and tackle pigmentation. Alongside the 10 per cent glycolic acid complex in this cream, Alpha-H incorporate nourishing avocado and jojoba oils.

Comments: 'My hands and cuticles looked a lot better from the first use; I started to use at night and hands quite smooth now' • 'fantastic results, with hands and nails a lot softer – it did sting slightly at first' • 'pretty perfect consistency and superfast absorption, fantastic results: hands looked plumped and felt super-soft overnight – the best hand cream I have used. Brilliant. Top marks!' • 'great sized tube for work handbag, cream absorbed really quickly, hands felt really soft and moisturised'.

Circaroma Replenishing Hand Cream

8.61/10 We're delighted to see that another group of testers has voted in this super-softening hand cream from a small aromatherapy brand that first appeared on Beauty Bible's radar some 15 years ago. Aromatherapist and founder Barbara Scott had long believed that organic was the way to go for her clients: Circaroma's range of face and body care was the result. The base features a bevy of skin-cherishing oils including sunflower, coconut, almond and jojoba butter plus cocoa butter, scented with damask rose, patchouli and rose geranium. NB: Testers implore her to offer a handbag-sized tube as well the dressing table-size jar.

Comments: 'Lovely thick cream that is perfect in every way: I only need to apply at night from the chunky jar for smooth supple hands that are as soft as my eight year old's' • 'this has been a bit of a miracle for my older-looking-than-my-age hands, which feel superbly moisturised and look younger now' • 'lovely subtle scent and left no greasy residue, hands look plump and well-nourished: I would buy this product for myself and as a gift' • 'my most favourite scent of any toiletry product I've tried' • 'perfect to use at night as it absorbs so quickly and waking up with rose scented paws is just lovely' • 'I've always thought of hand creams as a boring necessity but this is wonderful: skin looked smoother and the results lasted all day'.

♡ WE LOVE...

We keep tubes of hand cream in our handbags and by every tap, but late-night slathering is best for age-defying hand treatments, allowing them to get to work overnight. In Jo's handbag you'll find a tube of This Works Energy Bank Hand Makeover, a new arrival that seems to 'blur' the appearance of veins and lines on Jo's hands, while on her bedside table there is buttery Emma Hardie Hand and Nail Cream. For on-the-go, she loves lavishing on rich Lanolips Antibacterial Hand Cream, which satisfies her inner Howard Hughes. As well as Seven Wonders Miracle Lotion, Sarah is pretty well addicted to MV Organic Skincare Hand Rescue (see left), a rich cream that lives up to its promise of intensive hydration with its blend of scented oils including sandalwood and rosehip. Expensive but one pump is plenty and it lasts for months, even kept at the kitchen sink.

Nail treatments: our award winners

There are different formulas for nail-boosting treatments. Oil treatments soften the cuticle area and help to nourish nails at the base, making for stronger and more flexible nails. Specifically nail-strengthening (chemically-based) products are painted on like nail varnish, and work to harden nails. (We don't counsel the use of those for more than a month as they can make nails brittle and likely to snap.) Some of these products were trialled as cuticle treatments, some nail strengtheners (with plenty more tested for this very latest edition) – and here's the low-down

AT A GLANCE

Nails Inc Vitamin E Oil Pen

Dr LeWinn's RenuNail Nail Strengthener

Liz Earle Superbalm

Argan+ Precious Oil Elixir

Nail Magic Nail Treatment and Conditioner

Orly Cuticle Oil

REVIEWS

Nails Inc Vitamin E Oil Pen

9.4/10 A sexy-looking beauty accessory, this: a shiny silver wand-style product with a brush at one end, which you 'prime' by twisting to deliver nourishing vitamin E. It was trialled as a cuticle treatment but used over time you should also observe strengthening benefits, with nails becoming strong but flexible. You'd do well to keep it in your handbag – to put bored moments to beautifying use…
Comments: 'Brilliant having the pen because I have no excuse now! Glides on with no mess, trialled it on my left hand, and the difference is clear: moisturises immediately so cuticles are less obvious instantly, and now soft enough to push down; nails look much stronger and healthier: thanks to this I have now started taking much better care of my hands' • 'nails and cuticles now look uber-glossy and in good health: would absolutely buy' • 'fantastic for strengthening my dry, brittle nails, cuticles softer and easier to push back, easy to do on the move – I am addicted!' • 'I really love the sheer convenience of this brilliant nail wonder'.

Dr LeWinn's RenuNail Nail Strengthener

8.57/10 A stella mark for Dr LeWinn's hero nail product, formulated for weak, brittle, slow growing nails, prone to chipping and breaking. The brand promises 'long, strong, healthy looking nails in four weeks', if you follow directions to apply daily, removing weekly and starting over. They emphasise you should then move on to RenuNail Sensitive for two weeks before returning to this product – but no more than four times a year.
Comments: 'This gave amazing results. I was extremely impressed with strength and length of the nails on my right 'test' hand, even with gardening and housework' • 'Wow! A super generous size bottle, so additional value for money. Plus points are increased strength with no peeling or splitting, plus it can be used as a base or top coat' • 'strong smell on first application but only the once' • 'within two days I noticed a dramatic strengthening of the nail – then became stronger and harder' • 'it has improved my brittle weak nails dramatically' • 'the perfect product – I REALLY love it and am enjoying beautiful nails for a prolonged period of time'.

Liz Earle Superbalm

8.38/10 A seriously multi-tasking product (it glosses lips, smoothes heels, etc) – but here we trialled it principally as a cuticle treatment. Superbalm's rich texture comes from avocado, rosehip and shea butter oils, plus beeswax, fragranced only with pure natural essential oils of chamomile, lavender and neroli.
Comments: 'After a few weeks nails and cuticles much, much better' • 'also brilliant as a softener for

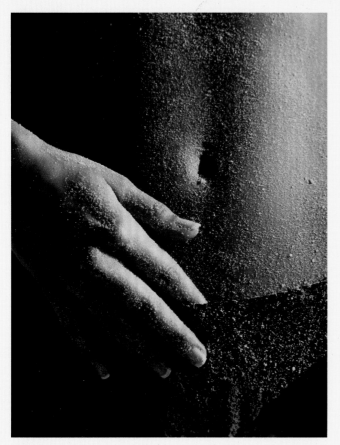

longer splitting: I have suggested my manicurist use this product'.

Nails Magic Nail Treatment and Conditioner

 8.14 10

Developed in 1960 by Oregon-based manicurist Martha Peterson for her clients' problem nails, this Beauty Steal lacquer is still a staple item for many fragile-finger nailed women, including Sarah (see right). Now with a toluene-free base, it lasts after opening for 12 months. You can use as a base and top coat 'sandwich', with a varnish middle, or two thin coats alone, removing twice a week for the first eight weeks, then once weekly.

Comments: 'my nails were absolute rubbish, very weak, wouldn't grow, flacky [sic] and damaged from false nails: I could see an improvement in strength, look and growth within a couple of weeks and after two months they are getting better and better' • 'excellent for nails – but not a cuticle softener – nails stronger, less prone to breaking' • 'my mum says this has made a massive difference, her nails look better than they have done in years'.

Orly Cuticle Oil

 8.12 10

This was tested as a cuticle treatment, not a specific nail strengthener – but again, if applied nightly, we believe it should be good for nail durability. There's a deliciously sweet, slightly citrus scent, thanks to orange blossom.

Comments: 'My dry, slightly brittle nails looked much healthier, did make a difference' • 'great product: very easy to apply, made my really dry, flaky nails and bad cuticles much stronger and healthier, and looked very hydrated' • 'I'm a nurse so wash my hands a lot, then put on lots of hand cream; this helped make my nails stronger so they don't break so much; you only need a drop per nail, so it lasts for ages' • very easy to apply' • 'my dry, scruffy cuticles are softer and in better condition, though nails no different' • 'love, love, love it!'.

dry, cracked heels' • 'nails have a lovely sheen after use – almost like a clear polish' • 'I was surprised: after a few weeks, nails have grown quicker and are healthier – no mean feat in a cold winter' • 'even after two days I noticed a difference between the treated and untreated hand; I'm glad I could compare as I wouldn't have believed how good this is!'.

Argan+ Precious Oil Elixir ❁❁

 8.28 10

Another multi-tasking product formulated with oils – principally Moroccan argan oil with a range of others – known to help all manner of skin, hair and nail problems by delivering intense hydration and nourishment. It's economical as you only need to massage in a few drops nightly.

Comments: "After a few applications nails now in much better condition and much less brittle, it puts real condition into the nails and nail bed' • 'loved the smell and this really helped nails and cuticles - they look moisturised not ugly and ripped: my manicurist says my nails look much better' • 'my cracked, split, dry nails look moisturised and are no

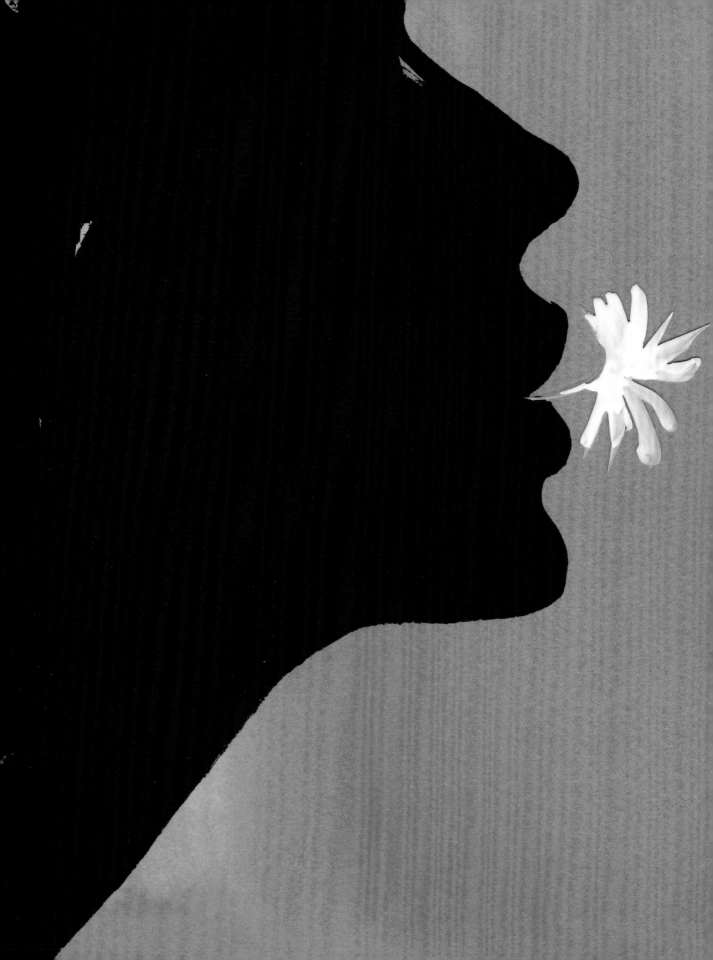

'Never stop
your *passion*.
Just keep going.
Be useful.
Stick up for what
you BELIEVE in.
Get *angry* about
what you
CARE about'

Jane Birkin

Learn a few lip tricks that put a smile on your face

'Feathering' – those first lines that appear around our lips – fills many of us with anxiety. But don't despair – there are ways to help you create a fabulous pout

We speak, we laugh, we eat, we kiss! – so the lip zone gets a lot of action. No wonder, then, that fine lines and wrinkles – starting off with 'feathering' – develop around the lip contour not long after they show up in the eye zone, often causing women we know quite some distress (and beware, it happens earlier – much earlier – if you're a smoker. Skin really doesn't like the free radicals contained in smoke, or that puffing action). Over the next few pages you'll find your 'lip action plan': the treatments, the make-up, the tricks to make your pout fuller,

smoother, sexier – and, in turn, maybe just a little smilier. So your lips won't tell the world your real age…

Brush lips with a toothbrush to remove any flakiness. For perfect lip colour, you need a smooth base. To achieve this, we suggest regularly using an old, soft toothbrush – which you keep for this purpose – dabbed in balm: make gentle circular movements to buff away flakes and really push the balm into the lip skin, because it has no natural moisturisation of its own.

Give lips back their natural, rosy hue. Lips – like so much else – tend to fade as we age, and naturally rosy lips are rare. (Though if yours are really pale, do get your iron levels checked.) So we believe in giving them some help. 'As you get older, slightly brighter lips are important,' advises Trish McEvoy, 'but they shouldn't be opaque or matte. Outline the lips (see lip liner tips below), then fill in with sheer or semi-sheer lipstick.' Mid-rose toned lipsticks are, most make-up artists agree, the most flattering for women of forty-plus – think of the colour that lips naturally are, only a tiny, tiny bit stronger. If you choose a really sheer lipstick, you can go a bit darker – it'll just leave a slick of colour.

Use a nude lip pencil for a crisp, youthful outline. Choose a rose-y nude, not a brown-y nude, which should be as close to the natural colour of your lips as possible – and then, explains Terry de Gunzburg, 'You can draw your lipline at the outer edge of your lips and actually increase the apparent size of both the top and bottom lips.' (You have to make sure the line dovetails perfectly at the corners of your lips, though. Otherwise the ghastly spectre of Ronald McDonald swims into the imagination…) There should, of course, never be a gap between the pencil and your actual lip – but you can use the pencil to 'extend' the contour of the top and bottom lips.

Lip pencil will help prevent 'feathering'. The waxiness helps stop moisturising or lubricating ingredients in a lipstick formulation from travelling into tiny lines around the lip line (and we all have those too…).

Try lip pencil and gloss, or sheer/semi-sheer lippy. No matt lipstick ever. Outline lips, then fill in with pencil; top with gloss or balm (tinted if you like).

Feel free to use your daughter's lip gloss. (Or your goddaughter's.) When it comes to many make-up items, we're recommending that you 'shift' your buying habits towards make-up ranges which specifically target more mature skins. But lip gloss? You can get away with pretty much anything, so long as it's not over-shimmery, or too intense in colour. (Or too sticky if you have longer hair – that awful feeling of strands being glued to your lips.)

Having said that, try adding just a touch of

shimmer to the centre of your bottom lip. This really does help make lips look fuller. Apply the shimmer (or gloss) with your finger, and pat it in. (Terry de Gunzburg's By Terry Or de Rose balm is also perfect for this, as well as for an overnight lip treatment: it has tiny shimmering particles of real gold, which look super-flattering.)

Between 45 and 60, give up the statement red lipstick, says Mary Greenwell. Mary remembers the time when she was walking down Fifth Avenue in Manhattan and saw a pair of red lips on legs coming towards her. Then she realised it was a mirror, and that's the moment she gave up her red lipstick. For now. 'Somehow, on a woman at that stage in her life, a geranium or poppy or pillar box red lipstick is all you see when you look at the face – and it doesn't look sexy. After sixty, you can take it up again – it becomes a glamorous "statement", a bit eccentric and rather divine.'

Also avoid shrieking orange or fuchsia, and very pale lipsticks, advises Barbara Daly, 'although pale gloss is fine'. But, says Barbara, 'bright, rich colour can look very chic at night'; she created silver-mopped fashion designer Betty Jackson's trademark soft, clear crimson especially for her. NB: The word is 'soft'…

TIP

Remember that lips need sun protection just as much as the rest of your face. So either choose a lippy containing SPF15, or apply a separate product (balms with sun protection are great, and widely available) before your lipstick. NB: If you suffer from cold sores, an SPF lip product may help prevent them.

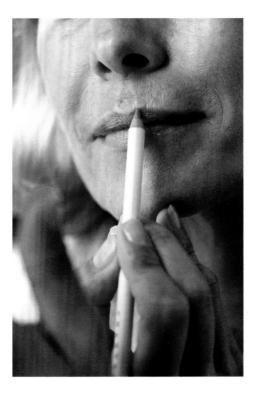

Lip gloss: our award winners

Ah, lip gloss. Gorgeous, glamorous, makes-you-feel-girly-at-any-age lip gloss. What's more, it's possible to use lip gloss not just for a slick of sexy shine, but to create the illusion of a fuller pout. At this stage in life you're almost certainly looking for something that stays put that bit longer than the rest. Look no further, say our panellists

AT A GLANCE

New CID Cosmetics i-gloss

bareMinerals Marvellous Moxie Lipgloss

Lancôme Juicy Tubes Ultra Shiny Hydrating Lip Gloss

Clinique Vitamin C Lip Smoothie

TIP

Applying lip gloss generously all over is fine for 15-year-olds, but there's a more age-appropriate technique for this stage in life. Add a dab to the centre of the bottom lip, swipe it side to side with your finger, and don't rub lips together – smack them like you're saying, 'Ma! Ma!' If you need more, repeat the process. (See our tips for applying lip pencil, page 133, as this gives gloss a base to 'cling' to and prevents gloss and lipstick travelling.)

REVIEWS

New CID Cosmetics i-gloss

 8.9/10
An awfully clever gizmo, this: at the touch of a button it lights up so that you can apply in the dark using a mirrored panel on the side of the wand (very useful for taxis). The colour which our testers received was Moonstone, a sort of holographic, crystalline pink, which is very fetching when lightly applied over a lipstick – but a bit too 'disco' if applied generously on its own.
Comments: 'Easy to apply, very glossy, not sticky, moisturising, colour is just right' • 'blown away by this glam glossy girlie high-tech product, wonderfully moisturising yet sheer; I've bought it for five girlfriends' • 'gorgeous, gorgeous, gorgeous! Loads of comments from girls asking what it was, and men saying how lovely my lips looked' • 'inbuilt light and mirror are fab inventions for lippy lovers!'.

bareMinerals Marvellous Moxie Lipgloss ❋

 8.57/10
With smoothing shea, avocado and murumuru butters, a revitalising 'infusion of minerals' and protective vitamin complex, this new entry certainly makes lips look more luscious immediately and, in an independent study, lip fullness actually increased in four weeks (doesn't say how many times you have to apply it though…). Our testers tried pinky-mauve Rebel, from 14 shades. NB There is an initial tingle factor, which some liked, others not so much.
Comments: 'Love this; more colour than your average lipgloss, glides on really well and not gunky or sticky; lips felt plump and moisturised; angled applicator so you avoid Clown Mouth even in a hurry with no mirror' • 'sexy lips without being in your face!' • 'absolutely loved this product which is very moisturising, made lips look fuller and better and actually improved them over time' • 'lasted well for a gloss, a bit left after a meal'.

Lancôme Juicy Tubes Ultra Shiny Hydrating Lip Gloss

 8.34/10
With their angled tip (for ease of application), Juicy Tubes have become a cult, with limited-edition shades and fragrances. Our testers had Melon 22, a classic sheer rose pink with a melon-y scent. Super-shiny – and often fruit-scented – Juicy Tubes are a love-'em-or-hate'em product; for our testers, it was a Juicy love-in… (Though some did find the stickiness a problem.)
Comments: 'Lovely sheer flattering colour, and it's so moisturising – gave dry, flaky lips immediate relief, also helped plumpness a little' • 'I like how instantly glam it makes me look' • 'impressed by the suitably scrumptious range of shades' • 'lasts well for a lip gloss: I'm never without it'.

Clinique Vitamin C Lip Smoothie

8.17/10
A particular favourite of ours – and another new entry: twist one end and the luscious, non-sticky gloss flows through the brush, conditioning lips with shea and cocoa butters. Although pomegranate and acai berry pack a powerful antioxidant punch, it's not 'fruit-flavoured' or scented. Tons of shades available but testers received Strawberry Bliss.
Comments: 'With one sweep of the brush I was transformed from dowdy housewife to foxy lady!' • 'a dream to apply: a couple of quick slicks and Bob's your uncle!' • 'amazed at my little lips appearing more "pout-y"!' • 'very moisturising: glossy, glam and enjoyable'.

Lip pencils: *our award winners*

A must for the more mature make-up kit. As we've said, lip liner defines the lips (which become more 'blurry' as lines arrive). It helps prevent 'bleeding' by creating a waxy barrier that stops lipstick travelling and gives any lip colour something to 'cling' to, helping it stay put. These were all sent to ten women and had them beaming

REVIEWS

Jane Iredale Lip Pencil ✿

8.06/10 A new winner from one of the first mineral makeup brands founded by make-up artist Jane Iredale in 1994 and now a best-seller worldwide. In 12 shades, this creamy soft-textured crayon proved to have lasting power, on its own and under lippy. Our testers trialled Spice, a suits-everyone nude, and the only extra they would have liked is a sharpener (you can use a simple pencil sharpener).

Comments: 'Great, smooth lip liner and the nude colour is fab, doesn't drag at all and hasn't bled into fine lines; made my lipstick last longer, and I also wore it alone' • 'went on like a dream, very easy to apply precisely, very versatile – best applied with a light hand' • 'lovely to use, very soft, creamy and moisturising, easy to apply; really does give my lips a more defined look and stopped lipstick from bleeding'• 'great lipstick base when applied over mouth, colour stayed even when drinking coffee'.

MAC Lip Pencil

8/10 The shade Spice, which was sent to our testers, is an absolute legend in the make-up world, probably the best-known lip liner of all time, as used by supermodels, super-make-up-artists, you name it… A perfect brown-y/pink lip colour, with vitamin E to condition lips, it glides on smoothly and stays put, too.

Comments: 'Soft creamy pencil which lined and filled in lips very easily, I loved using it all over lips with lip gloss, lasts for ages and makes the gloss last twice as long as normal' • 'smooth and easy to apply, looked good, and made other lip products

last longer so saving me money – always a bonus!' • 'delighted with this pencil and how natural it looked – excellent as liner and base colour'.

Korres Lipliner Pencil ✿

7.89/10 These more-natural-than-many lip pencils, a new entry from a popular Greek brand, are made from cedar wood (for true colour), and formulated with softening, nourishing jojoba and macadamia nut oils and vitamin E. In five shades, we tried Neutral Light, the most popular.

Comments: 'I was frightened of looking very '90s but this was soft, smooth and went on very easily; did need balm if applied all over lips – I would buy this product' • 'when I outlined lips then filled them in and put similar shade lipstick on top, it lasted six hours and through four cups of tea – very impressive' • 'no "bleeding" at all but the pencil did need sharpening often' • 'very realistic outline as the shade was a great match for natural lip colour'.

Sisley Phyto-Lèvres Perfect

7.66/10 From the luxury end of the make-up spectrum comes Sisley's winner: a deep rose/nude pencil (Rose Thé) enriched with kokum butter, aloe vera and jojoba oil for softness and hydration, plus beeswax for a long-wear finish. There's a brush at one end for softening the line you've smoothly created.

Comments: 'Simply the best lip liner I've ever tried; slightly creamy and goes on smoothly and precisely for a realistic outline; I used it as a lip liner, base and lipstick; the lip brush applicator at the other end was an excellent tool for blending' • 'nice smooth-textured soft pencil that went on easily and didn't smudge, the outline was not too hard so you don't look like an old woman!'.

AT A GLANCE

Jane Iredale Lip Pencil

MAC Lip Pencil

Korres Lipliner Pencil

Sisley Phyto-Lèvres Perfect

♡ WE LOVE…

Jo has a wide selection (Chanel, Benefit) and is fairly unfussy about the brand, so long as the shade is right – a truly nude tone, since she's almost as afraid of VLL (Visible Lip Line) as VPL (Visible Panty Line) from a too-dark liner. Sarah now uses Green People Instant Definition Lip Crayon in Praline, an earthy rose brown, which does double duty as liner and colour.

TIP

Do condition lips before applying lip liner: even the creamiest can be a bit drying on dry lips! Apply balm and leave to sink in for a few moments before putting on lip product. (Actually do keep lips conditioned anyway, lip liner or not; see page 137 for lip treatments.)

Lip-plumpers: our award winners

Nothing in a wand is going to give the plumping effect of something that comes in a cosmeto-dermatologist's syringe – but for millions of us who are happy to help nature along purely with cosmetics, a lip-plumper can be a useful addition to the beauty arsenal

AT A GLANCE

MAC Plushglass

L'Oréal Paris Glam Shine

♡WE LOVE...

The one that really works for Jo (so much that the tingle's almost painful!) is Valerie Beverly Hills Bee Sting Lip Plump, in a chic little silver mirrored compact which she can now (annoyingly) only pick up in the States. It's a cosmetic effect, rather than a long-term treatment – but definitely does make lips a touch more Bardot. She's also a fan of the wondrously-named Soap & Glory Sexy Mother Pucker Lip Plumping Gloss. Sarah almost never remembers to do it, but the Valerie lip-plumper certainly works – and it's fun!

True 'lip-plumpers' offer ingredients which actually increase the volume of the lips temporarily (such as capsicum, which works by bringing blood to the lips accounting for the tingle in the million or so nerve endings in the lips) – or for longer-term plumping contain ingredients to encourage the production of cushioning natural collagen in the lip area. Sad to report, this proved probably the most disappointing category in the book – and nothing we trialled for the new paperback edition knocked our socks off either (though there is one new entry, from L'Oréal Paris). Of more than 30 products we've now dispatched to our testers, just a couple proved worthy of inclusion – and reading testers' comments this was more to do with an instant optical illusion than any longer-term change. But do also see We Love…, left, and Lip Glosses on page 134: the message is that you can achieve a bee-stung look, albeit temporary (and rather a small bee…but better than a large trout we think).

REVIEWS

MAC Plushglass

7.66/10 A sheer lip colour with a high-shine finish, MAC describe this as delivering 'a cool-warm vanilla buzz to the lips'. It features vitamin E and lip-conditioning ingredients, and is available in 13 shades (our testers received Ample Pink, a soft neutral). As we said above, although this was popular and gained a few high marks, the effect was transient. Testers differed widely on what they felt about the tingling!
Comments: 'Very effective for instant illusion of fullness – gave my lips a plump shimmery, sexy look – and stays on for ever' • 'instant tingle but not unpleasant, I re-applied every two hours and felt my lips were genuinely fuller and looked plumper within minutes of applying' • 'pale pink shade was very natural and youthful, subtle and beautiful; I re-applied every two hours' • 'the tingling made me think it was plumping out my lips and I think it did make them look a little fuller, but I wasn't keen on the "thick" feeling of the product' • 'created a genuinely puffy lips look but I found the "stinging" sensation uncomfortable' • 'pleasant sensation and I think the gloss made my lips look and feel slightly fuller and more youthful: a make-up bag staple'.

L'Oréal Paris Glam Shine

7.6/10 This is also definitely a 'mere' lip gloss rather than the type of product which works by stimulating the nerve endings to 'pump up' the lip tissue – but it, too, out-performed designated lip-plumpers, in terms of results. Glam Shine is an enduring 'classic' within the extremely affordable L'Oréal Paris make-up range, with what they tell us is a high proportion of light-reflective, ultra-glossy oils – plus 'Crystal Shine' particles, to catch the light in all directions. Glam Shine comes in a really big portfolio of shades, finishes and textures: our lot had 400 Juicy Rose Glow (the sort of rosy neutral we always request from participating brands, as it matches almost everyone's colouring).
Comments: 'This is a comfortable gloss to wear which definitely made lips look shiny and full – although the results, as with most lip glosses, are pretty fleeting' • 'deliciously moisturising – feels like a balm, looks like a volumising gloss' • 'overall, I've enjoyed using this' • 'not exactly Brigitte Bardot or Angelina Jolie, but definitely my normally thin lips (which have further deflated with ageing) look a bit fuller' • 'comfy texture compared to most other lip glosses – not too sticky'.

Lip treatments: our award winners

For lips and the surrounding skin, a treatment product can be a boon. The winners here are mainly uber-lip balms, which condition lips (and some plump them out). Use them on your lips for daytime hydration and at night on your lips and lip zone to target feathering

Among the many, many lip treatment options out there, these earned the biggest smiles from our panellists (we've now trialled over 30 entries, in this growing category)…

REVIEWS

Avène Cold Cream Lip Cream

 From a well-known French pharmacy range, this new entry was an emphatic winner with our testers, who particularly liked the tube with little applicator nozzle. Formulated for 'severe dryness', ingredients include castor seed oil, also mineral oil, and sucralfate, used medically in wound healing.
Comments: '10/10. Very moisturising, left lips feeling soft and smooth; marked improvement in condition and the occasional cracks in the corner of my mouth, which medicated balms have not helped' • 'after three months, fine lines less visible, lip line more defined – a very effective product indeed' • 'really like this product, simple, effective and cheap' • 'has got ride of dry flaky patches on lips and definitely softened them'.

Clarins Moisture Replenishing Lip Balm

 Ingredients in this little tube of lip magic from the Clarins HydraQuench collection include essential rose wax, ceramide 3 (a super-moisturiser), shea butter and rice oil. It's not specifically designed to be 'anti-ageing', but Clarins submitted it for this category and the responses from our testers show it rose to the challenge.
Comments: 'Felt good and really delivered on performance: lips are smoother, softer and look more fulsome' • 'quite sticky to start with but soon absorbed and lips look healthier, plumper and more youthful' • 'healed my son's trumpet-playing sore chapped lips in 24 hours'.

Clarins Extra-Firming Lip & Contour Balm

 Unlike the Clarins product above, this comes in a glass jar that's more bathroom- than handbag-friendly. Silky-soft and lightweight, the balm features Clarins's lip-plumping Maxi Lip Complex, to help boost production of collagen and plump and smooth fine lines, plus vitamin E. The fragrance is attractive, with star anise, cardamom, cinnamon and vanilla.
Comments: 'Lip-plumping, moisturising and really hydrating – fab, fab, fab!' • 'my lips look plumper and healthier and there is a slight reduction in feathering around them' • 'a soothing balm with a velvety texture which improved the condition of my lips 100 per cent; lips moister and more kissable!'.

Dermalogica AGE Smart Renewal Lip Complex

And, golly, it is complex – (and quite costly…), boasting a patented polypeptide to condition skin and stimulate collagen formation and minimise fine lines, and prevent signs of aging caused by Advanced Glycation End products…plus more usual emollients including synthetic beeswax. Testers remarked on the teeny grains that exfoliated efficiently.
Comments: 'I liked using this product and the results: grainy effect helped smooth dry patches, would definitely use this regularly at night' • 'lips often very dry and flaky – felt hydrated and comfortable on application and since using this treatment dryness has completely gone; dramatic improvement' • 'very impressed; I used it on very dry cracked lips and it moisturised instantly and restored lips to normal quickly'.

AT A GLANCE

Avène Cold Cream Lip Cream

Clarins Moisture Replenishing Lip Balm

Clarins Extra-Firming Lip & Contour Balm

Dermalogica AGE Smart Renewal Lip Complex

 WE LOVE…

Ritualised several-times-daily use of a balm (our very own Beauty Bible Lip Balm, a real steal and all-natural too) goes a long way towards keeping our lips soft and supple, and Jo also applies Liz Earle Naturally Active Superskin Lip & Eye Treatment around the lip area, which she feels helps with any incipient 'feathering'. Sarah adores lip balms but isn't yet evolved enough to use another treatment – but she does smear her night facial oil over her lips, so perhaps that counts!

*L*Moisturising lipsticks: *our award winners*

Don't know about you, but we like our lipsticks dewy, comforting and lip-replenishing. (Since they lack oil glands, lips are prone to dryness.) However, at this stage in life a moisturising lipstick offers more than a mere feel-good factor: its softly sheeny appearance is infinitely more flattering than any matt lip look

Which to choose? You'd do well to start with these top-scorers, from well over four dozen we've now sent out to testers. (NB: The one downside of moisturising lipsticks is they often need more frequent slicking, as the richer and creamier a formulation, the faster it slides off lips. But we think it's worth it, for sheer comfort and flatter-factor.)

REVIEWS

Clinique Chubby Stick

 We did slightly punch the air when this big fat lip-slicking pencil triumphed here, because at Beauty Bible Towers we each own an indecently large number of shades. We personally love the fact they're completely goof-proof: so sheer in texture you can literally apply in the dark, as well as the lip-quenching texture – like a balm, really. Now available in an equally chubby number of shades (our testers received Mega Melon, a warm neutral).

Comments: 'This was really easy to use and very moisturising: my lips didn't dry out at all during cold weather' • 'had a cold when I first tried this and lips were cracked, but this has made them feel soft and they look better than with my normal lipsticks' • 'loved the giant crayon design' • 'very easy to use, natural finish and no "clogging" feeling you get with some lipsticks' • 'a great invention for when you want a pop of colour – I love the fact it's so moisturising and I sometimes wear it when I don't have any other "face" on; this product is always going to be on my wishlist now'.

Guerlain Rouge G Exceptional Complete Lip Colour

 At the really 'luxe' end of the lipstick spectrum: a hefty silver bullet which you slide the lipstick out of, so it flips open to reveal a double mirror. (Very Hollywood glam, this.) It offers lip-plumping vitamin A palmitate, hydrating wild mango butter, hyaluronic acid and wrinkle-filling Ayurvedic guggul resin. Of the 25 shades, we trialled 04 Gentiane, a subtly shimmering tea rose.

Comments: 'Left lips feeling soft; didn't dry them out as some lipsticks do' • 'smooth, rich and moisturising' • 'fantastically comfortable – really moisturising and stays on your lips giving the feeling it's continually delivering hydration – the nicest-feeling lipstick I've ever used' • 'using it made me feel I should have been on a movie set in the 1920s – wonderful, feminine packaging' • 'gorgeous!'.

Elizabeth Arden Ceramide Ultra Lipstick

This glam, gold-packaged lipstick really scores for the lip-quench factor, which is down to Tahitian Gardenia Extract, shea butter, the ceramides that Arden is famed for (a Ceramide Triple Complex here), plus antioxidant vitamins A, C and E. It also promises a 'lip-plumping' effect, thanks to a peptide complex called Volulip. You'll love the range of shades too – more than 15 to choose from (testers were sent a selection).

Comments: 'Lovely smooth velvet texture, I usually need lots of balm but my lips didn't feel dry while testing this product; the colours are great' • 'glossy, very moisturising, easy to apply – needs a lip liner if you want it to last' • 'a really luxurious product, made my lips look good and rather full, as well as

AT A GLANCE

Clinique Chubby Stick

Guerlain Rouge G Exceptional Complete Lip Colour

Elizabeth Arden Ceramide Ultra Lipstick

Clinique Colour Surge Butter Shine Lipstick

The scores referenced: 8.87/10, 8.83/10, 8.57/10

♡ WE LOVE...

The ranges Jo likes best offer a wide shade choice of lush-textured lipsticks: Clinique Colour Surge Butter Shine Lipstick (favourite shade Berry Blush, a terrific neutral), DHC Moisture Care Lipstick (an affordable brand which hails from Japan), and the wondrous winning entry here, Clinique Chubby Sticks – which Sarah's also addicted to – in a rainbow of pinks and reds. For daytime, lazy Sarah usually wears Lipstick Queen Medieval, a perfect rosy sheer (like 14th century saints, apparently...) or Chubby Stick as above. Lipstick Queen Poppy King's Saint Pinky Nude is wonderfully creamy and lip-loving.

feeling good' • 'the first real lipstick that has ever felt comfortable on my lips; gave a nice sheen and was very long-lasting' • 'really like this, feels lovely and would double as a lip salve'.

Clinique Colour Surge Butter Shine Lipstick

One of Jo's faves, this: really lip-quenchingly comfortable, with a beautiful glossy finish that lasts longer than most lipsticks, she finds. Its secret: special butters, moisturisers and modern waxes that melt at body temperature for a silky texture, plus high-shine 'gellants'. (A new word in beautyspeak!) Fifteen flattering shades (testers received 426 Perfect Plum, a soft mauve-y nude).

Comments: 'Really liked the glossy sheen; moisturising like a balm but with reasonable coverage and no lip gloss stickiness! Really pretty packaging. Not particularly long-lasting though' • 'very moisturising and creamy with a nice sheen' • 'smooth, velvety texture is absolutely lovely on lips, didn't leave my lips dry at all' • 'tube is gorgeous to whip out at a party and colour goes with almost everything in my wardrobe: *love* it'.

FINDING YOUR PERFECT LIP SHADE...

On younger women, paler-than-real-lip colours can look fantastic – but not now! And too dark shades can make an older mouth look harsh. Soft pinks, subtle corals and rosy-browns are the safest bet, subtly putting back the colour that disappears with age (because pigment decreases). Avoid opaque lipsticks: as you get older, solid colours can make the mouth look mean, while the drier matt formulas make lips look tiny and show every line. (That's why we've chosen specifically moisturising lipsticks here.)

Love your life

You can't freeze-frame life. It changes all the time, sometimes slowly, sometimes with chaotic speed. But what you can do is to adopt strategies to help you cope with the rollercoaster. How does that fit in with anti-ageing? A calm mind and taking joy in life make you look beautiful and live well. So laugh as much as you breathe and love as long as you live

Here are some of our favourite strategies, many of which are now used in healthcare.

Be loving to yourself. Sometimes loving and valuing yourself are very hard. That's when we're likely to cause ourselves grief, rely on others for our self-esteem, and make decisions – big and small – based on other people rather than what we really want for ourselves. You could start by just saying to yourself that you are a good person, not perfect – no one is (and please do give yourself permission to get things wrong, make a muddle, be imperfect in everything) – but you try your best. If you believe in spirituality, try thinking of yourself as 'a spark of the divine'. And above all, when you're faced with a decision, ask yourself what you really want to do. (And, of course, extend this loving way of thinking to everyone else too.)

The day starts better after a good night's sleep. We find we sleep soundly when we're glad and grateful. So when you go to bed, write down – or just list in your mind – at least three nice things that have happened. They can be as simple as hearing the birds sing, seeing the sun, or a phone call from a friend. Or praise at work. Or a great cup of coffee. A funny TV show… Then send blessings to the people you love. (And the world in general.)

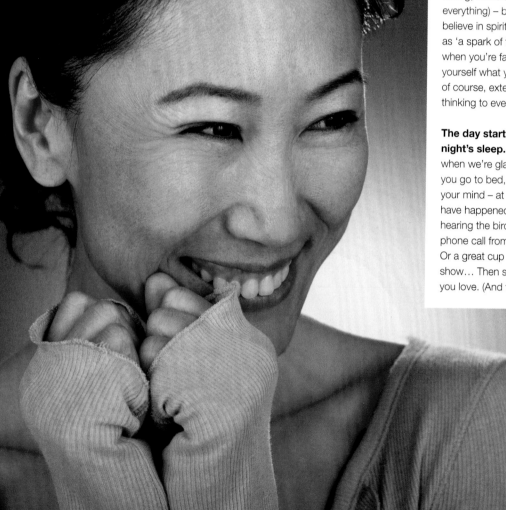

TIPS

Make things fun: wear a tiara when you're hoovering (try accessories or toy stores for gorgeous bargains); brighten tedious chores with your favourite music; trade help with a friend. Reward yourself with flowers, a movie, a good cup of coffee or tea with a friend.

Keep a Happy Box: collect mementoes of joyful times – letters and cards, emails these days! – inspiring photos, tickets from planes, boats, trains and concerts – and leaf through them when you're having a doleful day.

Don't make decisions in the middle of the night. Around 4am (when women tend to wake if there's something on your mind) is the dark hour of the soul, according to psychiatrist Dr David Servan-Schreiber, the late author of *Healing Without Freud or Prozac*. 'There's a fragile moment at the end of the first long period of deep sleep (about four hours into the sleep cycle) when we cross over into the lighter REM sleep [dreaming time]. Underlying anxiety – especially separation anxiety where we feel a threat to important relationships or a lack of fulfilling ones – manifests then.' Your brain can't process things then, he says, so please don't try: do the breathing exercise right, and if you don't fall asleep read a novel, do the ironing, listen to the radio or even watch a dotty DVD on your laptop.

When you wake up, decide that just for today your intention is that you will
be as happy as you can be. Whatever happens. This doesn't mean you won't notice difficulties – of course you will. It does mean you will try to live in the solution, not the problem.

Breathe. Inhale for a count of four, hold for seven, then exhale very slowly to a count of eight. Repeat four to six times, feeling your breath go in and out of your body. If you like, imagine your breath is like a wave coming up a beach, hovering at the top, then ebbing slowly out to sea. Do this whenever you can during the day, but morning and bedtime at least.

Think of someone you love and stretch out your arms to them – literally. (If they're there to hug in person, so much the better.) You will find you're smiling and your heart is warm. Carry that feeling through the day.

Stretch some more. Do some yoga poses if you know them (for more on yoga, see page 204). Or just stretch your arms and legs out, shake your feet and hands – feel the fizz of energy.

Make yourself look as gorgeous as you can. Especially if it's a grey day – weather- or mood-wise. Wear colours, put on make-up, brush your hair.

If you have a wobbly moment of any kind, do the breathing exercise again. Bring your attention to the centre of your chest and widen it – don't cave in. Feel your shoulder blades sinking back, down
and together. Then try saying 'yesss!', even 'thank you', and looking forward and up to a hill, a spire, the sky. (To understand why we suggest this, contrast it with looking down and saying 'no'.)

Never lose hope. If it seems to be slipping away, phone a friend but choose one who will support and encourage you – avoid the Eeyores.

Smile. Research has shown it sends feel-good hormones called endorphins rushing through your mind and body. You feel better. So does everyone else. Smiles make friends.

Examine the wobbliness. If you've done something wrong, put it right. Most likely you haven't and it's an old tape replaying in your head and body. Have a few drops of Bach's Rescue Remedy and count up the good healthy positive things in any situation. If the wobbliness persists, repeat again. If it is really troubling you, consider talking therapy of some kind and/or homeopathy.

Reach out to other people. Be nice – it's so much easier. Pay compliments. Listen, really listen.

Notice good things. Even tiny ones: store them up to remember at night and when things are difficult.

Never give up on passion. (We heard novelist Edna O'Brien say that, and she's now in her late seventies.) Yes, we do mean the physical sort of passion! And being passionately interested in people and things of all sorts. Be passionately creative too: paint, sing, play an instrument, garden, take photos – whatever you enjoy, do it!

Cultivate peace. We can't really tell you how – try seeing what makes you feel peaceful and doing more of it. Or it may be a case of 'being' rather than 'doing'.

Make yourself look as *GORGEOUS* as you can. *Wear colours*, put on **make-up,** brush your hair

Hang on to your marbles

Fewer lines and a trim waistline are all fine and dandy – but in the bigger scheme of things, nobody would question that keeping your brain sparky and your memory sharp(-ish) is going to do more for your quality of later life than pretty well anything else in this book

'Not fade away' is a BIG theme of *The Anti-Ageing Beauty Bible* – and it applies just as much to our brains, as well as to hair, complexion, eyebrows and so on.

Memory loss is probably the biggest brain-related anxiety we experience, once we hit a certain age. We're not talking about full-blown dementia, such as Alzheimer's disease – though that prospect can be seriously angst-inducing, especially if there's a family history – but about the Craft (Can't Remember a Flipping Thing) moments that strike everyone, usually kicking in around perimenopause. Naturopathic physician Dr Mosaraf Ali explains, 'Anxiety, depression, physical fatigue and anything which causes less blood flow to the brain weakens the ability to store or recall memories.' So: when you bump into someone unbelievably familiar but you can't remember their name (or how you know them), stress or exhaustion are the most likely explanations.

The good news is that, as experts agree, there are many, many lifestyle steps that we can all take to improve our memories.

Eat oily fish. It's rich in omega-3 essential fatty acids (EFAs), which researchers worldwide agree are vital for brain function; they have been shown to help depression and general mental acuity, as well as helping age-related memory loss and just possibly helping to prevent dementia (research is ongoing). These brain-friendly lipids can't be manufactured by the body, and must come from our diet. And the richest source of omega-3 EFAs is oily fish. So if you're vegetarian, like Jo, take them in the form of supplements (see page 180 for our suggestions). Everyone should also consume lots of dark green vegetables such as spinach, watercress, dried seaweed and spirulina (all of which also contain B group vitamins – see box opposite), walnuts, flax and hemp seeds and their oils, try these over vegetables and we like them stirred into baked beans... Phosphorus may also help the brain, and is needed for the body to absorb those vital B vitamins; it's found in oily fish and also in nuts (including walnuts, Brazil, cashew, peanuts, pecans and pine nuts), eggs, lentils, soya, wholegrains and – yay! – chocolate (the darker the better). You can self-test to see whether you are deficient in omega-3 EFAs with a simple at-home blood test (see DIRECTORY).

Do sudoku or quizzes or crosswords. And/or play a lot of Scrabble. All of these help with memory. The general principle is that exercising your brain with any different routines and new tasks is effective. Learning to play the piano (it's never too late), a new language, even finding your way around a new city – any new skill – gives the memory area of your brain a vital workout.

Train your brain with an App. Every day at 8am, Jo's iPhone reminds her: 'It's time for your brain training.' She spends five minutes doing online games (matching shapes, colours, etc) which improve attention and memory, and speed up thinking time. The App is Brain Trainer by Lumosity (www.lumosity.com) and is available via iTunes. Graphs help you chart your progress – and the alarm is a reminder to do the brain exercises. (Although as your memory improves, the hope is you won't need a prompt.)

Eat ten almonds a day. They contain an incredible array of nutrients and are the richest source of vegetable protein. Soak them in room-temperature water for 24 hours, peel off the skins, crush and eat with a teaspoonful of Manuka honey, to benefit from micro-nutrients essential for brain function. Or add to muesli.

Support your memory with supplements. Ayurvedic practitioner Sebastian Pole prescribes Brahmi Plus, which combines organic herbs including gotu kola and bacopa monnieri, which increase memory and enhance concentration; it also lowers anxiety, clears your mind and revitalises your intellect. (We're sold on it.) We're also considering taking phosphatidylserine (PS), a phospholipid which has been shown to improve memory and mental acuity, due to multiple functions which basically help your brain cells talk to each other. (We're told Memory Lane by Power Health is a good formulation.)

Massage your head, neck and shoulders. This not only helps quell anxiety, but boosts blood flow to the brain. We are particularly keen on scalp massage as stress shortens the muscles in the scalp, making the scalp all but immobile in very frazzled people. Firm pressure with the pads of the fingers is pretty darned miraculous – or better still, book in for an Indian

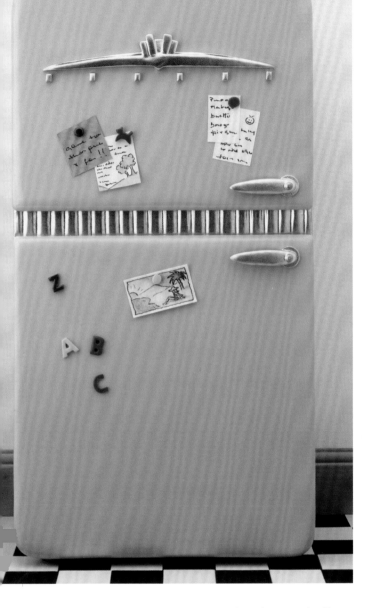

BE ON THE BALL WITH B VITAMINS

Over the past decade, research has increasingly shown that taking high doses of three B vitamins (B6, B12 and folic acid) can help age-related memory loss. These B vitamins help keep homocysteine (an amino acid) at a healthy level. Raised homocysteine may increase the risk of Alzheimer's and heart disease. Taking the vitamins probably won't help if you don't have a mild degree of memory loss but won't harm you and may help other things, eg, stress. If your brain is as sharp as a needle, we think it makes all-round good sense to eat plenty of foods containing these Bs. Find vitamin B12 in meat and fish, with folic acid and B6 in asparagus, lentils, most beans and leafy green vegetables (see our Supergreens Facelift Diet, page 176 – and combine the benefits for face and mind!). For specific supplements of the vitamins, see page 180.

yoga – nature's greatest anti-ageing wonder, in our opinion – see page 204.)

Avoid alcohol, coffee and cola-style drinks. Alcohol in particular is linked with poor memory (and not just in a where-the-hell-did-I-leave-my-keys-after-that-second-bottle-of-champagne way); if you are experiencing regular Craft moments, try cutting down or cutting out alcohol and seeing if that makes a difference, because it does affect the way brain cells communicate. (We're not suggesting that anyone becomes a nun. A special occasion is a special occasion, but for many people a few glasses of wine a day is a habit that's surprisingly easy to give up, once you've made the link with positive improvements.) Caffeine can exacerbate stress – and there's some evidence that, over time, the gradual increase of stress hormone (cortisol) levels in the blood can prevent the brain laying down a new memory, or from accessing existing ones.

Get plenty of sleep. We all know that when we're sleep-deprived, we can hardly remember our own names, let alone phone numbers and the fact we have to pick up our dry-cleaning. Sleep is the brain's way of processing events into memories. For more wisdom on better sleep, see page 208.

And if all else fails, write it down. Whoever said you were meant to remember everything: birthdays, anniversaries, shopping lists, To Do lists, not to mention matching every name in your bulging address book to a face…? Be kind to yourself: the pressure we put our brains under is unprecedented in the history of humanity. Try not to stress out when your memory fails you, or feel it's the start of a slippery slope – it only makes things worse. It happens to us all. Stop, take a deep breath and let your mind rest for a moment. And remember (little joke!) that's what pens, paper, diaries, iPhones and online reminder services were meant for.

Head Massage, which many massage therapists are trained in. Use Google to find someone near you.

Don't multi-task. OK, so for most women this is like telling you to stop breathing. (Men, of course, are another matter…) But studies have shown that memory-related tasks can suffer in the hands of multi-taskers. At the very least, focus on doing – and finishing – one thing at a time. Practise mindfulness (more on page 144). You can sit still to do a waking mindfulness meditation – heck, you can even practise it while washing up. It's all about bringing your consciousness gently back to what you're doing. Whether that's walking, daydreaming – or doing the dishes.

Practise Iyengar yoga. The Cobra pose, which enhances circulation, may be of particular help to your brain. (For more on

Be mindful of life's pleasures

Forget diets. It's time to enjoy your food, eat just the right amount through 'mindful eating' (and lose that middle-age spread effortlessly)

As the years go by, it's ridiculously easy for the pounds to roll on. For most women after the menopause, the evidence is probably lurking around your waistline (we tend to gather fat around our middles due to a shift in the ratio of oestrogen to testosterone). Clothes are tighter. Maybe there's a muffin-top that didn't used to be there. And suddenly, you get as excited over a new pair of Spanx control pants as you once did over frilly, skimpy smalls.

Traditionally, women have turned to extreme diets to combat excess pounds. Trouble is that diets tend not to work long term because they're hard to stick to (and some you shouldn't stick to 'cos they are just plain dangerous).

But there is new thinking that part of the reason we gain weight is that in our busy, stressful world, we're simply not paying attention to what we eat. Think on this. What did you last eat? What did it taste like? Smell of? Did you really enjoy it? Chances are you just don't remember… We're so used to filling our tummies with food like we fill our cars with fuel that we mostly do it on autopilot. Mindlessly. While we do six other things. (Multi-tasking can be a disadvantage sometimes.) The result is that, often, we eat far more than we need because we just don't notice what we're doing. And we pile on the pounds. Because we've eaten too much. Simple!

But it's also quite simple and fun to practise 'mindful eating' – as well as eating well, of course (it won't work if you eat mindfully mashed potato, pasta, cakes and puds for every meal). The bottom line is: it's all about loving your food! 'Mindful eating' is a new (well, old but rediscovered) approach, which is proving very helpful for people who want to lose weight on a permanent basis, not the see-saw of weight loss and gain that's so familiar from so many diets.

So: let's start again…

Go and make yourself something you really enjoy. Needn't be complicated but take enough time to make certain it tastes and looks delicious. Find your favourite place to eat, sitting at a table. Or treat yourself to a coffee or tea and lemon tart at your favourite patisserie.

Now…start by taking a few slow breaths to relax. Look at the food. Notice the colours, texture, smell. Then take the first mouthful. Don't do anything else at all. Just look and taste and smell. Swallow slowly, chewing thoroughly if necessary. Go on to the second mouthful and do the same. Finish your food in the same way, deliberately paying attention to it. That's what mindfulness is – being fully aware of what's happening. With food, it's the sensations and thoughts that occur as we eat. The colours, aromas, textures, flavours, even sounds of the food. And drink – think of the sensation as you taste the chocolate powder on a cappuccino, encounter the cool milky foam, the contrast with the hot, intensely-flavoured coffee.

If your mind wanders, just bring it gently back to what you're consuming. Sometimes it's helpful to say it to yourself, aloud or in your head: 'Now I'm biting into a peach, through the furry skin into the flesh, feeling the juice run down my chin…'

If you like to read or watch TV when you're eating on your own, try to do one thing at a time. So stop reading while you take a mouthful, taste, chew, swallow. Then pick up your book. You will focus on both more completely. (Ideally, ditch the book and switch off the TV.)

If you're eating with friends, it's still possible to be mindful. The key is to do it slowly – and lovingly. So often when you eat out, the food which your host/ess (or the restaurant chef) has cooked and cosseted like a baby is dispatched without anyone really appreciating it. Thinking and talking about each part of the meal is a compliment. So it's win-win!

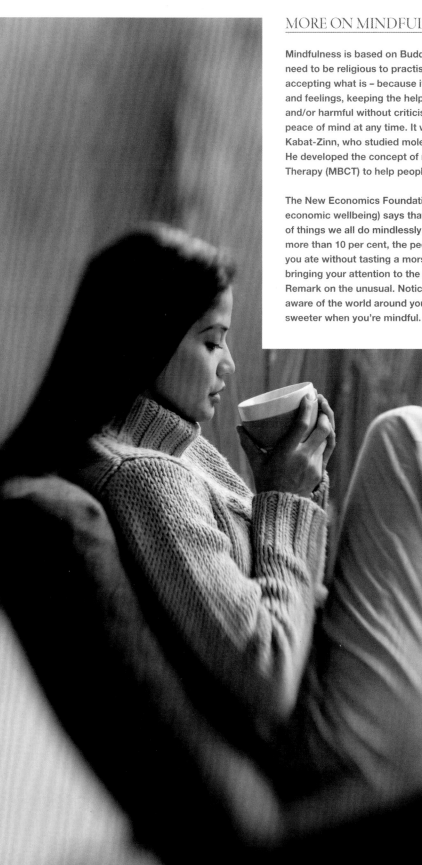

MORE ON MINDFULNESS

Mindfulness is based on Buddhist philosophy; it's not a religion and you don't need to be religious to practise it. It's the art of staying in the moment and accepting what is – because it is already here. It's a way of slowing thoughts and feelings, keeping the helpful ones, gently discarding any that are foolish and/or harmful without criticising yourself in any way. So that you can access peace of mind at any time. It was developed in the West by Professor Jon Kabat-Zinn, who studied molecular biology and also yoga and Buddhist studies. He developed the concept of mindfulness, and Mindfulness-Based Cognitive Therapy (MBCT) to help people cope with stress, anxiety, pain and illness.

The New Economics Foundation (an independent British think-tank focused on economic wellbeing) says that being mindful is 'noticing'. Look at the number of things we all do mindlessly every day: the article you read without retaining more than 10 per cent, the people you talk to without listening…and the meal you ate without tasting a morsel. You can shift that, suggests the NEF, by bringing your attention to the present: 'Be curious. Catch sight of the beautiful. Remark on the unusual. Notice the changing seasons. Savour the moment. Be aware of the world around you and what you're feeling.' We promise: life tastes sweeter when you're mindful.

Minimise those bad (facial) hair days

Stop yourself turning into a moustachioe-d lady – here's the lowdown on hair removal

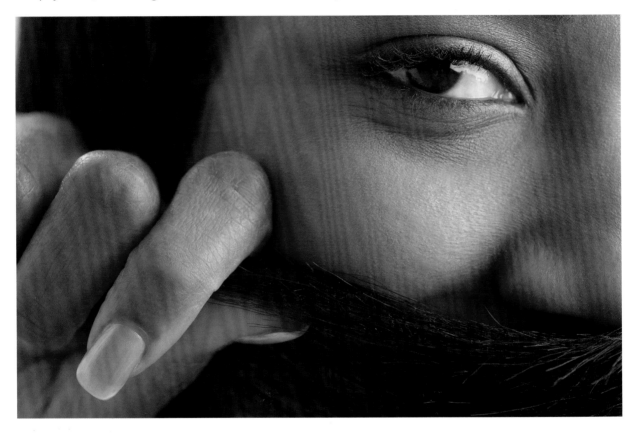

One of the most common questions we're asked is how to get rid of moustaches and, to a lesser extent, other areas of facial hair. We recommend having an appointed 'facial hair buddy' who will tell you when you're sprouting, and you can reciprocate. Mole hairs, in particular, make a break for it after menopause and, as eyesight fades, they can be easily missed.

Now conversely, one of the great blessings of ageing is that elsewhere on the body hair becomes finer and may even disappear altogether (hoorah!). But if you're still fighting excess hair anywhere on the face/body, here's a useful rundown of all the removal techniques you need to know about.

One warning with moustaches: depending on the density of down on the rest of your face (we all have it so don't have conniptions!), completely removing your moustache may leave an obvious hairless patch. In this case, electrolysis is a good option

as the therapist can just take out the coarser, more visible hairs. Alternatively, you could have the whole of your face threaded (but that's quite high-maintenance, so be warned).

Never shave your face. We differ about shaving for legs: Jo does, Sarah doesn't. (If you do, make sure to use a razor dedicated for just this purpose – Jo favours the Gillette Venus range.) But shaving a moustache leads to stubble, and you eventually end up having to do it every day, and fretting over someone feeling a bristly upper lip when they kiss you.

First try bleaching – not so much removal as a disguise. Many of us grew up with crème bleach, and for fine, sparse moustache hairs, it's still an option. However, some testers report that it can sting so much, particularly on your face, that you end up red-skinned, with varying shades of ginger facial hair because you've had to wash it off too soon. Bleach comes in different versions for face and body: get the right one! And please read and follow the instructions to the letter: do a patch test first, every time, don't use with Retin-A, or fruit acids of any kind, and only use on the areas it's listed as safe for.

Experiment with tweezing. Simple, cheap and great for eyebrows, but not recommended for more than the odd stray hair on the rest of your face as it may irritate hair follicles, causing sensitivity and even scarring.

Melt hair clean away with a depilatory cream. These relatively cheap products dissolve hair at the base of the follicle and are useful for legs and underarms (though you'll need to do it often), less so for the face as even dedicated facial versions may irritate sensitive skin, and may not remove all the hairs.

Find a good salon, and try waxing. With waxing, warm/hot wax is applied to skin, then ripped off with a muslin strip bringing the hairs with it. It's usually effective for upper lip and fine hair on the sides of your face, but not suitable for coarser hair on the chin. Never let the therapist use a metal knife for this: it may burn your skin – they should only ever use a wooden implement, and we like salons best which provide a hygienic pack in which every single spatula is used once only, rather than repeatedly dipped.

Get sweet on sugaring. Sugaring uses the same procedure as waxing except that the sugar tends to stick only to the hairs not the skin – so it can be more comfortable. It does need a skilled practitioner to be effective.

Or try threading. (We love threading.) This is an ancient method of hair removal practised in Asian countries. A pure, thin twisted cotton thread is rolled rapidly over untidy areas. As well as shaping brows, skilled practitioners can remove hair anywhere on the face, all over if desired. It's not painful in our experience, but not comfy (it 'pings'). Again it's temporary and needs upkeep.

For permanent hair removal, look at electrolysis. A fine needle conducting an electric current is inserted into the hair follicle, destroying it. You may need several sessions with some maintenance later, but it's an ideal option for a small number of coarse facial hairs, although it is impractical for larger areas, according to consultant dermatologist Dr Nick Lowe of the Cranley Clinic, London.

Laser hair removal is another option. Here, the hair follicle is effectively cauterised with a laser. It's a perfect choice for upper lip hair, says Dr Lowe. Advances in technology mean that any hair with pigment in it can be lasered. (Which usually precludes

treatment of white or grey hair.) There used to be a problem treating coloured skin but new lasers protect tanned, Asian or black skin from losing pigment. These newer modified lasers incorporate cooling technology, says Dr Lowe, who uses the Alexandrite 755 nanometre laser, which cools the skin with a high-flow jet of cold air.

Be aware: laser hair removal won't give you results overnight. (And it's expensive.) It will take between three and six sessions to get the optimum reduction of hair growth, depending on the thickness. And please note: reduction not permanent removal. 'None of the lasers will totally and permanently remove all hair, but this method will achieve up to 70 or 80 per cent in a lot of

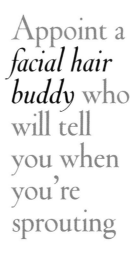

Appoint a facial hair buddy who will tell you when you're sprouting

patients, and patients can come back for maintenance sessions,' advises Dr Lowe. To help extend the time between maintenance (and minimise regrowth), he recommends a prescription cream called Vaniqa, which interferes with some of the proteins that form hair. On the positive side, Dr Lowe says laser hair removal usually works extremely well, and is also useful for ingrowing hair.

Don't go near lasers if you have pigmentation problems. Laser hair removal is not suitable for anyone with vitiligo (patches of de-pigmented skin) as it may stimulate new areas. Anyone with eczema, psoriasis, hives or urticaria should have a patch test first.

Beware of IPL. Many beauty salons offer treatment with IPL (Intense Pulsed Light), as do some cosmetic surgery clinics. However, Dr Lowe advises caution: 'I've seen so many patients that have had burns and blisters, loss of pigment and scars.' (Dr Lowe uses IPL systems for removal of thread veins, sun spots and for rejuvenating skin.)

And be very careful where you have any laser or IPL treatment. Dr Lowe cautions against booking laser hair removal at beauty salons: you should go to an experienced trained physician at a reputable clinic. We recommend you follow the same guidelines for this as any 'cosmetic tweak' such as Botox, etc, to optimise your chances of the best outcome – see page 46.

A final caution: very occasionally with these high-tech methods of hair removal, hair growth may be stimulated instead of reduced, due to the technology not delivering enough energy to the hair follicle; usually the problem can be overcome by switching to a different laser system. But it's another big argument for going to someone who is trained properly and experienced.

'The only real
ELEGANCE
is in the mind;
if you've got that,
the rest *really*
comes from it'

Diana Vreeland

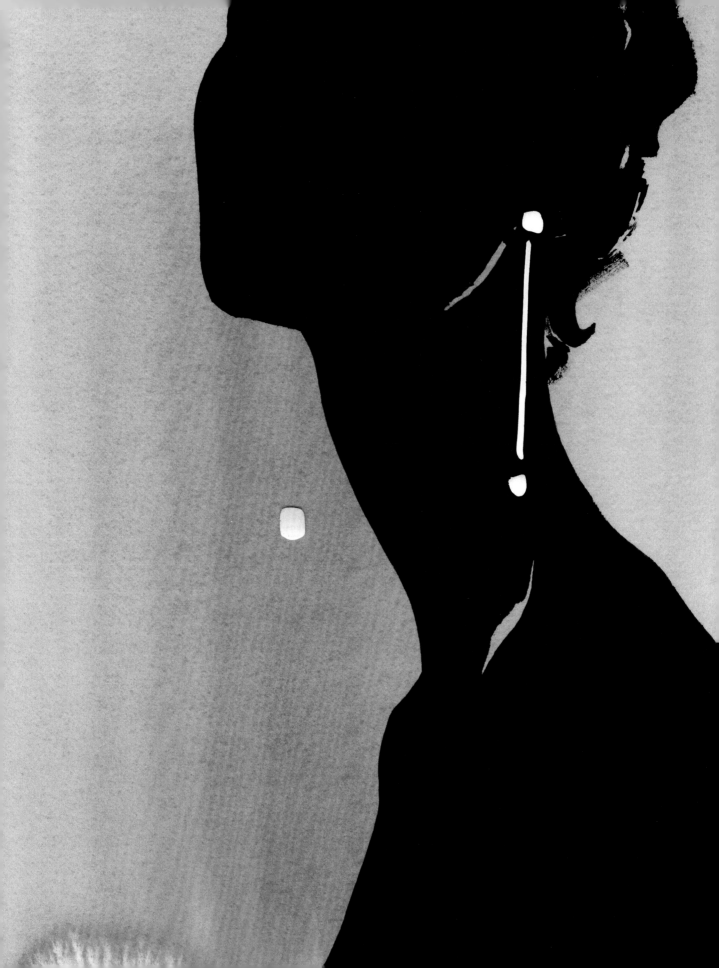

Nourish your neck (and keep it swan-like)

As our necks start to sag and the texture looks crêpey, our hearts begin to sink. The reality is that the skin is much thinner on the neck than on our faces, and thus more easily damaged. (And we do tend to overlook it.) So, no more neglect – just lavish it with loving care

To misquote Nora Ephron, don't feel bad about your neck.
We love Nora Ephron (screenwriter for *Heartburn*, *Julie & Julia*, etc), and author of the hilarious collection of essays, *I Feel Bad about My Neck*, in which she writes: 'One of my biggest regrets – bigger even than not buying the apartment on East Seventy-fifth Street, bigger even than my worst romantic catastrophe – is that I didn't spend my youth staring lovingly at my neck. It never crossed my mind to be grateful for it… Of course now I am older, I'm wise and sage and mellow. And it's also true that I honestly do understand just what matters in life. But guess what? It's my neck.'
We agree with Nora that necks can be angst-inducing. But we say: any neck – even 'turkey neck' (that unpicturesque term for a sagging neck) – can be improved, with targeted and diligent TLC.

Make like a Frenchwoman and 'double-moisturise'. One of the key issues with the neck is crêpiness, as the skin on the neck has relatively few oil glands and without moisture and lipids, it can start to look papery super-fast. Get into the habit of applying everything you put on your face right down to the bra-line. At the same time, sweep any body lotion up to your chin, so it gets twice the nourishment. Your neck and chest should be part of your 'cleansing zone', but avoid using a scrub on the neck, although a muslin cloth (used with cleanser) is fine.

And consider a targeted neck product. For our testers' favourites, and ours too, see overleaf.

Protect your neck with an SPF15 plus. As dermatologist Dr Nick Lowe tells us, 'The neck is easily damaged by sun exposure as the skin is much thinner than it is on other parts of the face, and its support structure is not as effective.' So the ceaseless battering of UV light breaks down collagen and elastin, leading to sagging. Any SPF you apply to your face – your first line of defence against ageing – should be applied to the neck, the chest and the décolletage, religiously. End… Of… Story. If you tend to 'miss' the sides of the neck because your hair's in the way, scoop it off your face pre-application. If you do have 'age spots' on your neck and chest, see our recommendations for treating these on page 190.

Avoid wearing perfume in the sun. Many a woman's list of neck woes includes pigmented areas either side of the neck. Certain fragrance ingredients – generally citrus-derived – contain psoralens, components which over-stimulate the pigment-producing cells. This produces localised brown patches (medically called Berloque dermatitis), that look like a streak of brown pigment rather like a raindrop running down a window pane. (Plus the alcohol in the scent dries out the skin.) The solution? If you want to enjoy a summer fragrance in the sun, try spritzing it on your clothing rather than your skin. (Check first, of course, that it doesn't discolour the fabric: you can try it on a tissue.) Or wear a ribbon around a wrist or your neck, drenched in scent, à la Marie Antoinette and her mob. Spritz a hankie with scent and tuck it in your bra – or your swimsuit, as long as you're not planning to get wet. And, of course, enjoy liberally after dark. Just be certain to cleanse away the fragrance the next morning with a wet flannel, before you go anywhere near the sun.

Take up yoga. One of the key reasons women develop 'turkey neck', double chins and those 'necklace rings' on the neck is because underlying muscles are weak. So neck firming is yet another reason to add to the list of why embracing yoga is a good idea (more on page 204). It's fantastic, fantastic, fantastic for strengthening the neck and the jaw and – as we've observed in previous books – we know seventy-something yoga devotees who have sharp jaw-lines and smooth, swan-like necks. And we want to be like them. It's not just us. Esteemed dermatologist Dr Karen Burke observes: 'If you do yoga you can postpone facelifts for years. People have those sharp jawlines because they're doing a total stretch.'

Raise the height of your computer screen. Whether you use a laptop or a full-size screen on your desk, you should make sure that it's high enough for you to look straight at it, rather than looking down.

Embrace polo-necks, pashminas, scarves and pearl chokers. If you really still feel Nora Ephron-ish about your neck, short of surgery/lasers (we'll come on to that), camouflage is your best option. These all hide a multitude of sins. Not everyone suits a polo-neck, but if you generally look better with a scoop- or a v-neckline, you can create a flattering optical illuson that draws attention downwards by hanging a necklace or rope of pearls over the top. Wear earrings, too, which distract the eye from your neck. But you have to trust us: nobody looks as unforgivingly on your neck as you do.

As a last resort, there's surgery. And fillers. And Intense Pulsed Light (IPL) treatments. We are going to point you in the direction (not for the first time in this book) of Wendy Lewis, who is the fount of all cosmetic surgery wisdom. In her book *Plastic Makes Perfect* (see ANTI-AGEING BOOKSHELF), she devotes several pages to all the options, which range from 'plastysmaplasty' (to tackle 'turkey wattle') to liposuction and the fillers Restylane and Perlane. But any procedure to do with the neck is A Big Deal (remember: your main artery and all the important nerves go through the neck); botched neck treatments happen. If you can afford any of these procedures, you can afford to talk to Wendy first: she is completely independent and not affiliated with any doctor, but knows better than anyone on the planet who's best at what.

And if you still feel bad about your neck, read Nora Ephron. Because at least there's someone who feels worse about hers than you do.

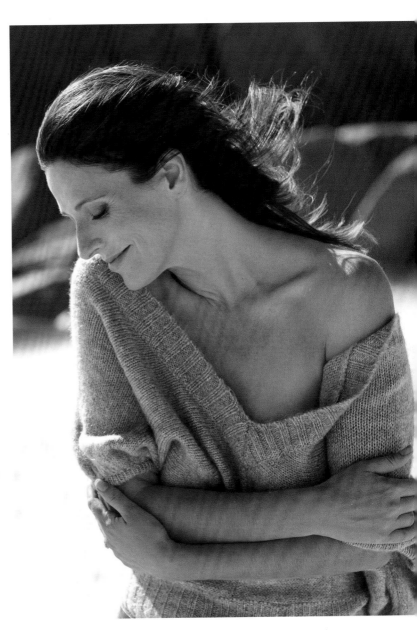

'I look forward to getting older when looks should become less of an issue, and when who you are is the point' Susan Sarandon

Neck treatments: *our award winners*

Why is it that so many women buy neck creams, only to leave them languishing on the bathroom shelf? Is it a fundamental belief that nothing can really make a difference to this notoriously hard-to-treat area? Certainly, the key with any neck treatment is ritualistic use – preferably twice a day (and do shield the area with an SPF15 during daylight, too) – and a high pleasure factor goes a long way to encouraging that ritual. If you follow our testers' recommendations and are religious with any of the following creams (from among more than 50 trialled), we hope you will be as pleased as our testers were

AT A GLANCE

Clarins Super Restorative Décolleté and Neck Concentrate

Clarins Extra Firming Neck Anti-Wrinkle Rejuvenating Cream

Guerlain Abeille Royale Neck & Décolleté Cream SPF15

Liz Earle Superskin Concentrate

RéVive Fermitif Neck Renewal Cream SPF15

Liz Earle Skin Repair Moisturiser Dry/Sensitive

REVIEWS

Clarins Super Restorative Décolleté and Neck Concentrate

8.89/10 This category is a bit of a triumph for French brand Clarins, which is still a family run business by the way. It was founded in 1954 by medical student Jacques Courtin-Clarins, who died in 2007 and was succeeded as chairman by his son Christian. This fluid treatment is instantly skin-firming, moisturising – plus it features a combination of plant extracts for specific, longer-term, age-defying power. Additionally, Clarins recommend a specific one-minute massage technique to enhance the effects (you'll find the instructions slipped inside the box).

Comments: 'Absolutely huge improvements: I have tried other (expensive) brands but I can now see benefits as never before. I had a real neck complex and grew my hair longer to hide it. Today I am considering a shorter bob!' • 'I haven't used a separate neck cream previously but I have now been converted and will make it part of my daily routine' • 'my favourite of the anti-ageing goodies I tried, skin looks noticeably softer, smoother and less crêpey, with definite improvements in tone' • 'my neck really does look tighter and younger, décolleté firmer and a little lifted: I am very impressed. Much better than just using my day or night creams'.

Clarins Extra Firming Neck Anti-Wrinkle Rejuvenating Cream

 8.88/10 A convinctin double whammy for Clarins with this second award-winner. Beauty Bible's diligent testers have confirmed Clarins' pre-eminence in neck rejuvenation. The texture of this product is different – a rich cream – and it features Clarins patented Extra-Firming Complex, as well as green seaweed extracts and sunflower auxins (plant growth hormones), which they say will soften, smooth and firm the neck and décolleté – and our testers agree.

Comments: 'I love this! Crêpiness reduced significantly after two weeks and continued to improve, neck looks younger and the skin plumper' • 'sinks in beautifully with no greasy residue, amazing texture and lovely smell' • 'skin was softer and smoother overnight, after two weeks my neck was tighter, firmer and less crêpey, and my décolleté plumper' • 'nice and light but still luxurious – seemed to melt into my skin leaving it looking lifted, and feeling silky, soft and smooth. I really saw a difference'.

Guerlain Abeille Royale Neck & Décolleté Cream SPF15

 8.57/10 This now legendary range from another much-loved French classic brand (testament to French women's longer history of taking care of their complexions)

harnesses the skin repairing power of royal jelly. Guerlain's research has established that bee products – in particular royal jelly – have a powerful effect on wrinkle correction and firming, so here you'll find it in a smoothing, lifting cream that also offers an SPF15 to prevent age spot formation.

Comments: 'I love everything about this product, consistency, absorbency, how soft it makes my skin feel – neck looks smoother and brighter and feels softer, and the crêpiness around my décolleté area looks much better' • 'my neck and décolleté were badly damaged through breast cancer treatment – skin feels soft, looks smoother and moisturised now, little lines are slightly less noticeable' • 'skin looked much more attractive and glowing; blemishes appeared reduced, lines and wrinkles less apparent, neckline firmer and smoother'.

Liz Earle Superskin Concentrate ✿✿

8.5/10 A high-scorer in previous books, a stellar performer in the facial oil category here, and a favourite of Jo's… Liz Earle sent another ten bottles of this to be trialled as a neck treatment, and they obviously knew what they were doing: the argan- and rosehip-rich oil, turbo-charged by vitamin E, came up trumps here too.

Comments: 'Very noticeable difference immediately; greatly improved smoothness, which continued with use; skin feels softer and smoother, the biggest difference is to fine lines which are far

♡ WE LOVE…

From being too lazy to use anything at all on her neck, full-on neck panic now has Jo veering between the serum-like Liz Earle Superskin Neck & Bust Treatment and Sarah Chapman's Skinesis Neck and Chest Rejuvenating Complex, a beautifully sensual-to-use cream that encourages diligent application. Sarah slathers all face creams and oils on to her décolleté, up her neck, jawline and practically into her hairline, always using an upward, then side to side, stroking motion with fingertips. (Although a specific cream may be a necessity soon, as she reads the comments!)

less noticeable' • 'neck felt and looked plump and smooth; healthier, fresher skin' • 'skin looks and feels beautiful, and younger because smoother' • 'Smells great, feels great and makes my skin look great! Neck is certainly less craggy, has eliminated all signs of crêpiness and dryness, lines finer and less visible, skin moisturised and supple'.

RéVive Fermitif Neck Renewal Cream SPF15

8.44/10 We often wonder why more neck creams don't incorporate an SPF, since the neck's so vulnerable to sun damage. Hallelujah: this one does (a chemical sunscreen, note), in a luxurious, softly rose-scented cream with special firming agents from wheat protein and barley extract, plus what RéVive call their 'youth molecule'.

Comments: 'Skin immediately lovely and velvety to touch, supple and plumped up; with regular use, everything is smoothed out and fine lines much more faded' • 'skin on neck and décolletage feels much firmer, softer and looks better – more supple' • 'skin looks glossier and firmer – just loved this product and think it does an amazing job'.

Liz Earle Skin Repair Moisturiser Dry/Sensitive ✿

8.41/10 Interesting! This everyday moisturiser from Liz Earle did well in previous books as a neck treatment, even though it's not specifically labelled as such. Once again, they sent us ten pots to be specifically trialled for this book. And guess what? Once again, Skin Repair got a great score from this entirely new bunch of neck-conscious testers. Packed with plant avocado and borage oil, echinacea, pro-vitamin B5, antioxidants – all the botanicals which are the signature of Liz's so-successful range, in fact.

Comments: 'Fantastic: the skin on my neck immediately became plumper, smoother and felt more comfy; neck looks much younger and healthier' • 'gave a kind of "soft focus" effect to lines' • 'skin felt instantly nourished by this rich, light cream, absorbs like magic, have never used a cream that made my skin feel so soft, supple and moisturised – would like to score it 12/10!'.

'Lift' your face – without surgery…

(Yes, it's possible.) Maybe you want to look your best for a special occasion. Or perhaps your face would love a boost after a stressful time. But you're not up for surgery, fillers, dermabrasion or lasers – so what's to do…? Here are the (non-surgical) fixes that we know really work

Try CACI. Over the years we've been in the beauty business, we've pretty much tried out all the non-surgical facelift systems. These mostly involve probes carrying low-voltage electric currents which are moved over your face to make the muscles jump around and work harder, giving a temporary lift – sometimes versions of these are used in tandem with facials. Of the many that have been launched over the past two decades, the one that has stood the test of time worldwide is CACI, which stands for Computer Aided Cosmetology Instrument. From the one original option (CACI Classic), there's now an almost bewildering range – which extend to microdermabrasion and ultrasonic peeling, and beyond the face to include CACI for bust enhancement, stretch

marks and cellulite. We honestly don't know how well all that works – but we do know that for a temporary (24 to 48 hours) boost, a CACI treatment can be rejuvenating. (And just lying still for an hour or so is a big bonus for many busy women.) For longer-term results, CACI recommend ten to 15 treatments and then maintenance sessions every four to six weeks. (Worth considering, we'd say, if you enjoy it, like the results and your budget permits.)

Find a great facialist. For our money, a good facial with massage by skilled hands can give some gorgeous instant results. (On page 79 you'll find our favourite facialists, but talk to girlfriends and investigate local talent – you might find a hidden magic-worker just around the corner. (Tell us if you do, at www.beautybible.com!) Some facialists undoubtedly have healing hands; indeed one of our fave raves Emma Hardie (who now has a lovely skincare line with products that regularly feature in our award winners) started out in the early 1990s with her own natural lifting and sculpting facial. Sarah wrote about it for *YOU magazine*, other beauty editors (including *Harper's Bazaar*'s Newby Hands) endorsed it – and Emma has become a legend in natural rejuvenation.

Get the needle! We swear by facial acupuncture. And believe us, the needles truly aren't scary. (The only version we did find too much to take was electro-acupuncture, where the needles carry a current which is progressively increased. You need to be made of sterner stuff than we are for that.) Sarah really loves a treatment from Annee de Mamiel, formerly a successful banker who studied acupuncture after recovering from cancer. Annee treats your whole body, explaining: 'Beauty is about being balanced on the inside, in every way – physically and psychologically. If you feel good about yourself, it reflects in the way you look. Dry, wrinkled, saggy skin mirrors what is happening in your body, so I look at the roots of the problems and treat those too.' For instance, the common problem of vertical lines between your eyebrows can relate to liver energy not flowing properly (frowning too much is a factor too!), so as well as needling the lines themselves, Annee treats the liver. As well as acupuncture, she makes up specially blended oils for each client plus a herbal tea to take home. Annee incorporates stimulating Tui Na Chinese massage (to invigorate the skin) and lymph draining massage and acupressure to relax you from top to toe. An increasing number of acupuncturists now offer facial acupuncture; ask friends for recommendations. (Jo sees a fab Hove-based therapist called Steve Mason for this.)

Just say 'ouch'. Much the most painful treatment Sarah has endured is having the muscles inside the mouth at the base of the tongue released by osteopath Vicky Vlachonis, now in Los Angeles, (who learned it from French obstetrician Michel Odent). As she wrote at the time, 'The results are extraordinary: any downward drift perks up and the contours of your face seem redefined – truly a non-surgical facelift moment.' And the pain is

TIP

If there's one low-tech gizmo we'd recommend for ironing out your face at home it's Sarah Chapman's Facialift, an odd-looking contraption with eight small knobbly cogs on a handle which rotate as you push them up and down your face. Good for massaging in product, or simply for stimulating the skin tissue and encouraging lymph drainage.

'BEAUTY is about being balanced on the inside. If you feel *good* about yourself, it reflects in the way you LOOK'

definitely worth the gain, according to Carine Roitfeld, former editor of French *Vogue*, who recently revealed that this internal facial massage is her secret for looking younger. 'They put on gloves and massage inside because all your stress is in your jaws. It hurts very much, but is my beauty secret,' she says. NB: If you want to try this do make sure you go to a practitioner who has really learnt this technique: you don't want to be a guinea pig.

Do it yourself. If you haven't got the time, budget or opportunity to have a treatment, you really can achieve wonders by yourself. Start by sipping some still room-temperature water, then spend a moment or two focusing on your breathing, as Annee suggests:

● Do this breathing exercise throughout the day: inhale through your nose to a count of three, exhale through your mouth for five, then pause for a second or two and let your body and mind go still and release tension.

● If possible, apply an instant face reviver (see page 212 for our testers' top-scoring products).

● Massage your face to relax muscles, allowing oxygenated blood to flow freely and toxins to be released, leaving you with a fresher, brighter complexion, less puffiness and fewer wrinkles. (See page 78 for guidelines.)

● Practise some yoga, or lie flat on your back for five minutes (more if you have it), knees bent, eyes closed (with damp teabags over them if possible). In your mind's eye, see blue sky – and as stray thoughts pop into your brain, convert them into clouds and let them float away.

Think nice thoughts. Your skin and face reflect your state of mind. If you're stressed, you run the risk of looking pinched and peaky. Try thinking of a couple of nice things that have happened to you today – remember someone you love and, if you're having an iffy day, that you never know what delicious thing might be around the next corner. Even if life is really tough (and it happens to everyone), there's almost always something positive. Gratitude and hope are great beautifiers.

Night treatments: our award winners

Here you'll find the treatments which – according to our testers – really do transform mere slumber into beauty sleep. Because of the body's repairing rhythms, most cellular patching-up happens while we're asleep, so that many 'miracle' treatments are specifically designed to be used overnight. And because we don't need to slap on make-up over the top, night creams tend to be richer. Here are the nighttime products our testers loved – out of over 90! – with some truly spectacular scores, and a couple of new entries for this latest paperback edition. (For day-time miracle treatments, turn to page 16.)

AT A GLANCE

Aurelia Cell Revitalise Night Moisturiser

Elemis Pro-Collagen Oxygenating Night Cream

Crème de la Mer Moisturizing Cream

Sarah Chapman Skinesis Overnight Facial

La Prairie Anti-Aging Night Cream

Lancôme Génifique Repair Youth Activating Night Cream

Clarins Extra-Firming Night Rejuvenating Cream

REVIEWS

Aurelia Cell Revitalise Night Moisturiser

9.5/10 Wow! This new award winner gained one of the very highest scores in Beauty Bible history. Aurelia Probiotic Skincare, which won our first Best New Brand award in 2014, uses ethically sourced 100 per cent BioOrganic botanicals, put together in scientifically-proven, evidence-based formulations. Like all the range, this rich cream contains anti-inflammatory probiotic technology with plant extracts – baobab, kigelia Africana and hibiscus, plus plant oils – borage and mongongo, vitamin E and shea butter, plus fragrant and relaxing flower essences – neroli, lavender, rose and mandarin – which testers all loved and commented on.

Comments: '10/10. Love it. 5 stars. My husband said "your skin looks nice today – plump and amazing" for the first time in 26 years of marriage… my skin looks radiant, feels firmer, fine lines plumper' • 'I saw a difference in my complexion after the first night, skin so much softer and smoother, silky and glowing' • 'the most divine night cream I have ever used, the smell is so gorgeous I looked forward to bedtime' • 'have already recommended it to others with sensitive skin' • 'people sometimes now refuse to believe I am 40 – a lovely, lovely cream'.

Elemis Pro-Collagen Oxygenating Night Cream

9.37/10 This outstandingly high-scorer is the night-time 'sister' product to a cream that's excelled in previous Beauty Bible books. Said to increase oxygen levels in the skin by 'up to 41 per cent', it combines an anti-ageing hexapeptide, marine extracts, antioxidants and Padina pavonica, a potent algae to boost firmness and elasticity. Luxuriously priced too.

Comments: 'My skin just drunk it in, skin was plumped up and very soft, helps with wrinkles because it's so hydrating' • 'does enhance radiance, dehydrated areas have improved dramatically and wrinkles greatly reduced' • 'skin looks better in every way, clear, soft and glowing, skintone more even and calmer' • 'this is the best night cream I have ever found – skin has never looked better'.

Crème de la Mer Moisturizing Cream

 Any doubting Thomasinas who are cynical about Crème de la Mer's anti-ageing powers can please be silent now. In our totally independent trial, this legendary rich cream – created by a NASA scientist to deal with severe chemical burns, and based on a 'Miracle Broth' including marine ingredients – has done incredibly well. Our experience is that it suits even the most sensitive complexions, but it's rich and best applied with a special 'pressing' technique.

Comments: 'Skin brighter, softer, amazing reduction in crêpiness round eyes and mouth; friends commented on how "well", "fresh", "been on holiday?" I looked' • 'cheeks more plumped up and less old and saggy' • 'I'm saving up to buy more!' • 'lives up to all the hype' • 'noticeable reduction in fine lines on treated side' • 'really impressed' • 'improvement in bigger wrinkles and grooves'.

Sarah Chapman Skinesis Overnight Facial

 We dithered a lot over whether to put this high-scorer here, or in facial oils – or even serums! It's basically a fusion of both, but designed to be used at night. So 'night treatments' is where we've parked this pump-action product, designed to deliver 'facial-like' effects overnight, with a blend of omega oils and powerful peptides, all deliciously scented with jasmine, rose, frangipani and tuberose.

Comments: 'My skin was particularly irritated and blotchy when I started but within a few days began to clear, becoming soft and less red – within a few days I was glowing' • 'my skin looked amazing after the first application, soft and plump, with visible difference in fine lines, with a real radiance; felt smooth and velvety' • 'sinks in quickly but stays on skin long enough for a good massage, love the dispenser too' • 'skin definitely looks fresher and young, fine lines more plumped and overall much improved'.

La Prairie Anti-Aging Night Cream

 Again, a luxe-priced winner – though not as pricey as some La Prairie supercreams. Rich in peptides, it also features an extract of green micro-algae (again, to help production of collagen and elastin), plus La Prairie's signature Exclusive Cellular Complex.

Comments: 'LOVED it! Inside the silver box is a silver jar with a spatula and when you apply the cream skin feels nourished and has a radiance' • 'my skin is glowing and silken, more toned, lines beside eyes less visible, and two rather large frown lines between my eyebrows have lessened' • 'my mature fair skin looks younger, definitely addressed fine lines particularly around my mouth' • 'most fine lines reduced, some bigger wrinkles too, and I am told I look younger'.

Lancôme Génifique Repair Youth Activating Night Cream

 The boffins in L'Oréal's labs harnessed ten years of research to create this light-textured, neroli-and-citrus-scented cream, which they claim 'revives the activity of the genes responsible for reinforcing the skin's barrier function'! They further promise 'one night's all it takes to obtain a more rested appearance…'

Comments: 'Really like sleep in the jar: I could tell the difference having used this: skin was soft, smooth, clearer, more radiant' • 'smoothed fine lines; skin felt and looked plumper, supple and with a healthy glow' • 'my husband has commented a couple of times on how great my skin is looking'.

Clarins Extra-Firming Night Rejuvenating Cream

Extra-Firming has been a 'classic' in the Clarins range, but sometimes, breakthroughs inspire them to tweak the formulation. This new version has won a place in our run-down of overnight sensations. Active botanicals include collagen-stimulating organic green banana extract, lemon thyme (to boost elastin production), and several peptides. It also features lotus extract to prevent the appearance of dark spots. (It's suitable for all skin types, but there is a version for dry skins, too.)

Comments: 'Face felt really soft and looked relaxed the next day' • 'my complexion looked less tired and brighter overnight; does enhance radiance, and balances any oily patches' • 'over time the dry patches I sometimes get have gone, remarkable considering its winter' • 'I will use it for the radiance and anti-fatigue benefits and because it is genuinely enjoyable to apply'.

♡ WE LOVE…

Years in, Jo still believes Liz Earle Superskin Moisturiser is the best moisturiser 'ever, ever, ever' - but she has switched to the new neroli-scented (rather than unscented but naturally fragrant) version: 'it's same outstanding nourishing and "plumping" cream, but with an even lovelier smell'. 'It's rich, nourishing and the "plumping" action is amazing,' she says. As well as a facial oil, Sarah happily strokes on MV Organic Skincare Rose Soothing & Protective Moisturiser, which suits her touchy skin wonderfully morning and night.

TIP

Many people we know swear by a silk pillowcase to sleep on, insisting that they wake up without the 'sleep creases' that can develop in skin as we slumber. Also a silk pillowcase – unlike cotton – doesn't absorb either your skin's natural moisture or the cream you put on, so you're giving your skin the benefit of any anti-ageing ingredients – not your pillowcase…

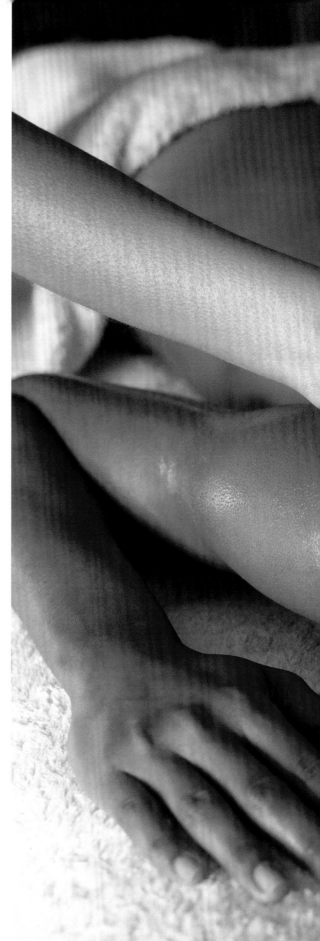

Give aches and pains plenty of TLC

We're not talking here about the sort of pain that comes with acute illness or injury. This is the general wear and tear that we're all prey to and which can make us look and feel older – so here's our prescription for kissing it better!

Two out of three people suffer neck and shoulder pain in their lives. Back ache is endemic, affecting eight to ten of us, the majority aged between 35 and 55. Then there are the usual headaches, not to mention sore feet (for more about them, see page 96). And none of them are beautifiers: we furrow our brows, the light goes out of our eyes, we stoop or slouch. (And left untended our joints may suffer irreparable damage.) So it's worth having strategies to deal with aches and pains. First of all, prevention – below you'll find the most useful tips we know for everyday stuff. And if despite your best endeavours you do end up in agony, see overleaf for advice.

Stand up straight. Improving your posture reaps heaps of benefits – preventing aches and pains, making you look slimmer, and even keeping you happier. Ears, shoulders, hips, knees and ankles should be in a straight line; pull your tummy button towards your spine. Breathe slowly. (See the box overleaf for more.)

Make sure you can see clearly. Having the right specs will help prevent that tortoise-poke-forward as you peer at a book, the

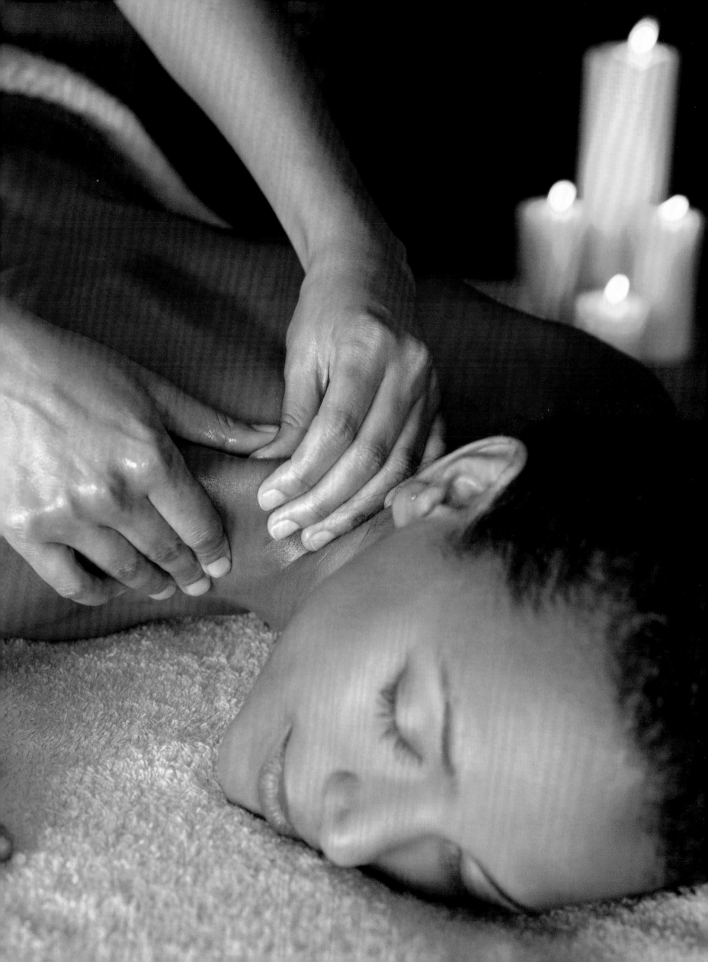

screen – or the road ahead (as well as stopping you frowning, which should save a few pounds on face creams). Have your eyes tested at least every two years, annually after the age of forty if you have glaucoma in the family (it can result in blindness, so this is vital). Check your lighting: if you're working at a screen, the main source should come from behind it to avoid reflections on the screen. If you're reading, the light source should preferably come from over your left shoulder; in the darker winter months, you will need stronger light than on a bright summer's day. (We like Serious Readers dedicated lamps.)

Keep moving. Our bodies were not designed to sit still for long periods. Neck, shoulder and back aches often come from sitting in a fixed position at screens (laptops are worst of all, see right) and also driving, lifting, etc. The golden rule is: get up and walk around every 30-40 minutes – more if possible. Sip a glass of water as you amble, and you'll be doing double beauty duty.

Position your head correctly. It's very heavy (about 12 pounds) and needs to sit directly on top of your spine rather than poking forward, straining muscles and causing injury. Aim to have your ears, shoulders and hips in a straight vertical line. Lifting your chest and letting your shoulders roll back and down helps; gently push your shoulder blades together (see exercises below).

Have your knees slightly lower than your pelvis when sitting. This helps put the spine into neutral position. If you don't have a chair with an adjustable seat, try putting a couple of folded towels under your bottom, and sit into the back of the chair.

Your screen should be at eye level. Have your forearms at right angles to your body and in a straight line to your fingertips. An arm rest may help. Your mouse should be easily accessible by swinging your hand round, to say 45 degrees maximum. You shouldn't have to lift your elbow or make a claw. RSI sufferers should choose a big 'elephant's foot' mouse or trackball.

Keep the documents you are working on at eye height to avoid squinnying at the bottom of the screen.

Do simple, gentle exercises to keep your circulation moving. A counter-stretch will reverse the hunched position, particularly after using a laptop; imagine you're 'opening like a flower', says Tim Hutchful of the British Chiropractic Association. Reach your arms out to the side, palms up, then open your fingers and turn your palms down to the floor; look gently up to the ceiling, push your shoulder blades together and hold for ten seconds. Follow with a 'chin tuck': pull your chin into your throat as if you are trying to make a double chin and hold for ten seconds. Also shrug your shoulders up to your ears and circle them back and forwards. (For a quick exercise programme for all ages, visit www.youtube.com and put Straighten Up UK! in Search – fantastic if you're feeling tired and/or looking peaky.)

POSTURE

Bad posture is to blame for all sorts of aches and pains. But here's an interesting thing: good posture can actually help to change your mood. If you feel low, you tend to look down, which keeps you feeling, well, low and down. Matters get worse if you hunch your shoulders and clasp your arms or hands in front. 'You're closing off your chest, which means you don't get as much oxygen in your lungs and your brain,' explains body language expert Robert Phipps. 'If you straighten up, open your chest and shoulders, look ahead and around keeping your eye movements horizontal, you start to feel better. Looking down connects with the emotional part of your brain whereas looking up and to the right engages with your future. You will notice your breathing changes, and your whole body lifts.'

Posture is also a vital component of social signalling: 'If you adopt a confident body posture, you project confidence. Barriers and defensive postures signal fear; uncrossing your arms and lifting your chin signals "I'm not afraid". Our minds and bodies are in a constant feedback loop, conveying information. Animals respond purely to body language; humans put a social veneer on behaviour but we always revert to animal instincts,' says Phipps.

A tip: on a first meeting or at an interview, mirror the person's body language for three or four movements, match their rate of talking and breathing, then sit back in your chair. 'At an interesting moment in the conversation, pause, lean forward and drop your voice slightly so they have to come forward to you. They are then mirroring you – through your confident strategy,' says Phipps.

Of course, posture isn't just about your social life. 'Good posture keeps your bones and joints in alignment so you can use your muscles properly and keep them fairly relaxed to avoid painful tension,' explains chiropractor Tim Hutchful. 'It should also prevent your spine being distorted into an abnormal position, which can lead to

LAPTOP KNOW-HOW

Laptop computers have liberated us in many ways but, according to chiropractor Tim Hutchful, the downside is that they can cause considerable damage to your neck and spine, resulting in lots of aches and pains including headaches. 'Because the laptop keyboard and screen are integrated, you risk compromising your neck, shoulders, arms and/or back when using one, so there's potential for problems in all these areas,' he says.

● Taking a small keyboard with you (pack everything in a rucksack so the weight is even) may seem like trouble but it can really help you avoid it.

● Try to work with your arms supported (on a train or plane table, or even on cushions if you're in the back of a car), to avoid neck pain from the muscles that hold up your arms.

T'ai chi helps many aches and pains, including knee osteoarthritis and fibromyalgia, as well as quality of sleep. It may also benefit bone density, and increase musculoskeletal strength.

pain in different parts of your body. Additionally, if you're evenly balanced, it helps to reduce abnormal wear and tear of joints. Remember that good posture is just as important when you're moving as when you're still,' he adds.

To support your spine, it's vital to strengthen the corset of abdominal muscles between the lower margin of your ribs and your waist, all round. Simply contract those muscles as you sit at your desk or stand at the bus stop. To create a 'cross bracing effect', try the Superman exercise: go down on all fours like a coffee table, arms and upper legs at right angles to your body. Raise your right arm and left leg to the horizontal, hold for five to ten seconds, then swap sides. Repeat five times. (Don't do this if it's uncomfortable.)

WHAT TO DO IF YOU HAVE ACHES AND PAINS

Spray on magnesium oil: it will relax the muscles in that area and should provide quick relief. You can use it several times a day, and before bed. Genius! (Try Magnesium Oil by Better You.)

Take an anti-inflammatory: we don't get on with conventional versions, so took the advice of integrated medicine guru Dr Andrew Weil and keep a stock of Zyflamend by New Chapter, a combination of plants that help reduce pain and inflammation in the joints (can also be used for skin).

Try Bromelain, an enzyme with remarkable painkilling properties, that's been extensively studied for use in digestive disorders (eg, heartburn, reflux and food allergies), also inflammatory conditions (arthritis, sports injuries and skin conditions such as eczema and psoriasis). (Bromelain by LifeTime Vitamins.)

Explore complementary therapies such as acupuncture, chiropractic (try McTimoney chiropractic if you don't like too much clunk-click stuff), Bowen technique, osteopathy and/or cranial osteopathy. Practise (gently) yoga, Pilates or t'ai chi.

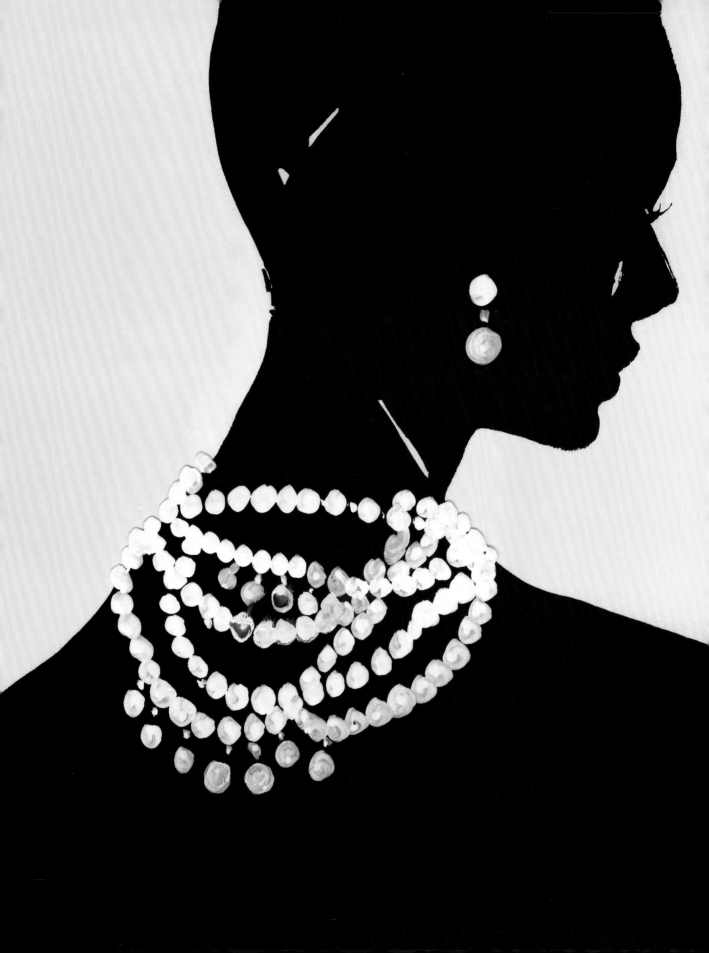

'Beautiful YOUNG people are accidents of nature, but beautiful OLD people are *works of art*'

Eleanor Roosevelt

Embrace pearls
(it worked for Grace Kelly)

We love pearls. Ropes and swags of them. As necklaces, chokers, bracelets and don't forget earrings. Real, cultured or plain fake. Sea or freshwater. Vintage or just-strung. Oversized and multi-stranded or neat, demure singles. White, pink, grey or black. With denim or satin, T-shirt, woolly or your most glam glad rags

Forget diamonds – we say: pearls are a girl's best friend. Why?

Because these lustrous baubles are just about the most fabulously flattering accessory for any mature complexion – whether your skin has warm or cool tones. (Michelle Obama looks amazing in pearls. So do Hillary Clinton, Oprah Winfrey and Elizabeth Taylor, which tells you everything you need to know about how they work for every complexion. Think of Coco Chanel, Audrey Hepburn, Jackie Kennedy Onassis, Princess Diana – all draped in them. And not for nothing have English and North American women traditionally been given a pearl necklace and earrings when they came of age.)

Pearls may swing in and out of fashion, but they are always miraculously flattering. Pearls distract the eye. They're lambent like moonlight, creating a sort of 'halo' effect when close to the face – bouncing light on to your skin and making it appear softer and more radiant.

A pearl collar or choker can disguise a less-than-fabulous neck. Dowager duchesses have

LUST FOR THE LUSTRE

Pearlised pigments and, in some cases, real crushed pearl (aka 'nacre') are also being incorporated into skin creams for instant radiance – great in a make-up primer, as it gives skin that 'halo' effect when foundation's applied on top. In make-up, these pearl-esque, light-reflective pigments really can create the illusion of softening fine lines, and minimising under-eye shadows or visible pigmentation.

always known that, but frankly it's a tip that many of us could make use of if neck-angst kicks in. You don't need a title or family jewels for this: Jo, in particular, is constantly on the lookout for great costume jewellery pearls, but also likes real baroque Indian pearls: she first found them in Anjuna Market in Goa, and while a practised eye might be able to tell them apart from much, much pricier versions, we're just not that snooty about our jewels. We just pile 'em on. Timeless. Classic. Minor-miracle-working.

And add a touch of pearl to your skin, too. Pearl is also a word – or rather, a texture – to bear in mind when it comes to creating a finish for your make-up. Applied judiciously – a touch on the browbone, for instance, or even on the eyelid – pearlised eyeshadow helps create a sculpting light-and-shade effect. Fact: too matt isn't good, after forty, because a face looks dry and dusty. You need a little sheen. But use 'the pearl test' when you're buying glimmering shades of any product, ie, does this have more shimmer than a real pearl? In which case it's probably too shimmery, whether you're looking at a lipstick or an eyeshadow.

'There is one piece of jewellery that is equally becoming to everybody, lovely with almost every ensemble, appropriate for almost every occasion and indispensable in every woman's wardrobe... Long live the pearl necklace, from our first date to our last breath!'
Geneviève Antoine Dariaux, *Elégance*

'Not for nothing
have women
traditionally been
given a pearl necklace
and earrings when
they came of age'

'We can't all look like the *wondrous* Carmen dell'Orefice (STILL a supermodel at 79) but we CAN look pretty damn *good*'

Look good in photos

(And feel better about yourself)

We used to think that a friend of ours – then editor of *Tatler* – was being so grand when she refused to be photographed before lunchtime. Now we absolutely understand what she meant. One of the commonest causes of those 'oh, damn!' moments – when we really feel like we've fast-forwarded a decade or two – is seeing ourselves in a hideous snap. 'Do I really look like that…?' Well, the answer is not really: in real life, people take in all of you (voice, smile, twinkling eyes) – whereas in a snapshot, it's so easy to see only your flaws.

So: we believe in positive reinforcement. It's possible to take a hideous picture of anyone (think of those 'drunken' celebrity shots which caught them mid-blink). But it makes all of us feel better if we can glimpse a photo and go, 'Actually, not looking so bad…'

This may be a cheat, but in the same way that famous people control 'official' images of themselves, we suggest that you only surround yourself with photos of yourself that you really like: from the photos on the mantelpiece to the pix you send to friends. And the photos on your Facebook 'wall', or in your online albums.

There's also a great deal more you can do to look your absolute best in photos than just simply say 'cheese'… We can't all look like the wondrous Carmen dell'Orefice (still a supermodel at 79 as we go to press) but we can look pretty damn good.

Don't be photographed before lunchtime. No, we really mean it: most of the early morning puffiness will have diminished by then – and eyes will appear more awake. (And it also gives time to get to the hairdresser, if required. You think we ever have our official pictures taken without hitting John Frieda first? No. Way.)

Remember: this is no time to go bare-faced. Make-up artist Bobbi Brown recommends a yellow-toned foundation and concealer (rather than anything with a hint of pink), as these look better on film. Use a mattifying foundation, rather than a dewy finish; apply with a sponge sparingly, and use concealer to even out any flaws such as broken veins, under-eye circles. Be aware, though, that pen-style light-reflecting concealers – designed to work on dark circles – can bounce back so much light if used with flash photography, they create a 'reverse-panda' effect. Brush translucent powder over the face and exposed skin on the neckline. Avoid shimmer, as any flash will exaggerate shine.

Use matt eyeshadows. Browns and greys look best in photos, with black or brown eyeliner, close to your lashes on top (and, if you like, bottom) lid. Use black or brown waterproof mascara, as any flash can lead to 'tear-ing', thus smudging your lashes.

Go for an enhanced lip-coloured lipstick. Something mid-rose, or a bit deeper – the colour of your lips only a bit more so. These are the shades we generally recommend anyway, but in pictures bright reds, corals and oranges look super-garish.

Stay out of strong sunlight. This creates major nose shadows and makes you squint. Outdoors, open shade is best – daylight under an awning or a tree. As model Lisa Snowdon says, 'Midday sun is the equivalent of looking at yourself in the mirror under an incredibly harsh spotlight, and is very ageing.'

Try 'the golden hour' instead. As Lisa adds, 'This is the first or last hour of sunlight of the day. This is the optimum time for photographs, when you cannot fail to look your absolute best.'

Pretend the photographer is your best friend. You'll be more yourself and your face will take on a more normal expression.

Relax your mouth. Make-up artist Tricia Sawyer recommends saying A-E-I-O-U to achieve this; to give the face a better shape and diminish a double chin, push your tongue against the back of your top teeth. Try not to crinkle your face into a big grin, as this will exaggerate lines around the eyes, but 'twinkle' with them.

Stand slightly sideways – and follow the beauty queens' advice. Angling the body slightly will make you look slimmer. Then put one foot in front of the other, which miraculously narrows the silhouette of the leg.

Never be photographed from below. This is the fastest-track to double chins and awful photographs. Instead, it helps if the photographer is positioned slightly above you: tilting your face up into the camera is hugely flattering (unless you have a long nose). Shots taken full-on can make a wide face look wider; try tilting your head slightly if the photographer is directly in front of you.

B-r-e-a-t-h-e. Many of us find it stressful having our photo taken, but if you hold your breath you'll look 'frozen'. Breathing out relaxes the face and body; inhaling raises shoulders and can give you a look of panic. So first take a few long, deep breaths.

And if all else fails, retouch. You think Hollywood stars REALLY look the way we see them? Online and on the high street you can get photos retouched. Or change to the more forgiving hues of black and white. Whatever it takes to get a photo you love is fine.

Don't let rosacea give you the blues

It used to be blushing that was embarrassing. Well, nowadays for getting-older women there seems to be an increasing problem with redness and rosacea. If you don't quite love your rosy cheeks (yet), here are some ideas

Although a fiery skin can sometimes affect young women, for others the problem starts as they get older. The causes of redness and rosacea are still pretty mysterious – basically something in the bloodstream triggers the swelling of blood vessels in the skin, causing inflammation (redness and soreness).

The triggers are notoriously individual, including food, alcohol, stress, pollution and perimenopause. There may also be inherited components which predispose people to redness: also it shows up much more on people with thin, fair skins.

However, there are some general guidelines which may help, as we learnt from Marie-Véronique Nadeau, the Californian former chemistry teacher who – after 'struggling' with rosacea from her early thirties – started her own skincare company (Marie Veronique Organics) to help people with problem skins. Here's her advice for dealing with inflammatory skin conditions:

Take turmeric faithfully. This Indian spice is a lifesaver for minimising flare-ups: take a 400mg capsule morning and night. It's hard to get enough by sprinkling it on your food, but do that too!

Use products with zinc oxide. As well as providing sun protection and helping wound-healing, this mineral is anti-inflammatory, so helps with most skin conditions including rosacea and also acne. Apply products which contain it (such as Marie Veronique Organics Everyday Coverage SPF30). Other helpful anti-inflammatory ingredients include emu oil, red raspberry oil and aloe.

Take specific supplements. In addition to a good anti-inflammatory diet (plenty of nuts and seeds, vegetables and fruit, oily fish if you're not vegetarian), Marie-Véronique says it's 'an absolute must' to supplement with vitamin C, vitamin D3 and omega-3 essential fatty acids. (See page 180 for more on supplements.) Rosacea patients may also need more of a specific and powerful antioxidant called SOD (superoxide dismutase), so add that in too. NB: Marie-Véronique advises avoiding iron supplements, particularly if you have severe rosacea, as iron may aggravate it.

Monitor your reaction to 'heating' foods. Caffeine, red wine, curries and so on affect redness-prone people differently (see Maggie Alderson's experience opposite). The only advice is to turn detective and track your own personal response.

Beware the sun (and sunbeds). Ultraviolet light and particularly UVA – the longer-wavelength rays that are linked to skin damage and also now to skin cancers – seem to affect some rosacea sufferers severely. Everyone should take care in the sun – ie, always wear sun protection and never fry your skin. But for anyone with skin sensitivity of any kind, it's wise to avoid sunscreens with a chemical sunblock since they are known to be more likely to cause irritation. Opt instead for sunblocks using minerals, preferably zinc oxide (see left). Additionally, avoid anything with citrus essential oils and any product at all with alcohol.

ROSACEA – WHAT WORKS FOR ME

Novelist Maggie Alderson developed rosacea in 2002, when she was in her early forties. Here, she describes her strategies for making the best of what can be a lifelong condition.

'Tucked away at the top of my bathroom cupboard I keep an insurance policy, in the form of a pack of antibiotics my doctor prescribed for my rosacea. I hate the idea of taking oral antibiotics for anything short of a life-threatening infection, but I keep them there just in case the day comes when I really can't live with the raised and angry red blotches on my face any longer.

'I came close to it last summer after using cheap chemical sunblock on holiday and ending up with cheeks and chin almost as red and sore as the worst sunburn, but I managed to get through it by binning the block in favour of hats and beach umbrellas – and giving up wine with dinner. After eight years with this progressively worsening condition, I have found that what you swallow makes as big a difference – if not more – than what you slap on. Coffee, white wine and spicy food are my worst triggers, but apart from sunblock, the other most aggravating factor is stress. Which is ironic, as having a face like an overcooked pepperoni pizza is pretty stressful itself.

'I have tried legion topical products over the eight years or so I've had the condition, from prescribed antibiotic creams to exotic blue potions from imported beauty companies. Some of them worked for a bit, but none of them will cure rosacea. There isn't a cure but one effective temporary treatment I've found is acupuncture, which can settle down a really bad episode – although I know it will always come back.

'So rather than wasting more time and money searching for the miracle, I've come to accept it and, like someone with a port wine mark, put my energy into concealment. You simply have to wear make-up every day.

'The best conventional base I've found is Giorgio Armani Designer Shaping Cream Foundation SPF20, used with Laura Mercier concealer, but more recently I've been exploring mineral

SUPPLEMENTARY BENEFITS

As well as increasing omega-3 essential fatty acids both in the diet and as a supplement, pharmacist Shabir Daya advises taking a probiotic supplement: 'These beneficial bacteria will help to rid the gut of potential toxins that inflame the skin but more importantly they may ensure that specific "bad" bacteria do not proliferate.' Also try anti-inflammatory herbs such as red clover and echinacea, plus yellow dock and dandelion, which have mild diuretic properties to help eliminate the troublesome toxins. A topical serum with pycnogenol (a powerful antioxidant and anti-inflammatory) may also help, he says: 'It immediately reduces redness and inflammation and also strengthens the collagen matrix and in doing so reduces the capability of these toxins to inflame the skin.'

> 'I've come to accept it and put my energy into concealment. You simply have to wear make-up every day'

make-up. It takes a bit of getting used to but once you get the hang of layering on the fine dust, the coverage is extraordinary, with a lovely dewy finish which doesn't look – or feel – too make-up-y.

'I'm also seeing signs of improvement to my skin. bareMinerals claim their products can help rosacea and mine has certainly calmed down significantly since I've been using it. The marks are still there, but they aren't nearly so raised and crusty.

'Most importantly, I know I now have a tool I can rely on to get me out of the house without embarrassment, even if I have the worst flare-up.

'One other tip: as well as the red weals and flaking spots, rosacea makes your facial skin as dry as a crocodile handbag. After sampling every miracle moisturiser on the market, the one that really makes the difference is Superskin Moisturiser by Liz Earle.'

Redness treatments: our award winners

We'll be frank: we didn't have incredibly high hopes for these. However, the products here – all of them trialled by panellists who put themselves forward because they have redness or mild rosacea – out-performed our expectations. We are seeing rapid growth in this category of products: redness has suddenly been identified as a 'boom' area by the beauty industry. Do remember that inflamed conditions are notoriously individual, so what works for some may not work for all

AT A GLANCE

Murad Redness Therapy Recovery Treatment Gel

Avène Anti-Redness Day Protective Moisturising Cream SPF20

Darphin Intral Redness Relief Soothing Serum

Dermalogica Redness Relief SPF20

NB **These products are (mostly) not designed as moisturisers, and many women will need to use them with, not instead of, day and/or night creams.**

REVIEWS

Murad Redness Therapy Recovery Treatment Gel

 8.14/10

Uber-antioxidant goji berry is the key anti-inflammatory agent in this gel (goji has 500 times the vitamin C of oranges, and more beta-carotene than carrots, FYI!). It accelerates the healing of dry, flaky skin, and the light gel also features soothing zinc oxide, azaleic acid, vitamin K and peppermint leaf extract, to reduce sensitivity. Dr Howard Murad helped pioneer the whole category of dermatologist skincare, and this is one of a capsule range within his brand specifically to target redness.

Comments: 'Sank in so quickly and left no residue, and I can't tell you how happy I am with this: my redness has demised, and my acne-enraged nose is a distant memory; my skin looks how it used to before all this started. I had become so self-conscious I hated going out even for the school run; I have spent a lot of money on creams before finding this – it's cleared up a lot of the problem with only the odd blip which is gone really quickly and without stress' • 'nice almost milk-like texture and it worked!' • 'left my face a lot less red than it was before – I now use every morning and will buy more' • 'lovely to use and very good results' • 'rosacea is definitely calmed, the broken veins are the same but I flush much more mildly, less red and less often – the only product I have really seen a difference with'.

Avène Anti-Redness Day Protective Moisturising Cream SPF20

7.89/10

If you've ever set foot inside a French pharmacy you'll be familiar with this range, which has a particular soothing thermal spa water at the heart of every product and specifically targets 'intolerant' skin (think: sensitivity, hyperkeratosis, rosacea, etc). From the 'anti-redness' collection, this daily moisturiser offers a high concentration of butcher's broom (Ruscus aculeatus) extract, renowned for its constricting action on blood vessels. There's a useful SPF20: redness-sufferers don't always realise that sun protection can play a vital role in easing this worrisome problem.

Comments: 'My skin is now much more even-toned – after a few days skin felt less "angry", more settled and resilient' • 'I hadn't heard of this brand before but now will be trying some of their other products' • 'the pale green colour – to counteract redness – doesn't show up when applied; gave skin a glow and made it soft to the touch' • 'although there's an SPF20, it has none of the grey tint/film I'd associate with that, which is a bonus' • 'skin looks more even and is less greasy, too' • 'fewer spots in the area where my hair touches my face'.

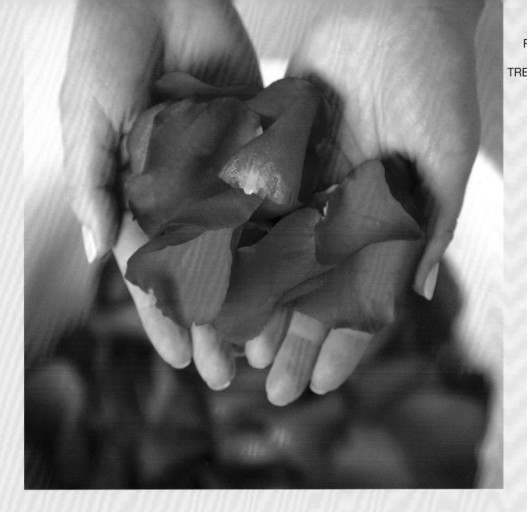

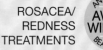

ANTI-AGEING
AWARD
WINNERS
BEAUTY BIBLE

Darphin Intral Redness Relief Soothing Serum

7.81/10 This is part of a recently introduced range from Darphin for sensitive skins, created to help strengthen skin while diminishing the appearance of redness. Calming botanicals include grape extract, antioxidant resveratrol, chamomile, hawthorn and peony extracts, in a gentle baby-pink serum.

Comments: 'After two minutes, my very red sensitive cheeks with thread veins felt soothed, and smoothed; moisturiser glided on; I looked forward to applying this every morning as it cooled my skin and took the extreme redness from my cheeks; skin more even and hydrated and I didn't have to use so much make-up to cover. Colleagues and family have noticed the improvement, which is lovely' • 'finally found something that's gentle and effective, will be investing in the accompanying products. Very, very pleased!' • 'skin looks healthy and not as red' • 'I loved this product, it worked brilliantly – 10/10!' • 'after two weeks my skin was less prone to redness'.

Dermalogica Redness Relief SPF20

7.69/10 A new award winner from skin therapy brand Dermalogica's Ultra-Calming range, which was formulated to relieve visible symptoms immediately and also to address deeper causes. This contains anti-inflammatory oat and plant actives plus hydrated chromium oxide, a natural earth mineral. It gives a sheer but concealing green tint, which blends in easily to neutralise the appearance of flushing. With chemical and physical sunscreens (essential for redness sufferers), this can be used as a spot treatment, all over as a primer or mixed into a prescribed moisturiser.

Comments: 'I suffer from rosacea and this left a matte finish which was a perfect base for foundation; skin looked clearer and more radiant and even on a hot day I didn't show any redness' • 'my redness was reduced a lot after using this for several weeks; my husband said my skin was clearer: I am very happy with this product' • 'takes a few rubs to sink in and was very soothing to my red areas, a great neutraliser, very effective at concealing the redness plus it made my skin very smooth and primed for make-up'.

TIP

A friend with flaming cheeks divulged that her secret soother is a spray of organic Pukka Rosewater which she takes everywhere. (It's in a glass bottle but not too big or heavy for most handbags; at home do keep it in the fridge for maximum effect.)

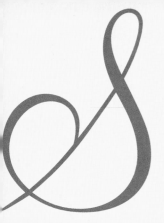

Serums: our award winners

Serums are hot anti-ageing beauty news. A week never goes by now without several new serums landing on our desks: there's a real anti-ageing 'beauty buzz' about them. The reason is that it's possible to concentrate higher levels of active ingredients in a serum – so potentially they can deliver impressive results. And you don't have to give up favourite day or night creams because serums are usually designed to be layered with them

AT A GLANCE

Darphin Predermine Firming Wrinkle Repair Serum

Dermalogica Multivitamin Power Serum

Pinks Boutique Anti-Aging Serum

YSL Forever Youth Liberator Serum

TIP

Allow serum to absorb for a few minutes before applying your moisturiser. Pay attention to areas where skin is thin and easily damaged, such as your neck and décolletage.

So: do the benefits live up to the serum hype? Or are serums just another way to get us to part with more hard-earned cash? They can be very pricey – right up to a heart-stopping £1,500, though these winners were significantly less expensive. Our testers were certainly impressed with the following, and we trialled dozens more for this very latest edition – with two new very high-scoring entries from Darphin and Dermalogica. Just remember, more is not more with these products – like facial oils, you need three to four drops for your whole face.

REVIEWS

Darphin Predermine Firming Wrinkle Repair Serum

8.79/10 From an iconic French brand, which specialises in products for older skin, this new category winner features Darphin's innovative Smart Firming System. This uses naturally derived molecules acts to stimulate collagen production, then to reorganise and restore elastin, giving complexions smoothness and bounce back. (The formulation does not contain parabens, mineral oils or animal based ingredients.) It's designed to apply in the morning, with a second application in the evening if your skin really needs a bit more support.

Comments: 'A dream to use and skin looked much smoother, lines and wrinkles were much softer. After two weeks, the lines appear less prominent and skin looked much brighter' • 'lovely light texture, after 24 hours there was a noticeable difference in my skin tone and brightness, overall it looked plumped and felt hydrated. After two weeks I saw an improvement in crêpeyness round my eyes and noticeable improvement in brighteness and tone' • 'brilliant results, my skin has definitely improved in softness, brightness and plumpness' • 'I LOVED this, sank straight in leaving my skin feeling like silk. It really blurs the fine lines, which are much less noticeable and great improvement on crêpey neck too. I can't remember having such noticeable results from anything and so quickly. After finishing the bottle, the difference is very noticeable'.

Dermalogica Multivitamin Power Serum

 This high-tech formula from a multi-award winning brand, which sells through skincare therapists, is desinged for ageing skin and offers a new 'skin-friendly' form of vitamin A plus other antioxidant vitamins and a new retinoid ester to 'intercept' the first signs of ageing and support

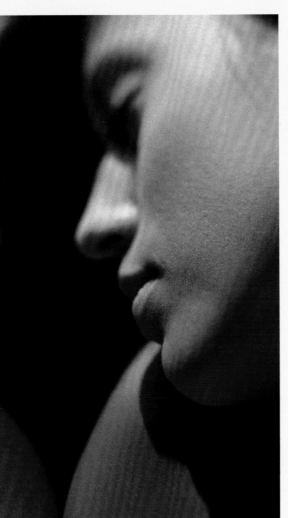

 Pinks Boutique Anti-Aging Serum ❋ ❋ ❋

8.57/10 Intended ideally for use under night cream or balm, a Soil Association-certified blend of rosehip, avocado, camellia and jojoba that's packed with antioxidants and sun-damage-repairing botanicals. British-born Pinks Boutique is one of the few organic 'spa' brands around and if you're a wannabe-natural beauty, their website is worth checking out for salon locations.

Comments: 'Skin immediately looked a bit more radiant, with a bit more colour in my cheeks, and after two weeks, crow's feet less noticeable, with overall plumpness and healthy glow. I love, love, love it, definitely improves my complexion and makes it looks less tired; plus my big frown line has magically reduced! I've become slightly obsessed with it…' • 'bottle goes a very long way as you only use a few drops, skin looks brighter and healthier' • 'noticeable difference with the side I applied it to – softer, smoother and plumper – and the other side of my face!' • 'skin looked much more nourished, brighter and younger after just two weeks – woo hoo! Lots of fab comments'.

YSL Forever Youth Liberator Serum

8.56/10 Trust us: you virtually need a PhD in Chemistry to decipher the press release that seeks to explain why this serum – from YSL's super-duper-high-tech range – is effective. Apparently it's all down to glycobiology (which has somehow been involved in seven Nobel prizes), and a trademarked ingredient called Glycanactif. But really, this is where we think Beauty Bible's value lies: our testers' comments – based on what they saw with their own eyes after months of use – will tell you more than marketing spiel ever, ever can.

Comments: 'Smooth silky luxurious feeling serum that glides on and sinks into skin. Within 24 hours, my skin was softer and smoother, after two weeks, skin was much plumper and brighter' • 'I look more alert, less tired and that dull washed out look has gone; skin doesn't look as thin/fine as before' • 'my skin looked brighter and fresher, and lines around eyes reduced so I feel more confident wearing contact lenses' • 'instantly brightened skin and gave dewy look; after two weeks, I noticed an improvement in crow's feet and lines from nose to mouth are softer and less deep, upper eyelids definitely less crêpey and firmer so eye make-up looks better' • 'a really great product'.

collagen and elastin. It's meant for daytime use, although one tester also used the serum – more like a 'paste-like cream', she said – at night and was very happy with it (as were the others).
Comments: '10/10! Gorgeous silky soft texture that sank in instantly, luxurious without being too rich; immediate smoothing and softening effect; a month into using it my skin looked brighter, toned and fine lines smoothed' • 'I applied to one side of my face first and was amazed to find how smooth my skin felt; after two weeks my skin felt and looked smoother and fine lines round my eyes minimised, skin continued to look brighter' • 'I took a photo of a large wrinkle on my forehead before starting and compared it at the end of the tube – it has definitely subsided. Previously Botox was the only thing that made a difference – indeed one of my friends thought I'd sneakily had Botox as my skin has been looking so smooth (I haven't)' • 'has a noticeable smoothing effect and skin feels tighter and firmer'.

♡ **WE LOVE…**

Two, for Jo, who now uses a serum almost religiously as part of her anti-ageing regime – and alternates one month with This Works, the next with Sarah Chapman. (To avoid boredom, mostly!) This Works products feature heavily in Jo's life, in this case No Wrinkles Wonder Essence: super-lightweight but with a heavenly rose smell. ESPA Skin Radiance Intensive Serum has a deliciously silky texture that Jo actively looks forward to using at night. Sarah is a big fan of Aurelia's Revitalise & Glow Serum, which does exactly what it says on the bottle. (Pop a drop of serum into your foundation for instant radiance.) For month-long boosts, she is impressed by Bioeffect 30 Day Treatment, which contains a barley-derived epidermal growth factor and claims a cumulative effect. (Costly though.) For a beauty steal, she favours Trilogy CoQ10 Booster Serum.

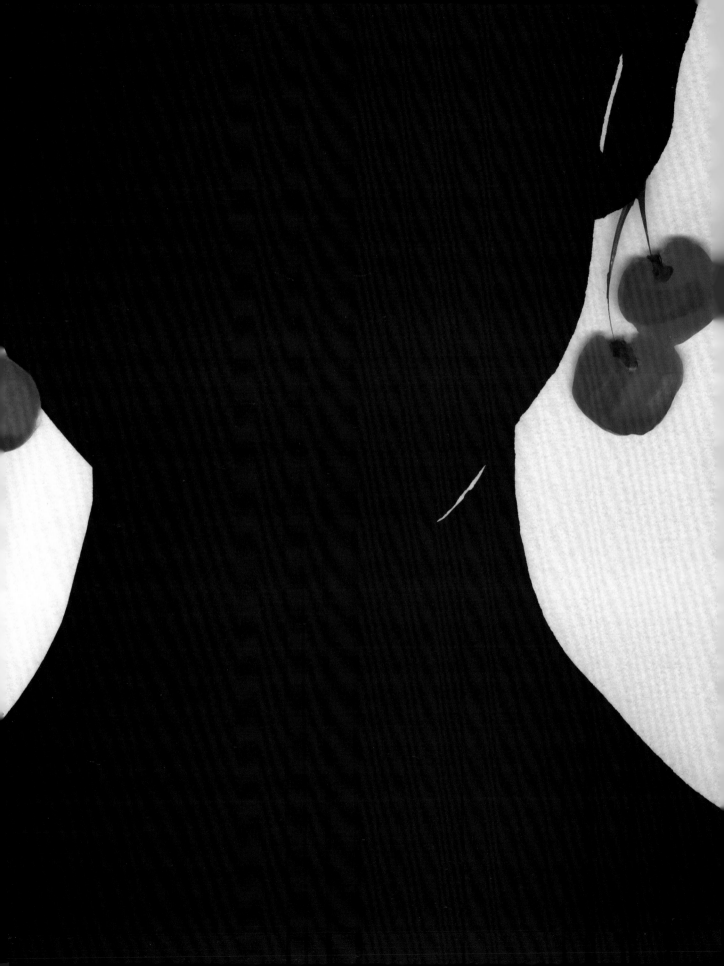

'Don't hold on to *anger*, or *regrets* – it's AGEING. Kindness is GOOD for the skin'

Marie Helvin

Supergreens Facelift Diet

Give yourself a natural face (and body) lift with this plant-loving diet

We could write a whole book about healthy eating (maybe one day we will). And by now you probably know the basics of what you should and shouldn't be munching for general health maintenance. (And if weight has become an issue, you can read all about a different approach to help you shed pounds in our section on middle-age spread and mindful eating on page 144.)

But here's something wonderful. We truly believe that you have it in your power to slow down the process of ageing (or speed it up, of course, if you do the wrong things). We're not talking about delaying the ravages of time with cosmetic surgery but by what you eat. (As well as other lifestyle steps such as sleep and exercise.)

There are two big processes that cause our skin (and indeed all the cells in our body) to age: dehydration and inflammation. You know the culprits! A poor diet, smoking (you don't, do you?), sun and alcohol, plus late nights, psychological stress, a polluted environment and not enough exercise. But eating plants – mostly fresh greens (mostly raw) – helps to hydrate every cell in your body. And that keeps your skin plump and moist. Add in lifestyle shifts such as more sleep, sun protection and exercise, and your skin will 'bounce-back' – as they call its suppleness capacity – like a Duracell bunny!

Chlorophyll-rich greens are packed with amino acids, which are the building blocks of all protein. Unlike animal protein (where the body has to work to break apart the protein into the separate amino acids), green plants offer you instantly absorbable amino acids to transform into protein.

We learned about this concept by trying a green food supplement called Sun Chlorella from Japan. This superfood settles your gut into a state of delicious calm and efficiency. And when that happens, it helps to 'lift' your face and peachify your skin (Sarah couldn't believe it when she first noticed the transformation after taking Sun Chlorella for a month or so).

The reason? Your skin is the mirror of your digestion and, according to Traditional Chinese Medicine practitioner and nutritionist Nadia Brydon, there are two pairs of energy (Qi) lines called meridians running down your face. If your gut is unhappy, the lines droop and so does your face. Stabilise your digestion and whoosh! The energy is replenished and everything goes upwards.

It's not just your face that sags, says Nadia, because the same meridian runs down through your breasts and stomach. 'When we eat too many foods high in calories and refined carbohydrates and low in micronutrients, we're hastening the sagging in these areas too; eat foods high in micronutrients and low in calories – such as fresh greens – and we help to tone, contract, firm and pull up the droops from the inside.'

The Supergreens Facelift Diet (see overleaf) cleanses the skin from the inside, toning, feeding, hydrating, lifting, moisturising, reducing puffiness and wrinkles – and putting back your glow from top to toe! In fact, the very best face and body lift we can give ourselves is to eat more greens in our diet every day, starting with an anti-ageing supergreen smoothie (see box overleaf). Then do the Supergreens Facelift Diet for two to three days once every three months (minimum).

Try following this diet for two days to start with, preferably over a weekend when you can rest as much as you want to. Do some gentle cardiovascular exercise for at least half an hour a day: walking is fine – dancing if you prefer, or jogging, swimming, hockey. Whatever pleases you.

Do remember this is not meant to be a penance. Make sure you have lovely clean fresh bedlinen, bath towels and nightie; your favourite music and DVDs, a stack of glossy magazines and whatever else you enjoy! Go out if you want to – lead your normal life, just stick to the diet.

It's often fun to do these things with a partner, so ask a girlfriend – or lover/spouse if they're game. But choose someone where there's no tension attached.

> 'If you starve yourself to the point where your brain cells shrivel, you will never do good work' Cate Blanchett

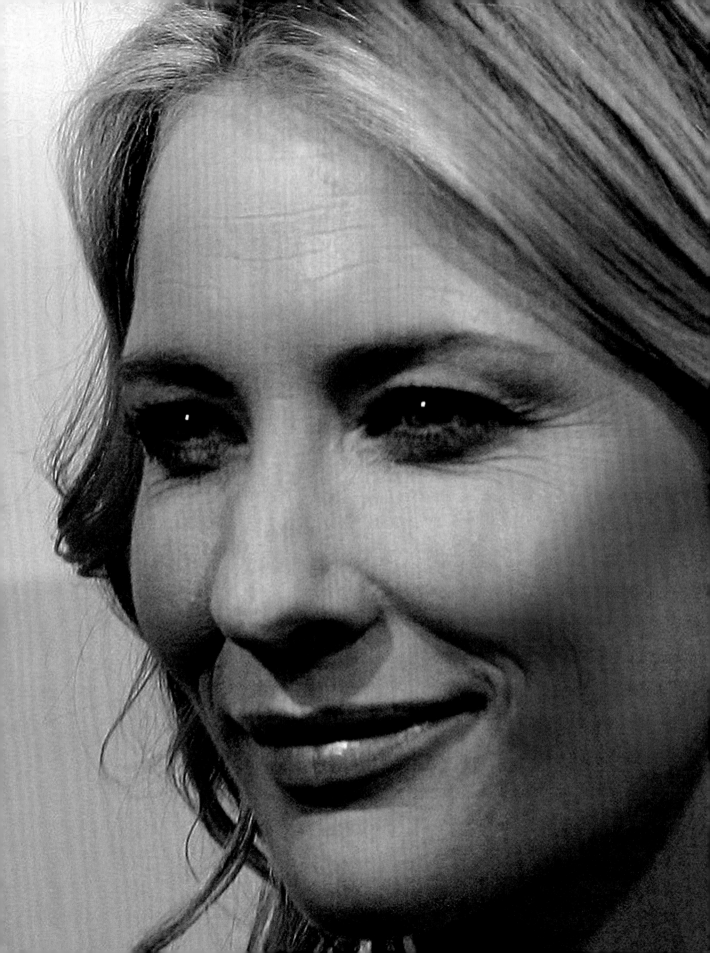

FRIDAY NIGHT

Prep for your weekend by eating a light evening meal between 6pm and 7.30pm. Always leave at least two hours between eating and going to bed. And do plan for an early night.

SATURDAY/SUNDAY

- First thing, drink a large glass of room-temperature water, with a slice of lemon if liked.
- Follow with half an hour of yoga stretching and meditation, or a walk. Salute to the Sun will start your day beautifully whatever age/fitness you are; for easy-to-follow instructions see www.yogasite.com/sunsalute.htm.
- Apply a hair mask before starting, if you wish.
- Brush teeth and tongue, gargle with slightly salted room-temperature water and splash face with cold water to wake up and contract facial skin cells.
- Before showering, body-brush your whole body with a soft, natural brush or mitten to help stimulate and detox the skin and lymph system. Brush from extremities towards the heart.
- Take a shower, ending with hot and cold hydrotherapy water treatment: alternate hot and cold water for half a minute each, repeat seven times in all. End with hot water before bed, cold water in the morning or before a night out. This contracts and relaxes every cell and moves the circulation, so helping to eliminate toxins.
- Shampoo and condition your hair in the shower.
- Moisturise from top to toe.
- Fill 2 x 1 litre bottles with natural spring (or filtered) water, and sip through the day.

THE DIET

Breakfast
Drink half your Supergreen Smoothie (see recipe right)

Mid-morning snack
- Sip half your remaining Supergreen Smoothie
- 50g soaked almonds and 100g white grapes or raw peas, carrots/cucumber sticks

Lunch
- 100–175g steamed or grilled fresh fish of any sort (just not tinned or frozen)
OR 100–175g fresh tofu
OR half an avocado
- 200–400g mixed salad: make a big salad with some or all of the following: torn leaves of lettuce, rocket (arugula), watercress, basil and spinach; chopped red pepper and cucumber; grated carrot and beetroot, radishes, spring onion; 110g living sprouting seeds, eg, alfalfa, pulses, mung bean shoots; 1 teaspoon pumpkin and sunflower seeds. Dress with 1 tablespoon extra virgin cold pressed olive oil and lemon juice, with salt and freshly ground black pepper to taste
- Pudding: 200g mixed berries
OR 100g papaya
OR 100g apple/pear/grapes
- Sip 350ml natural spring water (more if wished)

Mid-afternoon snack
- Drink remainder of anti-ageing/anti-inflammatory Supergreen Smoothie
- Apple or pear or 100g grapes
- 350ml natural spring water (more if you wish)

Evening meal
- 100–175g fresh organic chicken
OR fresh tofu
OR avocado
OR roasted/steamed vegetable medley seasoned with fresh herbs
- Mixed salad and pudding, as above
- 350ml natural spring water or more if desired

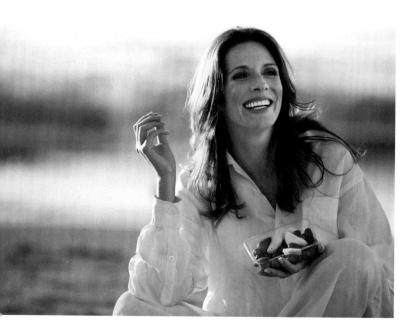

SUPERGREEN SMOOTHIE

Pure rocket fuel! This will help reduce your appetite, rejuvenate your skin and whole body, plus give you endless energy. Drinking it in the morning reduces your appetite for sweet tastes so it helps balance blood-sugar levels. Always store in the fridge in a screw-top jar (or wide-necked vacuum flask) and make fresh daily.

Makes about 1 litre in all. All measurements are approximate, so don't fret about being exact.

Blend together
● 600ml still mineral water
● ¹/₂ chopped cucumber with skin and pips
● ¹/₄ peeled avocado
● 1 chopped celery stick
● juice of ¹/₂ lemon or lime
● ¹/₄ teaspoon unrefined salt
● small double handful of mixed green leaves (60–80g) from the following: spinach, chicory, watercress, rocket (arugula), Savoy cabbage, chard, lettuce, kale, bok choy (Chinese cabbage), sprigs of mint, parsley, coriander, basil, etc (you can often buy bags of organic mixed green leaves)

● 5–15 pillules Sun Chlorella A (if not used to greens in diet, use 5 tablets for the first 3 days, then build up to 15 over the week)

Plus, optionally
● 1 clove garlic
● 1-2 slices of fresh ginger (5-10g)
● 1 small chopped spring onion
● ¹/₂ apple or ¹/₂ pear or 100g papaya, mango or melon to sweeten slightly

If you are constipated
● 1 tablespoon fresh flax oil or ground flax seeds

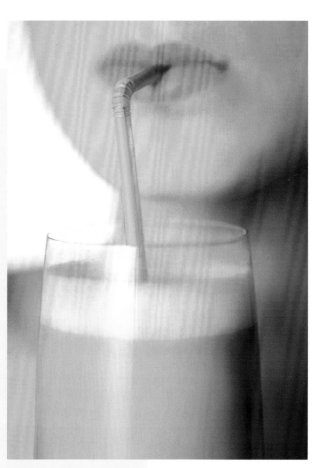

'Eat food. Not too much. Mainly plants'

Michael Pollan's 'Food Rules'

LOVE THESE FOODS

Organic where possible
● Fresh vegetables, freshly made veggie soups and juices
● Fresh salads
● Sprouted seeds and pulses
● Fresh fruit
● Nuts and seeds (soak nuts for 12 hours at room temperature)
● Fresh fish including sushi
● Tofu
● Lean meat/game
● Hot water with slice of lemon
● Spring water
● Herb teas eg, ginger, fennel, peppermint

REDUCE THESE FOODS

● All processed sugar and sweeteners
● Processed and tinned foods
● Junk foods
● Dairy products
● Wheat products (especially 'industrialised' bread; if you want to eat bread, look for long-fermented sourdoughs from artisan bakeries)
● Red meat
● Crisps and peanuts
● Pasta and pizza
● Any foods with E numbers and additives
● Sweets/chocolate
● Tap water
● Coffee
● Fizzy drinks
● Alcohol

Discover the supplements you really need

You could spend a fortune on supplements. Or you could miss them out altogether. Neither are good options for optimal health and beauty, we feel…

Consider investing in these basics. Leading experts worldwide consider these the ones you really should include.

● **Multivitamins and minerals:** research shows that even people eating the best diet possible nowadays are deficient in some essential nutrients. Result: you feel and look under par, you're more likely to get ill and you have less energy all round. Invest in a good product, food state if possible for maximum absorption (and value).
Try: All Natural Perfectly Balanced Multinutrients, which contains vitamins, minerals, antioxidants, green foods (including blue green algae, chlorophyll and spirulina), plus liver-cleansing herbs and probiotics (to keep your gut in great order).

● **Omega-3 essential fatty acid:** our bodies don't make essential fatty acids, of which omega-3 is the most important. We need it for pretty well everything in our bodies, including keeping our skin plump, soft and supple. It fortifies hair and nails too. If not veggie try to eat two portions of omega-3 rich oily fish a week, and consider a supplement. Look for a product with EPA and DHA, either based on fish oil, krill or the plant echium.

Try: Ideal Omega 3 by Ideal Omega, a particularly pure form of fish oil, but for those who don't like fish, or are veggie, try Echiomega from the plant *Echium plantagineum*.

● **Vitamin D:** research suggests that at least 50 per cent of adults are deficient in this 'sunshine' vitamin, particularly as we get older. It's vital for your bones, muscles and the immune system, among other functions. It also helps to ward off low mood and depression. Scientists now suggest taking 1,000-2,000 IU daily.
Try: D Lux 1000 spray by Better You – it tastes of lemon and is absorbed rapidly.

We think it's worth adding in these too: you probably won't need or want to take all of them, so read through and see which seem most relevant to you.

● **Phyto-oestrogens:** we don't take HRT (though we're totally sympathetic to women who've tried everything else and feel it's worth the risks), but we do like plant oestrogens which help to mimic our natural hormones and help with hot flushes, night sweats and vaginal dryness.
Try: Sage Complex by Food Science of Vermont, which contains sage, wild yam, dong quai, red clover and a bunch of other herbs including Siberian ginseng, hops, pomegranate extract, fenugreek seeds and kudzu.

● **Digestive enzymes:** as the years pass, our natural supply of digestive enzymes to process food declines, leading to bloating, wind, bad breath – oh dear!
Try: Extrazyme-13 by LifeTime vitamins – a capsule before a meal should do the trick.

● **Hyaluronic acid:** the latest compound to be dubbed the 'fountain of youth' – and with some justice. A protein that can hold 1,000 times its own weight in water, it plumps up skin cells, so helping to erase fine lines and wrinkles. Levels decline with

> 50 per cent of adults are deficient in 'sunshine' vitamin D, particularly as we get older

age: as much as 50 per cent by the age of forty.
It's also a key factor in keeping joints lubricated
and working smoothly. And another thing (or
two): it may help dry eye syndrome and also
vaginal dryness.

Try: Hyaluronic Acid Capsules High Strength by
LifeTime Vitamins, one to two capsules daily.

● **Co-enzyme Q10 (aka Co-Q10):** this vitamin-
like compound, which also declines with age, is
essential for keeping your muscles (including your
heart), gums and immune system in good shape,
and it's vital for anti-ageing in all ways, as well as
helping with energy generally. NB: If you take a
statin (to lower cholesterol), it's important to take
Co-Q10 too as the statin can block production of
Co-Q10 and this may create problems in itself.

Try: Super Ubiquinol by Life Extension – ubiquinol
is the active form of Co-Q10. Most products are
formulated as ubiquinone which is then converted
into ubiquinol; taking this supplement as ubiquinol
tends to suit people with any sort of digestive
problem such as IBS (irritable bowel syndrome) or
sluggishness. Take one daily with food.

How to fade your stretch marks

Most women have looked down their body at some point and gasped as they saw the zigzag lines embellishing their skin. We can't really pretend they're gorgeous, so if you can't learn to love them (or at least live with them), we have ways of making them less…

Stretch marks shouldn't be called stretch marks at all – they're really 'hormone' marks. They may happen at puberty (when hormones kick in), pregnancy (ditto) and even sometimes at menopause (which seems especially cruel, if you ask us, considering all the other stuff we have to deal with). It's a bit of a hormonal lottery as to whether you'll get them, but women (and some men) do also get them after weight loss and weight gain (that was Sarah). And the bottom line is that however stretch marks appear on your body, they can cause some distress. So: what to do? Below you will find some general tips – and overleaf, the products our ten women tester panels voted the most effective (and somewhat to our surprise, some really were).

Do as they do in the Mediterranean. Oil yourself. Liberally. Regularly. Olive oil, cocoa butter, shea butter, rosehip oil (which has shown great skin-healing results): all manner of rich and lavish oils will lubricate and nourish the skin. So: anoint your stretch marks at bedtime with oils. When skin is well-nourished, the marks are less obvious. It will also feel smoother and sexier, and more strokeable generally. We're all for that.

Eat foods rich in vitamin K, and plenty of essential fatty acids (EFAs). Vitamin K is a fantastic 'skin-healing' vitamin, found in leafy green vegetables (Brussels sprouts, broccoli, spinach, parsley, okra, mustard greens, peas, artichokes), lentils, kidney beans, plums, liver (if you're not vegetarian) and dairy products. To preserve the vitamin K, all the vegetables should

ideally be consumed raw, or very lightly cooked (save the water for a soup or stock, to reclaim its nutritional value). See page 180 for more about EFAs and their sources.

Live a more holistic lifestyle. This is pretty much the advice that you'll find scattered through this book (because when it comes to looking and feeling fabulous IT WORKS), but eating a good diet, exercising regularly and maintaining a stable weight may have another benefit: it may just help fade your stretch marks. OK, so this is just us speaking (not some doctor with a string of initials after his name), but Sarah used to have shiny stretch marks zigzagging up her hips on either side of her belly. After several years of healthy living – and oiling her body (see left) – she realised the marks had literally vanished. When Jo read this in the answer to a reader's question to www.beautybible.com, she decided to check out her own ancient stretch marks and discovered – to her astonishment – that they had faded too. Not a sign. We can only attribute this to consistent healthy living, and a diet that incorporates plenty of EFAs (plus supplements) and literally mountains of the types of veggies mentioned left.

Try HealGel. Anecdotally, HealGel has had remarkable results on many different types of scarring (including tough-to-treat keloid scarring). Developed by leading plastic surgeons with a biochemist, this treatment – which also works on sprains, sunburn and bruising – can be worth a shot. You need to apply it two or three times daily, and although you only need a titchy bit, that could prove an expensive option. For other options, trialled by our tester panels, see overleaf.

Buy a tankini. It's tummy stretch marks that really seem to upset the women we know. (Despite the fact that the marks are usually a proud badge of motherhood.) If the one thing standing between you and baring your stomach in public is a network of stretch marks, consider a tankini: the vest top of this style of two-piece swimsuit can be rolled up when nobody's looking, so you get the glorious feeling of air on your skin (and a touch of sun) in the privacy of your back deck/garden, or rolled down in company. Your bikini days may be over, but your tankini days needn't be.

If they really distress you, consider laser or IPL treatment. This works best with pigmented stretch marks; pale or flesh-toned marks don't respond so well to treatment – although there are now re-pigmenting lasers that can help with this. The Lux1540 laser has been approved by the FDA in the US for the treatment of stretch marks, but is only available in a handful of locations. We would certainly suggest only going to a 'master' of laser surgery (local clinics may promise the earth to get your bucks, but as with all high-tech treatments we advise major caution). Be sure you are armed with all the right questions, as per Wendy Lewis's advice on page 46. You may want to consider a pre-treatment consultation with Wendy herself (Wendy works in the US but you can contact her via email and she does consultations on Skype – see DIRECTORY). Beware: this will be expensive, and at this stage in life it's unrealistic to expect to go back to your smooth-skinned former self.

STRETCH MARKS: THE SCIENCE BIT

Stretch marks – as many of us know – start as fine red or brown lines (sometimes raised) and can deepen to purple on some people. But it's the legacy of stretch marks that causes so much heartache: they fade to a white or silver colour (usually lighter than your natural skintone), but the skin can be much (much) slacker – so it folds and, yes, hangs differently. They're most common on the abdomen, breasts, thighs and buttocks. As well as reproductive hormonal changes, why are stretch marks also linked with gaining and losing weight? According to Dr Eric F Bernstein (Clinical Associate Professor of Dermatology at the University of Pennsylvania School of Medicine, and head of the Scientific Advisory Board of www.stretchmarks.org), 'When people gain weight, our hormones are metabolised by fat cells. Hormones resemble fat and cholesterol, so when we gain and lose weight it affects the hormones in our body – and also the hormones in our skin.' Normal skin is 80 per cent collagen and just 4 per cent elastin, but that elastin is oh-so-important for skin resilience – and stretch marks are basically damaged elastin fibres. According to Dr Bernstein, 'Elastin fibres are the single hardest thing to repair in skin.'

SCAR GAZING

Beat-generation poet Fran Landesman, who's still writing and doing readings in her eighties, wrote a poem called 'Scars' – and it applies just as much to stretch marks (except that wouldn't sound so poetic…). Fran has had grateful fanmail from women who she's helped to come to terms with their scars. You can find the whole thing on www.franlandesman. com – do look. Here's a snippet we love:

Don't be ashamed
Everybody's got scars
From our various wars
On the way to the
    stars
So I'll show you my
    scars
If you show me yours
In the streets and the
    bars
Everybody's got scars
On their way to the
    stars
Everybody's got scars

SKIN TAGS

Skin tags: these tiny little growths, which may be flesh-colour, or sometimes look brown or purple-ish, are not harmful but are often unsightly and can be irritating if they are near or on your eyes, or where clothes rub. An old-fashioned DIY method was to tie a piece of cotton tightly round the base, blocking the blood supply so they eventually dropped off (ligation). However, this carries a risk of infection, so do consult your family doctor or dermatologist who can remove it with a minor surgical procedure. The most common options are cryotherapy (where very cold liquid nitrogen is applied directly to the area), cauterisation (heat is used to burn off the tag, called electrolysis), and excision (the tag is cut off with a scalpel). Your doctor will use local anaesthetic if necessary and provide an antibiotic ointment to prevent infection. If the tag is very close to the eyelid, the procedure may need to be done by an ophthalmologist.

Stretch mark treatments: our award winners

Stretch marks are a concern for expectant mothers but as the collagen and elastin in skin break down with ageing, they can be even more anxiety inducing in later life. For some women, stretch marks make an unwelcome appearance at menopause, since they're linked with hormonal upheaval rather than 'stretching'. This was one of the toughest challenges in the book: can anything lessen or reverse stretch marks? Our testers were rather pleasantly surprised overall (and so, to be honest, were we). There is a new entry by Weleda for this updated edition

AT A GLANCE

Aromatherapy Associates Renewing Rose Body Oil

Weleda Stretch Mark Massage Oil

Shiffa Healing Balm

Bio-Oil

TIP

One tester trialling the top-scoring cellulite product Thalgo Crème Thalgomince (page 38) noticed that it had a double-whammy effect, not only greatly improving cellulite but also helping to fade her silvery stretch marks. Result!

REVIEWS

Aromatherapy Associates Renewing Rose Body Oil ❀❀

8.75/10 Fascinatingly, Aromatherapy Associates resubmitted this rose, orange blossom and evening primrose-based light oil for the previous paperback – and in an incredibly tough category it came out top once again, scoring an identical mark of 8.75/10! So here are our testers' most recent comments. They just adored the all-round benefits of this oil.

Comments: 'I have some old stretch marks and new ones especially at my arms where I've lost some weight; the new stretch marks seem to be less angry/visible – but overall it helps perception of them as you feel you're "making a difference"'
• 'marks less prominent and it helped to fade the smaller stretch marks; has a lovely fragrance'
• 'used it on my stomach and marks look softer and skin feels smooth' • 'has a lovely, feminine smell that's almost a substitute for perfume; I also used it on elbows – which have "split" skin – and saw an improvement almost immediately' •
'reduced redness and also crêpiness on body'
• 'though no effect on long-standing stretch marks, I suffer from arthritis in my back and have trouble sleeping. I used this as a massage oil for my back; it helped me drift into a lovely relaxing sleep and I would purchase this again and again just for that!'.

Weleda Stretch Mark Massage Oil ❀❀❀

8.5/10 Although this pure natural formula from a favourite long-established British brand was intended to help prevent stretch marks in pregnant mums (for which it has garnered awards), our ten testers tried it on existing stretch marks. And although old silvery stretch marks were stubborn, testers said they softened their appearance – and testified that newer ones showed signs of fading, resulting in the high average score. Based on almond oil and fragranced with a mix of essential oils – geranium, lavender and orange – this rich blend also contains organic arnica to help improve skin's elasticity and tightness.

Comments: 'What a revelation! My skin was immediately really soft and smooth, not at all sticky or tacky, and the newer stretch marks on my arms much less noticeable after a couple of weeks' •
'so lovely I used it all over my stomach and breasts too – I'm having to stop myself wearing plunging necklines all the time!' • 'wondrous result on my skin, which looked more hydrated, toned and significantly smoother' • 'some of my stretch marks appeared to benefit and skin looked smoother overall and more toned'.

Shiffa Healing Balm ❀

 8.28/10 A multi-tasking luxury balm created from a blend of organic butters and oils (plus a few synthetic ingredients) by a Dubai-based doctor, this balm was specifically submitted for assessment of its action on stretch marks. To be frank, those results were a bit up-and-down: some testers saw great improvements in stretch marks, others none – but they did generally completely fall in love with the balm's fragrance, texture, and its effect on both mood and dry skin. We say: even if you're unlucky enough not to see an improvement in your stretch marks, you'll enjoy its fall-back position as a face balm/hand cream/foot treat.

Comments: 'I would marry this product if I could; my "white" stretch marks are definitely much better – much less noticeable and I can hardly "feel" them any more' • 'stretch marks are less evident – not totally faded, and although I don't believe there's a product that can magically ease them they are certainly far less noticeable' • 'made stretch marks look better as they were well-moisturised, but all-round my skin was much smoother and healthier after a week – I also used this to treat my son's eczema and it immediately reduced itching and inflammation' • 'my hands were raw and parched from frequent hand-washing – and this really turned the corner for them' • 'a slice of decadence, with multiple uses' • 'once I opened the jar and smelled the balm I was a goner…'.

Bio-Oil

8.21/10 Bio-Oil is something of a beauty legend, with many women we know swearing by its effect on scars and stretch marks, as well as an everyday (or rather, everynight) facial oil. We'd never managed to put it through its paces till the trials for this book, and it performed very well in this challenging category. We do need to knock one myth on the head, though: there's a common misconception (echoed in their marketing) that Bio-Oil is 100 per cent botanical, when the key ingredient is mineral oil. (That does happen to be amazing for helping to maintain skin's moisture.)

Comments: 'Lovely fresh smell and after a few weeks, old scars have begun to fade considerably, some gone completely, skin is smoother and less crêpey' • 'also very good on eczema on hands and boobs' • 'absorbs easily and no residue on clothes, skin now looks smoother and improvement in general texture; stretch marks still visible but my C-section scars have nearly vanished!' • 'I've used this as a preventative during my pregnancies and through diets and had very few stretch marks, which have faded by now. This is great'.

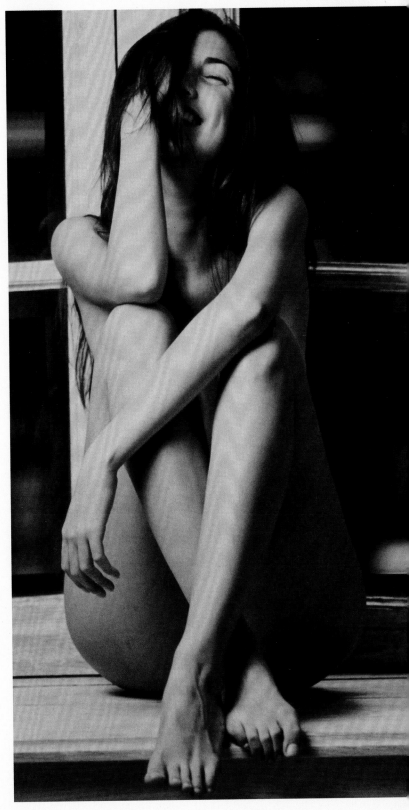

Put sun spots in the shade

Age spots. Liver spots. Whatever you like to call them, they're something we can all live without

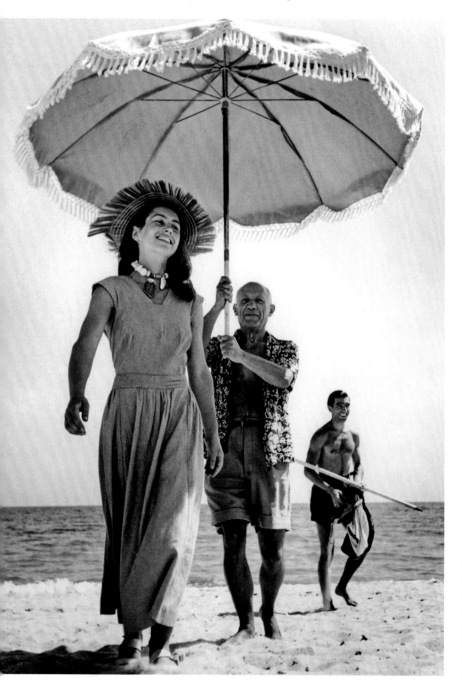

Lines we can live with. (Just.) But according to research carried out for Clinique, the problem of uneven pigmentation can be more distressing than wrinkles. The research also identified that from the perspective of a stranger looking at your skin, pigmentation issues ('dark spots', 'sun spots', 'age spots' – or to give them their formal name, 'solar lentigines') can increase your perceived age. Ironically, according to Dr Daniel Yarosh (who is Senior Vice President and Chief Technology Advisor at Estée Lauder), 'Today, these spots are appearing in people decades before their first senior moment. That is a dangerous sign that sun worship is out of control.'

It's fair to say that tackling the problem is one of The Big Beauty Challenges Of All Time (which is one reason we're so tub-thump-y about sun protection everywhere in this book) – but on the upbeat side there are steps you can take if you're troubled by uneven pigmentation.

Never venture out without an SPF30 or over. And please Start Right Now! This is non-negotiable; it should prevent the spots you have from getting any worse, and may actually go some way towards slightly fading them. If you aren't affected by age spots so far? A daily SPF15 (or higher) will go a long way to preventing their future appearance; for a rundown of the daily sun-protective moisturisers which our testers liked best, see page 188. Hand creams with a built-in SPF can be super-useful on the backs of hand/forearms. If you tend to spend a lot of time outdoors, apply regular sunscreen to these vulnerable zones, and remember to repeat after hand-washing (advice which we echo in our HANDS section, page 122).

Wear a hat. If you have sun spots, or seek to avoid their appearance, we also advise: get yourself a fabulous, stylish collection of fairly tightly-woven straw hats, and keep on a peg near your door/s, for easy grabbing when you go out on a summer day (not a baseball cap because the brims aren't big enough, plus they miss your ears which are very vulnerable). Sometimes anti-ageing solutions can be wonderfully low-tech. Wide-armed, large-lensed sunspecs also help.

Try a specific 'age spot' treatment. A vast amount of cosmetic research dollars is currently being channelled into this area of skincare. Dermatologists in some countries can still prescribe hydroquinone for the problem, but in others this skin-lightener has been banned (research showed that it caused mutations in DNA in animal lab tests – though we totally disapprove of those). And even in the US, where its use is popular, treatment with prescription 4 per cent hydroquinone is restricted to a maximum of 12 weeks. We would suggest one of the alternative over-the-counter cosmetic options – and for a shortcut to the most effective, see what really works on page 190.

Apply the product very carefully – don't slap it on before reading the directions. Be aware: most of these treatments take some time to kick in, and there are no overnight miracles here. (You're probably looking at three months minimum, which is longer than most 'miracle' wrinkle treatments take.) Be aware, too, that some are for all-over skin application, and others are literally 'spot-targeted', requiring the use of a cotton bud to apply precisely. Get out your magnifying glasses and read the instructions before throwing out (preferably recycling) the box. Another tip is to apply a thin amount to dark areas at least one

THE SCIENCE BIT

Sun spots, explains Dr Daniel Yarosh, are a direct result of accumulated sun damage, which triggers melanin-producing cells in the skin to lose control and produce too much pigment as a defence mechanism – on the face and chest, in particular, but also the arms and backs of the hands, where they're harder to conceal. Fairer skins are more susceptible – and against a paler background, age spots show up more, too. Jo had one of those 'oh s**t' moments when a dermatologist told her that the dark patches on the side of her face were sun spots, not – as she'd thought/hoped – beauty marks. Which goes to show how easy it is to miss the edges of the face and the outer jaw-line when applying sunscreen. So be sure to smooth your morning SPF into the whole face. Many botanicals have proven pigment-lightening actions, including azaleic acid (from barley and wheat), kojic acid (from fermented mushrooms), retinoic acid and retinols (vitamin A derivatives which are also famously effective against lines), magnesium ascorbyl phosphate (a stabilised form of vitamin C) and liquorice. They all work by inhibiting the melanin-producing enzyme tyrosinase.

KEEP AN EYE ON YOUR MOLES

Most people have ten to forty moles, some many more. Most moles are benign but it's always worth doing a mole check every month or so from top to toe, including your back. If you notice changes in colour (especially if moles are bi-coloured), size, height or shape, or they bleed, ooze, itch, appear scaly, or become tender and/or painful, consult your doctor or dermatologist.

hour before bedtime; this will let it fully absorb into the skin so it won't slide into your eyes when you press your face into the pillow. (Although the products are mild, skin-lightening ingredients can still sting eyes.)

Use make-up to conceal the spot. Once you've got an age spot, what's to do? For a quick fix, turn to make-up. As we explain on page 88, after your primer, dot on a matt, yellow- or peach-based corrector or concealer (deeper peach for women of colour), with a little brush,

then press it in with your finger – don't sweep it on. If needed, top with cream or liquid foundation or brush on a mineral powder base.

Be careful with fragrance. Certain perfume ingredients – particularly some derived from citrus (such as bergamot) – can interact with sunlight to cause permanent pigmentation problems, in the form of 'staining' of the skin, with dark streaks or patches – typically on the neck and chest, where perfume is spritzed or splashed. We counsel: in summer, it's safest to apply perfume to skin for evening only rather than daytime, or put it where the sun won't strike directly. (So long as there's no risk of staining your clothes, fabric is a wonderful 'carrier' for scent, too; more on page 102.)

Zap 'em. The super-high-tech solution is laser treatment, which can disperse these patches of pigmentation, literally 'zapping' the melanin into oblivion. It's painful. It's expensive. If you really decide to go down this route, turn to page 46 and arm yourself with all the advice that you need to shop around to optimise your chances of a safe, effective treatment.

Sun protective day creams: *our award winners*

In recent years, many beauty companies have added sun protection to their day creams, and some other products such as foundations. We applaud this, as most of us tend to forget that even incidental exposure – ie when we are trotting around shopping– can damage our skins. That extra bit of protection is a valuable aid in keeping our skin healthy

Remember though, that helpful as these SPF-containing cosmetics are, they should not be your only protection against solar rays. The SPF defends the skin from UV rays for a couple of hours, not more. Make sure that the label details UVA and UVB protection. UVA penetrate deep into the skin, play a major part in wrinkling and ageing, and are implicated in skin cancer. UVB is for burning, inflammation and – via those routes – ageing. But please don't think these will be adequate protection if you are sunbathing or in the sun all day.

REVIEWS

No7 Protect & Perfect Intense Day Cream SPF15

9/10 In this category, the products had to perform well as an ordinary moisturiser plus give some sun protection. This product proved a convincing new award winner. It promises advanced protection from the ageing effects of the sun and environment plus their skin-firming ori-retinol complex. Some of our testers worried that because it is targeted at 'young skin to delay the first signs of ageing' it wouldn't be potent enough. But they still liked it a lot.

Comments: 'Loved the flowery powdery smell, and it went on like a dream. I felt it made my skin look radiant and had a visible line blurring effect' • 'didn't burn after two days sunshine' • 'left skin looking smooth and fresh, somehow both matte and dewy ie not shiny' • very effective moisturiser and make-up went on really well after' • 'a great all round moisturiser with the bonus of an SPF – now a must-have' • 'I always apply an extra SPF but this does contain the famous Protect & Perfect antioxidant complex as an additional safeguard against the environment'.

Clinique Superdefense SPF25

8.88/10 Another impressively high score for Clinique, who've done very well in this book. Their thinking is that 'stress ages skin, making it dull and lifeless' (we agree!), so alongside the broad spectrum sunscreen, there are 'skin de-stressing' ingredients, including a rare red microalgae extract. It's lightweight and – being Clinique – hypoallergenic and fragrance-free.

Comments: '10/10: sank in easily, gave dewy effect and kept skin moisturised all day; good base for make-up and skin doesn't dry out after foundation/powder are applied' • 'skin felt soft and moisturised all day, looks radiant • 'love it! Moisturises very effectively, absorbs very well with no residue, it didn't aggravate my acne and was a very nice base for foundation' • 'you use very little so it lasts a long time' • 'moisturised really well, the best I have tried; sank in well leaving dewy glow'.

♡ WE LOVE...

For a couple of years now, This Works In Transit Skin Defence has been Jo's go-to SPF for summery days: it's a great make-up base, light and skin-quenching (with an SPF 30). For winter, it's Sarah Chapman London Skinesis Dynamic Defence Anti-ageing Day Cream SPF15. Sarah too has several favourites including Clinique Superdefense SPF25 and Zelens Daily Defence Sunscreen SPF 30, actually a proper sunscreen but so moisturising Sarah uses it for double duty.

Vitage Advanced Antioxidant Skincare Skin Defence SPF 30

 8.75 / 10

Vitage is a British brand that trumpets the high levels of antioxidants in all their products. In a skin-protective daily moisturiser, that's particularly useful – and here, they underpin it with an SPF30 broad spectrum cream, delivering UVA and UVB protection. Hyaluronic acid ensures optimum moisturisation, while aloe vera soothes and quenches. It's lightweight, with a matte finish, and therefore ideal under make-up.

Comments: 'I am really impressed with this product, it glides on, absorbs quickly and foundation went on very well after applying it' • 'brilliant product: you get a teeny hint of sunscreen whiteness but that disappears to leave a youthful radiant glow. Foundation went on beautifully too. I love it' • 'made skin look very dewy and soft, really calm feeling too; great moisturiser and skin had lovely healthy glow' • 'my skin lapped this up, fantastic moisturiser'.

Estée Lauder DayWear Advanced Multi-Protection Anti-Oxidant Cream SPF15

8.69 / 10

We're long-standing fans of this product, with its cool-as-a-cucumber scent and equally cooling, melts-into-skin texture. Lauder was really the first brand to share research with beauty editors into the important defensive role antioxidants play; in this updated favourite day cream there's a state-of-the-art blend that neutralises free radical damage, as well as UVA/UVB protection. It is lusciously skin-quenching yet we've always found it a good base for summer make-up. As we've recommended this to readers countless times, we're gratified DayWear makes an appearance here.

Comments: 'Smooth, gorgeous consistency, providing a good level of moisture all day' • 'love it! If you've ever mashed an avocado to use as a face mask and put slices of cucumber over your eyes, the scent of this will be familiar' • 'I've been very happy with how my skin looks while using this' • 'lovely texture – soothing and smoothing'.

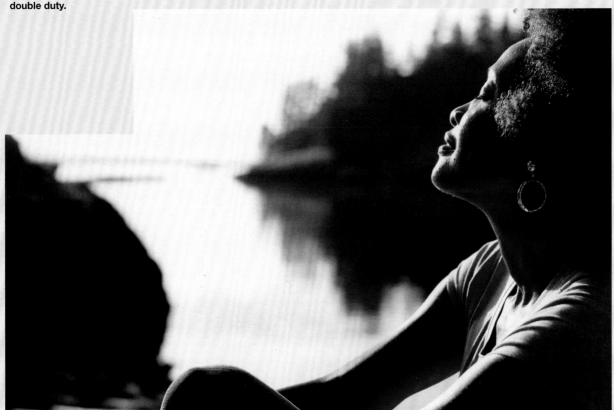

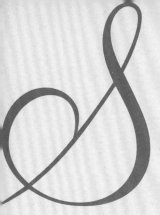

Sun spot treatments: *our award winners*

In recent years, the beauty industry has declared sunspot (aka brown, liver or age spots) Public Enemy Number One, with lots of launches targeting hyperpigmentation. Bold claims are made – but as we know (somewhat to our surprise) from the first edition of this book, some products really do improve pigmentation. The award-winners here put on a very impressive performance – and there's two new entries for this edition

REVIEWS

Darphin Orange Blossom Aromatic Care ✿ ✿ ✿

8.12/10 From a French aromatherapy brand snapped up some years ago by the Lauder empire, this Ecocert-certified facial oil blends seven specifically radiance-enhancing, skin-brightening ingredients including powerfully antioxidant cranberry, lavender, lemon, carrot, bilberry and liquorice (to boost natural radiance) – plus orange blossom, a key ingredient in the aromatic scent that testers loved. Five drops should be applied before your regular moisturiser at night.

Comments: 'Lovely citrussy smell; I like the intense moisturising effect and the fact it's encouraged me to massage my face' • 'I've noticed texture, elasticity and tone of my skin has improved – in one sentence, my skin looks clearer' • 'skin clarity improved and I shall be buying more the minute it runs out – though that'll be a while as it's very long-lasting; my complexion looks much more clear and even after using this as instructed: morning and evenings' • 'after two weeks, age spots (albeit not too significant) were less noticeable' • 'clarity and tone were improved and skin had a fresher, healthier colour; a family member I hadn't seen for months commented on my lovely skin, which was really nice to hear!' • 'I have no sun spots on my face but some small ones on my hands; the treated spots faded so much that after four weeks of using this lovely oil, they were barely visible' • 'luxurious and pampering, quick and easy to use'.

L'Occitane Immortelle Brightening Essence ✿

8/10 A new award winner from this French natural brand's Brightening Skincare collection, this light serum, dispensed via a dropper in the lid, contains its signature immortelle essential oil plus a wild daisy extract, which they promise helps regular melanin synthesis and so reduce hyperpigmentation. An effectiveness test carried out on 55 women showed that 75 per cent felt their skin was immediately brighter, with nearly all saying it became smoother and more even-toned, with an average reduction in the appearance of the dark spot surface area of 41 per cent after eight weeks.

Comments: 'I used this all over my face and on my large age spots – on both cheeks – which definitely appear lighter after two weeks. My whole face looks brighter. I am really pleased with this serum, which has a lovely scent and sinks in beautifully' • 'my skin looked clearer and brighter with a lovely glow – sometimes no need for any moisturiser or make-up!' • 'at the end of the bottle, my skin has improved dramatically: a friend told me that it looked fantastic. The age spots on my face have disappeared and only one of the areas on my neck is still slightly visible; also my skin is smoother and the fine lines improved' • 'my mum noticed that my pigmentation had reduced in size: I am really pleased with this lovely product'.

AT A GLANCE

Darphin Orange Blossom Aromatic Care

L'Occitane Immortelle Brightening Essence

Spotner

Elemis Advanced Brightening Even Tone Serum

Spotner

8/10

Age spot treatments don't always have to be applied all over: this comes in an 'Appli-pen' for (age)spot-targeted use. The key active ingredients include alpha-hydroxy acids (AHAs, or fruit acids) – and there is mallow, mint, yarrow and lemon balm extract in there too. Dermatologically tested, Spotner can be quickly and easily applied to individual marks – twice daily, ideally – and allowed to dry before you layer it with other products such as moisturisers and sunscreen, although Spotner features a high-level SPF50: the very best way to ensure marks don't get any worse.

Comments: 'I had some large spots on my hand, and a few smallish ones on my face: after two weeks, the more prominent spots have definitely started to fade and the small slight ones are disappearing; it left skin comfortable and moisturised where I applied it – I love the convenient pen applicator and am very happy with the results' • 'my skin tone has improved and the fading marks are much easier to deal with and cover up' • 'on the treated side, there is a slight reduction in the density and colour of the pigmentation, and I feel long-term regular use may help' • 'I was sceptical but my age spots are nowhere near as dark as they were, plus it was easy and fuss-free to apply' • 'a small red spider vein has definitely diminished' • 'this is a really great product, I no longer have to wear concealer on this area'.

Elemis Advanced Brightening Even Tone Serum

7.75/10

This intensive brightening serum is clinically proven to reduce the appearance of uneven pigmentation, also brightness, evenness and clarity, in just 28 days with the results improving at 56 days. With Elemis' hallmark marriage of nature and science, it contains daisy and pea extracts plus a Bio-mimetic peptide to block tyrosinase, the enzyme responsible for melanin production so it helps to prevent future darkening.

Comments: 'Love the product and am very impressed: skin is smooth and is well moisturised, looks slightly clearer, slight fading to pigmentation, general improvement in clarity and texture' • 'my sun spot on my forehead near my hairline and the outer tip of my right eyebrow have faded by about 50 per cent: I am thrilled. Clarity and tone have gotten better, even my thread veins less noticeable.

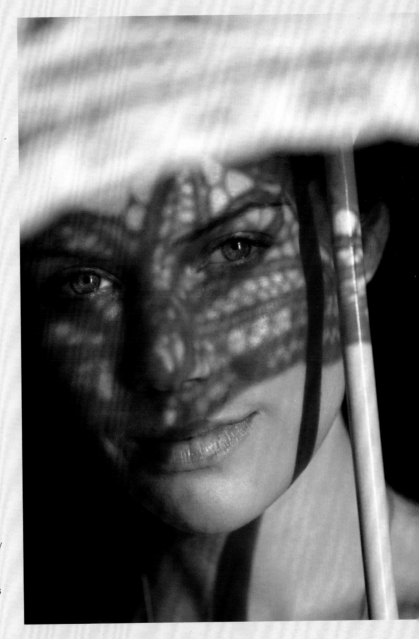

Yay!' • 'no difference in age spots but it is doing something to improve clarity and skin feels a lot better overall: I love this for its skin brightening properties' • 'no dramatic results but I did see some fading of my age spots, particularly noticeable in the large one above my eyebrow where I only applied the serum to one half and could see a difference in the pigmentation. Serum also brightens, tightens, smoothes and clears skin so it does look younger'.

Brush up on tooth wisdom

The thing the majority of people remember most vividly from a first meeting is your smile. (Why do you think Julia Roberts became galactic?) OK, as the years go by, flashing a Californian-babe beam may look out of place but long term, caring for your teeth (and gums) is vital for your appearance, confidence – and your general health

We've become a bit obsessed about our teeth and gums. We're both lucky in that we have quite strong teeth and, partly because we eat well, they aren't discoloured or stained. (Though Sarah had veneers applied in her thirties because of brown stains and shortened teeth due to tetracycline antibiotics as a child.) But we want to keep them that way, and also keep our gums in good shape so that teeth don't get loose. (The thought of putting them in a glass at night is a powerful incentive.) Plus, your whole mouth structure is so important for literally holding up your face – if that gets slack and/or you lose teeth, your cheeks cave in, and that really does age you in a trice. So we're going to spend a bit of time in this section of the book giving you expert advice from London-based holistic dentist Dr David Cook, who has transformed the mouths (and in some cases lives) of several people we know.

So, what ages your smile?
- Stained, discoloured or mismatched teeth.
- Gum disease, which causes gums to recede so teeth look long and horsey; gaps like black triangles often appear at the gum line; loose gums mean teeth may fall out.
- Tooth loss (also grinding, see below) can lead to the lower part of your face looking 'caved in', appearing pinched and shorter with more lines and folds, as well as having gaps (obviously).
- Grinding your teeth at night (bruxism) wears them down, making them shorter and squarer, which distorts the proportions and makes them look less attractive when you're smiling.
- Grinding also causes jaw muscles to bulk up so you get a square-jawed look (not very feminine).

Can the state of your teeth affect your health? In a word, yes...
- Gum disease (aka gingivitis) increases the risk of heart disease, stroke and, in women of child-bearing age, low-birthweight babies. There is also increasing evidence of a link with osteoporosis, type 2 diabetes, Alzheimer's disease and other inflammatory conditions.
- The bacteria that cause gum disease can be passed to others, so partners, children and grandchildren are at increased risk. (Kissing babies is a bad idea if you have gum disease.)
- Poor oral hygiene and gum disease are the primary causes of chronic bad breath (halitosis) and the sufferer is often unaware of the problem.
- Tooth wear and loss can lead to the collapse of your ability to bite down on food – this means your jaw muscles and joints have to work harder, putting strain on them and causing pain and further bite problems.
- Grinding your teeth at night can cause poor sleep patterns, with all its related problems.

WE LOVE...

Holistic Dental Tooth Powder, a minty fresh blend which contains a bunch of herbs to help clean teeth, maintain healthy gums and freshen breath, as well as gently abrading tooth surface to remove plaque and stains without damaging the enamel.

'Nothing makes a woman more beautiful than the belief that she is beautiful'

Sophia Loren

So what exactly is going on?

Read Dr Cook's advice on common problems and how you can treat them.

Brighten stained and discoloured teeth

As teeth age they tend to get darker, due to stains building up on the surface of the teeth and also penetrating the surface through micro cracks and porosities. Tea, coffee, red wine and tobacco are the main culprits here, and surprisingly herbal and fruit teas are notable culprits too.

A twice-yearly professional clean by a hygienist can work wonders. Once all stain and surface discolouration is polished away you may be surprised at how good your teeth look. After that, using whitening toothpaste with a sonic toothbrush can be very effective at reducing the rate of further stain build-up. (You may need advice from your hygienist on how best to use a sonic toothbrush; also see box page 198.)

Teeth that are badly discoloured or have lost their sparkle and vitality can be rejuvenated with whitening (aka bleaching), using hydrogen peroxide gels which work all the way through the teeth and actually change the colour. Gel concentration and safe application time varies widely, so this should definitely be done under the supervision of a dentist. Provided that tooth whitening/bleaching is done professionally, it is safe, very effective and has few side effects apart from temporary sensitivity. Over-the-counter (or internet) whitening products are usually ineffective and may be damaging due to high acidity, so they should be avoided.

MATCH UP YOUR MOLARS

Misshapen, damaged or worn teeth can be enhanced with porcelain veneers, crowns or onlays to give a beautiful and functional appearance. These techniques can also be used to restore a severely worn or damaged bite, which returns facial balance and gives support to cheeks and lips – (that's why it's sometimes known as the 'dental facelift').

FIX CROOKED TEETH/ BAD BITE

A crooked smile or bad bite can be corrected with braces, and modern techniques are quick, comfortable and can be virtually invisible.

Love your gums

Gum (periodontal) disease is a chronic bacterial infection of the supporting tissue of the tooth (gums and bone). As the body tries to ward off the infection, inflammation develops; over time this leads to bone loss around the teeth. Often this happens with few external signs and little or no discomfort until quite advanced, which is why regular dental visits are so important. If the reversible early stage of gum disease (gingivitis) is allowed to continue into periodontitis, the bacteria and inflammatory cells can leak into the bloodstream and be carried around the whole body contributing to the problems highlighted on page 192.

What you can do:

● Brush your teeth! The first line of defence is hygiene – meticulous, thorough, regular cleaning with a toothbrush and floss will remove bacteria, reducing inflammation and aiding healing. Aim for twice a day at least.

● Regular visits (usually twice-yearly) to your dentist to monitor disease progress, and to the hygienist to clean the mouth thoroughly and advise on effective homecare – every mouth and person is different, so homecare needs to be tailored to individuals.

● Don't smoke – smokers are more prone to gum disease and once established it will progress much faster than in a non-smoker.

● Eat well: a diet low in all forms of sugar with healthy levels of antioxidants is beneficial. There is growing evidence that supplements of vitamin C, coenzyme Q10 and zinc (antioxidants which also act against inflammation) are also helpful. Natural live yoghurt which has both calcium and lactose bacteria appears to help prevent gum problems.

● Take exercise – it can help to reduce inflammation.

● Try to avoid stress as this leads to a higher risk of disease.

● Drink lots of still water (but not fizzy! See page 197).

● Gum disease runs in families, so be extra vigilant if there's a family history. Women are more likely to suffer, which is probably related to reproductive hormones.

● If you have another inflammatory disease, such as diabetes, keep tight control on blood-sugar levels.

● Brush your teeth! Again!

MAKE UP FOR LOST TEETH

Losing teeth at an early age affects your appearance as well as the way they function (or don't…), plus other teeth can drift around the jaw, leading to bite imbalances. Replacing lost teeth as soon as possible helps prevent more complex problems. There are three basic options to replace missing teeth, all of which can work well.

1 **Implant:** screwed into the bone, this is effectively a like-for-like replacement which can last a lifetime and is considered the gold standard.

2 **Bridge:** this uses adjacent teeth to support a replacement unit but can involve damage to the supporting teeth and commonly needs replacing after several years.

3 **Denture:** this is removable and allows easy cleaning, but can be uncomfortable.

Deal with tooth grinding and bite problems

The wear caused by teeth grinding at night and/or from a 'bad bite' (where your teeth are misaligned so they don't meet correctly when you bite) can cause the structure of your teeth to be badly affected. This can lead to problems such as sensitive teeth, receding gums, and broken teeth or fillings.

Grinding your teeth can actually lead to bite problems because of the damage to tooth structure. The whole thing can become a vicious cycle, causing pain in addition to the other problems above.

Additionally, persistent grinding at night prevents the jaw muscles from relaxing and can lead on to muscle spasm, cramps, head and neck pain, even migraines. Night grinding also disturbs sleep patterns, which can lead to tiredness, stress and so more grinding…

What you can do:

● Have your bite, jaw muscles and joints assessed regularly to catch any problems early, before too much damage occurs.

● Many people with a problem will benefit from a night splint – a custom-made appliance worn over the teeth when sleeping to position the jaws so as to allow muscle relaxation and better-quality sleep, and to help prevent further damage.

● If the damage is more advanced or symptoms are severe, your dentist may advise some form of bite reconstruction (potentially surgical); when done correctly this can not only restore appearance but prevent future problems. NB: This needs an expert practitioner.

● Tension in the head and neck due to a bad bite can be relieved by skilful use of complementary therapies such as physiotherapy, osteopathy and chiropractic. Simple exercises and home massage of the jaw can help greatly (as Sarah knows from personal experience).

A colleague who was prescribed a 'bite splint' says:

'From the first night, I slept more deeply than I had in years. I felt better, looked better and people started asking whether I'd had a holiday'

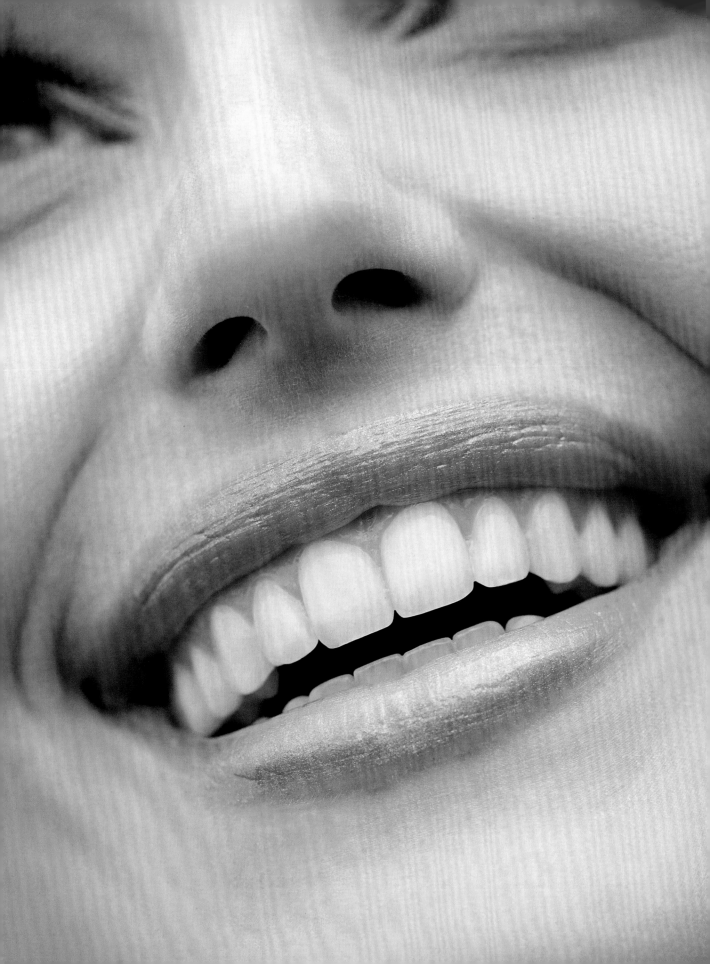

Learn about dental decay – the great enemy for teeth

We all know that sugar is a big problem food in tooth decay. But it's not just eating candy and cake, modern processed foodstuffs often contain hidden sugar, which is tricky to detect. What's more, from a dentist's perspective, natural sugar sources such as fruit and honey are just as problematic. And don't let's even mention fizzy drinks – yet…

To understand what's happening, the all-important link between sugar, acid and tooth decay and what to do about it, we need to know a little bit about the science. (It's riveting, promise!)

Here's Dr Cook's explanation: 'The human mouth is full of bacteria, happily living in the microscopic nooks and crannies and most of them causing no harm – in fact, some give us protection from more dangerous organisms. But certain types love to feast on sugar and the more sugar they eat, the more they multiply. The problem for your teeth is that as the bugs consume sugar, they produce acid (as a waste product) – and that's the agent which attacks and weakens teeth. The acid environment in your mouth also encourages more bacteria, so more acid is produced, and so on…and on…

'The body's defence against each sugar dose is saliva, which neutralises the acid. But this process takes about 45 minutes, during which the acid launches an attack on your teeth, dissolving some of the hard mineral coating of the tooth [demineralisation of the enamel]. Once the saliva has neutralised the acid, the minerals it contains begin to repair some of the acid-damaged enamel [remineralisation]. But if another dose of sugar comes along too soon – continuously sucking sweets, say, through the day, rather than in separate "hits" – effective repair is impossible and the weakened enamel begins to break down and dissolve again. This creates a protected home for more bacteria which can't be completely cleaned off – and a cavity becomes established. The sugar also forms a gungy residue called plaque, which sticks to the tooth.

'But there's an extra threat to your teeth in the shape of acidic foods and drinks, notably carbonated drinks, tea – including fruit teas, coffee, vinegar, alcohol, salad dressing and ketchup.'

What you can do:

● Clean away as much of the bacteria and plaque as possible – brushing and flossing thoroughly, ideally after every meal but at least twice a day.
● If you have snacked on something sugary or acidic (see next point), wait 30 minutes before brushing to allow the acidity in your mouth to become more neutral.
● Remember: the main offenders are sugary foods (including most fruits and fruit juices) and acidic ones (including fizzy drinks, tea, coffee, alcohol, vinegar, ketchup and most salad dressings).
● It is the repeated frequent acid attacks that cause the major damage, so if you want something sugary/acidic, eat it all in one go. Best of all, go for nuts or unsweetened natural yoghurt as a snack.
● Help the naturally protective saliva by chewing sugar-free gum after a meal, preferably one sweetened with xylitol (eg, Trident sugarless gum). This speeds up the neutralisation of acids and the xylitol – a natural sweetener and proven tooth (and bone) strengthener – helps stop the plaque from sticking to teeth.
● Drink plenty of water – this helps flush away acid and keeps saliva flow high.
● End a meal with a little cheese or unsweetened yoghurt: this helps speed up acid neutralisation.
● If you've had a lot of fillings in the past or some of the enamel has been demineralised, you can use a remineralising paste, smeared over the affected areas and left overnight or held in a custom-made tray. This can significantly increase the chance of reversing very early decay (water-based, sugar-free GC Tooth Mousse from your dentist is the most effective).

Know your fillings

Amalgam is a mixture of mercury with silver, copper and tin, which forms a strong, relatively stable material when set. It's been in use as a filling material for over 150 years and continues to be used today, largely because it's inexpensive and requires little skill to place quickly and successfully. So why the fuss? Because mercury is a known poison and extremely toxic. While the majority of the mercury in a dental filling is stable within the amalgam, small amounts are continuously released. If this were anywhere other than inside someone's mouth, it would be classified as an environmentally contaminated zone… Over the past decade, concern about toxicity from mercury in amalgam has increased and many countries restrict the use of mercury-based products.

As a patient, potentially the biggest exposure to mercury is when you are having old amalgam fillings removed. This can be accomplished safely. Check that your dentist understands the risks (you can afford to be blunt). Ensure that a rubber dam will be placed around the tooth to isolate it from the rest of your mouth. Dr Cook normally advises swallowing two activated charcoal tablets before treatment (these mop up any debris that slips past the dam). For more sensitive patients, a clean air supply during the procedure may be advisable, plus specific nutritional supplements afterwards. Once the amalgam is removed, there's a range of options as replacements:

● **Porcelain:** this is very aesthetic, strong and can be used anywhere.

● **Gold:** very noticeable (so unaesthetic), but the strongest and can be used anywhere.

● **Composite resin:** this looks very good and is durable in small- to medium-size cavities, but it is not suitable for back teeth unless they are small.

In Dr Cook's opinion, 'The aesthetics of porcelain outweigh the slightly better strength of gold – particularly "Emax", the latest generation material which is incredibly strong and looks fantastic. But any of the options above can perform very well. However, to get the best out of them requires meticulous technique and is time-consuming, so the procedure will be more expensive than amalgam.'

KEEP YOUR TEETH BEAUTIFULLY CLEAN

The reality is that it's less about what you use and more about how. The basic equipment of a toothbrush with a small to medium head and dental floss is all most people need – if they use it correctly. Having said that, electric brushes, particularly sonic ones, are very effective and there's a wide selection of different brushes specially developed for cleaning between and around teeth and gums.

Every mouth is different, and the correct tools and technique need to be tailored to each individual, so the best advice is to ask your dentist or preferably your hygienist to advise and demonstrate a personalised cleaning routine. Also have it checked after a couple of months to make sure you are managing it correctly. This is probably the best investment of time and money you can make and could save you many times the investment in the future. (For general guidelines, see box left.)

Mainstream toothpastes are all effective (although specific smokers' pastes and powders can be very abrasive and damaging). Fluoride is a naturally occurring element which is incorporated into tooth enamel, making it harder and more resistant to decay. Fluoride toothpaste has been shown to reduce the level of dental decay, so unless your diet and hygiene are perfect, not using a fluoride toothpaste may mean you need more dental work.

The evidence for a protective effect when fluoride is swallowed (in the water supply or as a supplement) is less clear and it can have toxic side effects, so using fluoride like that is controversial. However, if fluoride is applied as a toothpaste in the correct and tiny amount – a pea-size for an adult and half a pea of an appropriate product for a child – and not swallowed, the benefits can be great and the risk is probably negligible. (This is Dr Cook's opinion, which we respect – though we prefer to use natural fluoride-free toothpastes ourselves.)

Another controversial toothpaste additive is sodium lauryl sulphate (SLS): this is a chemical foaming agent common in many household products – shampoo, bubble baths, detergents, etc. It has been shown to cause skin reactions and ulceration. SLS-free toothpastes are available: Dr Cook's favourites are Tom's of Maine Clean & Gentle Care, and Sensodyne Total Care Gel. (We like the Green People and Weleda ranges, which have peppermint-free options suitable for people taking homeopathic remedies.) If you suffer from mouth ulcers, it's worth trying an SLS-free toothpaste.

TEETH-CLEANING TECHNIQUE

Brush your teeth outside and inside for two to three minutes twice daily (at a minimum), after meals, and follow with flossing. If you use a sonic toothbrush, all you need to do is hold the head steady against each tooth where it meets the gum – counting to six on each side. If you're using a manual brush (choose a soft one), hold the brush like a pencil and go round and round gently in little circles on the chewing surfaces of each tooth. The brush should be at a 45 degree angle towards your gum so that the tufts are pressed into it.

TIP

Toothbrush heads harbour bugs, so do change them regularly and particularly after you recover from any infections.

ANTI-AGEING
AWARD
WINNERS
BEAUTY BIBLE

Brightening toothpastes: *our award winners*

A first, for us: we've never trialled toothpastes before. But since a brighter smile can be instantly 'de-ageing', we figured: why not trial brightening, whitening toothpastes alongside all the beauty lotions and potions? With tooth-bleaching procedures more popular than ever, these are the low-tech, daily-use alternative. So: is it possible to brush your way to a brighter smile…? The averages here aren't spectacular but tend to reflect the fact that for some testers they worked really well, while others didn't see much difference. Still, if you're looking for a shortlist of where to head first when looking for a whitening toothpaste, we suggest you start here.

Aquafresh Iso-Active Whitening

7.5
10

A unique 'foaming-gel' – featuring a special ingredient that activates the gel as you brush – this 'directly targets bacteria to fight a key source of oral malodour'(!), and within the Iso-Active range this is the tooth-brightening option. In a pump-action dispenser (which testers mostly disliked, on the score there was too much packaging and the nozzle didn't work that well).

Comments: 'You apply this just like ordinary toothpaste but thinner, rather like Pearl Drops; teeth feel extra clean and mouth very fresh, better than a normal product, so I would buy though not certain if teeth actually whiter' • 'thick paste that really foamed up when applied, very minty but not so much that it stung, teeth felt really fresh and clean after, my slightly stained teeth look much brighter: did get compliments! I love this and won't be without it from now on, lasts a long time and my mouth feels so much cleaner as well' • 'after ten days of using this, two people in two days asked whether I had had my teeth whitened, so they obviously noticed a difference – though to start with I didn't…' • 'I was very sceptical but I have to say my teeth did look much whiter – I was impressed!'.

Beverly Hills Formula Total Breath Whitening

7.21
10

Beverly Hills Formula were pioneers in whitening toothpastes, and promise 'whiter teeth in one minute' from what is now a wide range of formulations. This particular toothpaste features an antibacterial formula to help fight plaque (and bad breath) – leaving breath fresher for up to five times longer than a regular toothpaste, so they say.

Comments: 'Nice light toothpaste with minty aftertaste and I definitely saw a difference, my teeth were much whiter and my family noticed; I tried the tip about leaving it on the tongue for a bit before brushing for freshness and this worked well' • 'my teeth do look good and don't feel rough to the touch as they did at first' • 'I have started drinking green tea without milk and noticed how much it stains the cup: I think it would have stained my teeth but this has kept them looking clean and bright' • 'I enjoyed using this and my teeth did look a little bit better'.

AloeDent Triple Action Toothpaste

7.11
10

AloeDent takes its name from the soothing aloe plant, a key ingredient in this natural toothpaste range, which also combines tea tree oil and green tea extract to fight against bacteria, plus Co-Q10 for healthy gums. The naturally whitening mineral silica is significantly less abrasive, they promise, than conventional stain-removing ingredients.

Comments: 'Really nice taste, no difference in amount of foaming, my teeth felt really clean after' • 'definitely makes my slightly yellow teeth whiter, difference showed up pretty much the first time of use; teeth feel very clean after using too' • 'I thought aloe vera would be horrid but I'm a convert! Teeth feel really clean and mouth fresh' • 'loved the taste – teeth and mouth felt clean and invigorated; though I didn't notice any difference in whiteness, I love this product: it may cost a few pence more but it's really worth it'.

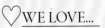

AT A GLANCE

Aquafresh Iso-Active Whitening

Beverly Hills Formula Total Breath Whitening

AloeDent Triple Action Toothpaste

♡ WE LOVE…

Jo uses a natural toothpaste with no specific brightening promises… Sarah is excited about PerioBrite Natural Whitening Toothpaste with CoQ10 and folic acid, which is fluoride and preservative free. She also likes (more expensive) BOCA herbal formulations for Day and Overnight, which contain home-grown propolis. BOCA is supported by medical and dental organisations.

TIP

Once you've brightened your teeth, keep stain-causing liquids from reversing the improvement by using a straw. (You can do this for hot drinks but it takes a bit of getting used to!)

Tinted moisturisers: our award winners

Tinted moisturisers are absolutely brilliant for evening out skintone without making a face look over-made-up. Some, though, are just too moisturising (and so shine-inducing), while others aren't quite dewy enough, so they go on patchily (and need a moisturiser underneath). With a long line-up of products to trial for this new edition, we asked our panellists to help us identify which really are 'the business'. Read on for lots of high-scoring entries, all of which feature an SPF – providing more useful protection against UV damage

AT A GLANCE

Bobbi Brown SPF15 Tinted Moisturizer

Aveda Mineral Tinted Moisturiser

Estée Lauder DayWear BB Anti-Oxidant Beauty Benefit Crème SPF35

Estée Lauder DayWear Sheer Tint Advanced Multi-Protection Anti-Oxidant Release Moisturizer SPF15

REVIEWS

Bobbi Brown SPF15 Tinted Moisturizer

8.81/10 A heck of a score for this new top-slot tint, which comes in a wider-than-most choice of seven different shades. (Testers put Light Tint through its paces, which is third-from-palest.) A lightweight formula targeted at normal and dry skins, it does feature skin-conditioning jojoba oil and other emollients to leave skin feeling supple; if you're prone to shine, there's also an oil-free version (though we didn't trial this).
Comments: 'Previously I'd always used foundation; though it doesn't cover quite as much, it give me a more natural, youthful-looking product – amazing' • 'impossible to go wrong with this: you can't apply too much' • 'gives complexion a bit of a boost while evening out thread veins, open pores, pigmentation – blends into the face a treat, and doesn't "settle" into fine lines' • 'skin looks healthier, more glowing' • 'my 18-year-old daughter asked to borrow it as she thinks it looks so natural and makes my complexion radiant' • 'the first tinted moisturiser I've ever liked'.

Aveda Mineral Tinted Moisturiser

8.64/10 Although this new entry (also a favourite of Sarah's) is oil-free, testers found it very moisturising down to the naturally-derived emollients (coconut and jojoba seed). With antioxidant resveratrol to help protect skin, plus mineral sunscreen (titanium dioxide), it also contains Aveda's signature tourmaline for radiance. In six shades, our testers trialled Sweet Tea.
Comments: 'Great results on my skin, sheer coverage with a satin dewy smooth sheer – 'no make-up' – finish and moisturises very well' • 'very easy to blend, goes on evenly every time; very sheer with one layer – giving just a little bit of colour and coverage; with a second layer it's more like a sheer foundation, which I prefer' • 'no settling into lines and I am told I look "very well"' • 'smoothed out open pores and reduced age spots, fine lines around lips much softer' • 'Like a silk film across my face: very light coverage but everything looks better: the best tinted moisturiser I have used'.

Estée Lauder DayWear BB Anti-Oxidant Beauty Benefit Crème SPF35

8.48/10 We're going to let you in on a little industry secret about BB creams, which have been A Big Beauty Buzz lately. In reality, many would previously have been categorised as tinted moisturisers: we've even seen one product hurriedly relabelled with stickers, to reposition it in the hot 'BB' category. Some – as in this case – do contain a higher-than-usual dose of 'light-reflecting pigments', which work to blur imperfections and boost skin's radiance and glow. For those concerned about the sun's ageing effects on the face, this BB also features a higher-than-average SPF35 plus mega-antioxidants, and has the signature cucumber-y scent we personally know

♡ WE LOVE...

Jo is now wedded to Chanel les Beiges All-in-One Healthy Glow Fluid SPF 15, which offers six shades including two pales. As well as the new Aveda award winner opposite, Sarah opts for a DIY approach to get a perfect shade, mixing a few drops of This Works Energy Bank Sunflash – a fab vitamin-infused bronze serum – into Suqqu Frame Fix Liquid Foundation SPF 30, which is so feather light it hardly resembles a foundation, especially when mixed with Sunflash.

TIP

Mary Greenwell insists that tinted moisturiser should be viewed more like a lightweight foundation than as something to change the underlying tone of your skin. She prescribes the same colour-matching technique as for foundation: apply to just below your jaw to find the shade that will blend in seamlessly. If you're very pale, you'll need to check out one of the ranges which now offers a selection of shades – many tinted moisturisers are one-shade-fits-all options, and one shade DOESN'T fit all.

and love from the rest of the DayWear range. In two shades; testers had the 01 Light.

Comments: 'Blends extremely well compared to my usual product, which just sits on my face' • 'velvety product delivering a healthy glow and colour, worn on its own' • 'the perfect holiday product: does the job of a whole shelf-ful – sun protection, foundation, moisturiser, primer' • 'skin looks younger when I'm wearing it – which makes me feel younger'.

Estée Lauder DayWear Sheer Tint Advanced Multi-Protection Anti-Oxidant Release Moisturizer SPF15

8.3/10

We can't help but be impressed when of dozens of products submitted for trials for this book, two contenders from a single brand make it to the winners' podium. This is an old and oft-recommended favourite of ours, with a touch of magic about it: the light, suits-all-skintypes cream that emerges from the tube is a kind of mauve-y/grey, but then is transformed on contact with skin to a customised shade on every single skintone. Alongside the SPF15 is DayWear's usual cocktail of skin-shielding antioxidants.

Comments: 'Considering I'm 47 this is impressive as it manages to cover all blemishes and fine lines – so light I don't feel I'm wearing any make-up' • 'velvety, smooth texture – so easy to apply' • 'throughout the day skin felt moisturised and looked bright, and I feel it has anti-ageing benefits' • 'did well covering up sun spots'.

Say goodbye to spider veins!

Thread veins, spider veins, broken veins: whatever you call them, they're a body woe (and a face angst) for many women. However, there are fixes. And camouflages

When a truly gorgeous-in-every-way friend in her early fifties was deserted by her (daft) husband, part of her fresh start was to tidy up the 'hated spider veins which creep in at various places up my legs and fan out over my thighs', as she put it. It isn't just legs that can be affected: many women are troubled by the appearance of thread veins on their face (cheeks, forehead, eyelids and around the nostrils), also neck and upper chest. They're particularly noticeable in people with pale thin skin. (And, says Jo, 'certainly the curse of my beauty life – the price for an English rose complexion'.)

The technical name for these clusters of tiny dilated blood vessels (capillaries), which appear just under the surface of the skin, is 'dermal flares'. They're incredibly common and while not serious, they are unsightly. On the legs, they can also lead to heavy aching legs and even pain. 'Little nerves in the veins can be painful if the veins get stretched,' explains consultant vascular surgeon Mr John Scurr of the Lister Hospital in London (our long-time 'veins' expert). They may be worsened by fluctuating levels of hormones, pre- and post-menopause, as well as standing up for long periods. (Men get them too.) Before treating leg veins, Mr Scurr explains that it's vital to have a scan first to check that there are no underlying problems, such as varicose veins (or, at the worst, deep vein thrombosis) – and be aware that varicose veins need to be treated before treating dermal flares. The following two treatment options are Mr Scurr's preferred choices.

For spider veins on legs, consider microsclerotherapy. Getting rid of these 'dermal flares' can be simple – but it's likely to be time-consuming. Mr Scurr recommends a process called microsclerotherapy, where each capillary is injected with a very fine needle containing a 'sclerosant' solution that expels blood from the vein, and leaves the walls of the vein stuck together so the blood can't return.

The sessions last about 20 minutes and are usually carried out by a nurse. Veins may sting a little but shouldn't be painful. A cylinder of tightly rolled cotton wool is stuck on each injection site immediately after to minimise bruising, and legs are wrapped in a light bandage before you leave. Both bandage and cotton wool can be taken off three hours later. Legs may ache slightly for a few days.

If you have a number of flares this process can take several weeks. And while microsclerotherapy is the most effective for legs, it's not appropriate for faces, where laser is the best and safest option.

Electrolysis is another option. In this treatment – suitable for faces as well as legs – an electrical current is passed through a fine needle to cauterise the vein so the blood is absorbed back into the body. (See right for more about facial thread veins.) Electrolysis is available at beauty salons, but you should always have potential 'deep veins' on legs checked out by a doctor first. Make sure you go to an experienced therapist who has the back-up to deal with potential problems, such as infection.

Schedule treatment for the tights season! Microsclerotherapy (and sclerotherapy which can be used for some varicose veins) can leave legs looking a bit battle-scarred so, if possible, time your treatment when you can cover up with black opaques. The process is definitely not a quick fix but, says our friend, it's worth it: 'Wonder of wonders, I now have unblemished thighs and legs. For the first time in years, I can leave the sarong behind when I walk to the pool.'

Remember dermal flares may stage a comeback. Mr Scurr warns that those pesky flares may return and need further treatment. Natural products, either to take internally or rub on, may help. Try Diosmin Complex by LifeTime Vitamins, a combination of natural compounds, or Zinopin Daily, a natural blend developed to prevent DVT for air travellers. Spider Veins Cream by Provenance features glycosaminoglycans (GAGs) that may help repair the damaged capillaries and possibly toughen the outer cell layers, minimising the appearance of spider veins. (Find a source for these in DIRECTORY.)

FACE YOUR THREAD VEINS

Cosmetic dermatologists treat unsightly thread veins on your cheeks and face with state-of-the-art lasers. Individual broken capillaries can be treated with walk-in-and-out lunchtime therapy which doesn't cause any bruising. (But you must, absolutely must, wear a sunblock for at least three months after.) Why not sclerotherapy? Experts including Dr Nick Lowe of the Cranley Clinic, London, and Dr Andrew Markey, say that while sclerotherapy is the gold standard for treating leg veins, they disapprove of using it on the face, because injecting the wrong vein may provoke an emergency and, in the worst-case scenario, lead to loss of vision. (Plus we've heard from a woman who had it done – unwisely – around her nose, that it's agony.) However, if you have developed thread veins during pregnancy, try waiting a few months after the birth because they may disappear on their own. And if you have acne rosacea with inflamed skin that looks like thread veins, you should probably be treated with antibiotics first. (For more on rosacea see page 168.)

In any case, please do make sure you consult a qualified and experienced dermatologist – it is your face after all! We recommend following Wendy Lewis's checklist of questions to ask, even before something which seems as minor as veins treatment (see page 46).

For us, a little bit of concealer (see camouflage suggestions right, and also top concealers on page 91) plus topical treatments minimise the problem very satisfactorily, without recourse to expensive treatments. Also see page 170 for products that have done well for facial redness. And do avoid scrubs or using anything scratchy on your face.

PS Sarah had more veins on her cheeks and round her nose in her twenties than she does now, and can only put that down to taking more care of her skin – with plenty of nourishing moisturiser in cold/windy weather and lots of anti-inflammatory foods and supplements, notably oily fish and omega-3 essential fatty acids (again!) – and leading a calmer life generally. Oh, and not drinking alcohol!

OUR TOP CAMOUFLAGERS

Products we know work include Estée Lauder Maximum Cover Camouflage Make-up for Face and Body and Vichy Dermablend Ultra-Corrective Foundation Cream Stick together with the same brand's Setting Powder. Laura Mercier Secret Camouflage can be very effective for faces, too.

TIP

Visible facial veins often come as a result of sun damage so – once again – please can we remind you to slap on the SPF! And avoid roasting and frying in the hottest parts of the day. And while we're at it, please avoid sunbeds too – they're a short cut to ageing and pose a significant risk of skin cancer. Remember: when it comes to tans, fake it to make it!

Take up yoga. Just do it, please

For us, this is almost the most important advice in this book. If you do it already, you will know the absolutely miraculous results of an hour or so's practise (sometimes just five minutes is enough to turn you round). Done regularly long-term, yoga can transform your life

We find yoga THE perfect exercise for a more mature body – and for ironing out any wrinkles in our minds. If you've never done it before, it can help enormously with flexibility – and bone strength, too. And there is nothing – repeat nothing – we've found that's better for stress, and for making us feel like we're on top of the mountain of different things we have to juggle. Plus it makes you look fabulous! At the end of a long day – or if you get up in the morning feeling and looking exhausted – the most effective way to go from tired and drab to glowing and gorgeous is to do some yoga. (Just try it.)

Take up yoga for your bones. As yoga teacher Jan Maddern, author of *Yoga Builds Bones*, observes, 'Yoga creates a balanced harmony between the ovaries, adrenal, parathyroid, pituitary and pineal glands, ensuring that the body receives a steady supply of the right hormones for maintaining bone strength and maximum health and wellbeing. The regular practise of weight-bearing hatha yoga postures offers women everywhere a safe way to build bone strength.' There is even some evidence that yoga can help people who have already developed symptoms of osteoporosis: according to Dr Andrew Weil, the world's leading expert in integrated medicine, two studies have shown that elderly women who took part in regular yoga classes, two to three times a week for between three and six months, saw a slight reduction in curvatures of the upper spine ('dowager's hump'). In one study the control group who didn't practise yoga actually saw an increase in upper spinal curvatures. In another study, older women who did a nine-week yoga programme gained a centimetre in height.

Take up yoga to balance your hormones. Consultant gynaecologist Michael Dooley recommends yoga to all his patients, particularly any going through the hormonal roller-coasters around menopause. Teachers have always held that certain postures can reduce hot flushes and night sweats as well as promote calm and restful sleep, and this was confirmed by researchers in India. (It also sharpened mental function – yippee!) During the long, slow asanas (postures), certain glands in the body are gently pressurised and depressurised, helping to stimulate and control the hormones produced by those glands. Yoga for menopause should place an emphasis on moving slowly and smoothly.

It is never too late to take up yoga, but

REACH A STATE OF UNITY

Yoga means 'union' in Sanskrit, the language of ancient India where the system originated more than 3,000 years ago. It unites body, mind and spirit through a combination of breathing, meditation, stretching and postures (asanas). There are different ways of practising yoga, varying from slow (eg, Hatha yoga) to dynamic (eg, Ashtanga) which suit different personalities. Iyengar yoga (a fairly recent development by BKS Iyengar) set out to be therapeutic and focuses on bodily alignment. Some people see yoga as a spiritual practice but it is certainly not a religion.

it's also never too early: as Suza Francina, a teacher who writes books about yoga for women (rather than babes) points out, 'If you practise yoga before the menopause, all the poses that are useful for coping with uncomfortable symptoms are familiar, and you can reach for them like an old friend. If you are familiar with restorative poses, then you have the best menopause medicine at your disposal.'

If you Google 'yoga for menopause' you may even be lucky eough to find a specific class in your area, as some teachers are starting to offer this type of yoga specifically (it's a baby-boom thing). Failing that, it's important to explain to your teacher if you have hot flushes, because they can guide you through the more restorative and cooling postures. The use of supportive props such as bolsters, blankets and blocks can help adapt postures so that you avoid gripping or straining, which can cause over-heating. Specific postures that are recommended during menopause include:

● Legs-up-the-wall pose (viparita karani), which is great for grounding.
● Head-to-knee forward bend (janu sirsasana) and seated forward bend (paschimottanasana) for irritability.
● Plough pose (halasana) and Shoulder Stand for hormonal balance.

The Shoulder Stand is known as 'the posture for eternal youth', but we would certainly recommend that shoulder stands are always done in a supervised class, unless you have been practising for some years.

LESS PAIN, MORE GAIN

Research by the US National Institute of Health revealed that taking regular yoga classes can reduce chronic back pain and enhance flexibility. In a 12-week study, volunteers who took 90-minute yoga classes twice a week showed 42 per cent reduction in pain and therefore reduced their dependency on pain medication. NB: It's vital to find qualified and experienced teachers who specialise in backs, however, as practising the wrong postures can make things worse.

OUR TOP YOGA PICKS

The accessories and websites we find helpful…

● **prAna Yoga Mats.** Nicely non-slip, with good 'give' (which helps wrists). If visiting a studio, we lay our mat on top of the mat provided, for extra support (whipping it away during balancing postures, when less 'squish' helps).
● **Gossypium yoga pants.** The Cropped Foldover Trouser is genius as the small amount of Lycra in the super-wide foldover waistband keeps the trousers (and your tummy) in place, without any restricting elastic. (As a close second, we also like prAna yoga gear.)
● **Beech sandals.** An important exercise in yoga is learning to stretch the toes so that the body is perfectly 'grounded'. These help: they contain built-in 'toe-separators', which help to train the toes to spread naturally, and help with balance and body alignment.
● **Yoga Journal iPractice App.** For iPhone users there is now no excuse not to practise when you're away from home: this app from the iTunes Store (put together by *Yoga Journal*, probably the best magazine about yoga published anywhere) features sequences put together by respected teachers – and you can set the speed at which you follow them.
● **www.lotusjourneys.com.** A holistic travel agency which arranges wellbeing holidays worldwide, including an excellent selection of yoga vacations and destinations.
● *Yoga for Beginners* **DVD with Patricia Walden.** A practical introduction which is precise and easy to follow if you can't get to a class.

Take up yoga for flexibility. There's a famous concept in yoga philosophy that a person's age is determined by the flexibility of his spine, not the number of years he has lived. (And recent research suggests that stretching the body may help prevent age-related stiffening of the arteries – we'd rather have ours flowing freely.) The improved balance and flexibility that come from regular yoga practise can also help prevent – or reduce the impact – of falls: a stiff body goes down like a ninepin, which is more likely to lead to bone breaks and fractures. And, of course, it's great to hang on to the ability to reach down to your shoelaces or up to a jar on the top shelf, because (even if this seems a long way off) it helps us remain as independent as possible for as long as possible. But we also very much like this quote, frequently repeated by one of Jo's yoga teachers: 'Flexible spine equals flexible mind'. The more we do yoga, the more we find we can roll with life's punches – going with the flow and adapting to change, as well as accepting that change is inevitable.

Take up yoga to tackle your wrinkles. Marie-Véronique Nadeau – who we met when she was visiting from Berkeley, California – is in her sixties, and she's her own best advertisement: almost line-free and with plumped-up, resilient skin. Marie-Véronique (who also has her own skincare line, Marie Veronique Organics) has put together a programme called The Yoga Facelift which we recommend if you feel you can make the commitment to facial exercises. As she says, 'The adage "If you don't use it, you lose it" really applies to the muscles of your face.' Women we know who practise yoga into their later years have sharper jaws and more defined facial contours, as well as glowing skin (it's the improved circulation). We also have a theory that the amount of time you spend 'inverted' helps hair growth, by boosting blood flow to the scalp. (Completely unsubstantiated, but we both have hair that grows like grass.)

Take up yoga for clarity, balance and to quieten 'monkey mind'. In the Yoga Sutras (sacred writings), there's a wonderful phrase: 'Yoga is the ending of disturbances of the mind'. We both find it gives us amazing focus, improves memory – and, when faced with a problem, shows us a clear way to deal with it for a positive outcome. We could cite endless scientific studies to back this up (and explain why), but we can also just tell you: it's true.

So we say, just take up yoga. Don't fret too much about which 'style' of yoga – but we would suggest that Hatha, Iyengar and Scaravelli yoga (which are more gentle) would be most appropriate. We recommend that peri- and menopausal women avoid Bikram (heated) or fast Ashtanga yoga, as these focus on creating heat within the body – and at this phase in life, that's something many of us are trying to avoid. The most important thing is to find a class/classes that fit with your schedule, as you're more likely to go, and the closer to home (or work) the better.

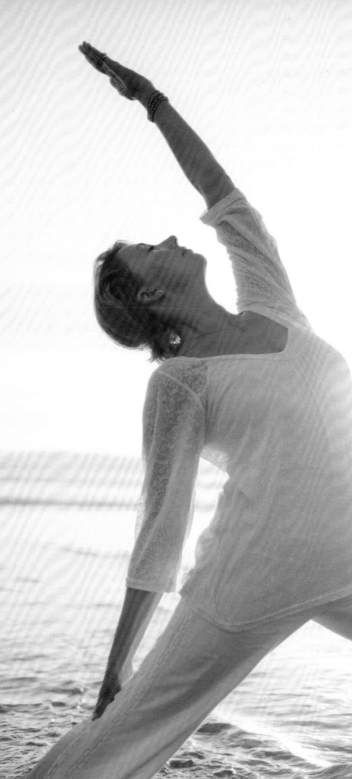

TIP

As well as helping with hot flushes, 'yoga postures and breathing techniques can help reduce general anxiety', comments Michael Dooley. 'If patients are worried about having cervical smears, for instance, I get them to do retention breathing.' (Inhale through your nose to a count of four, hold gently for seven, then exhale slowly through your mouth for eight; repeat five or six times twice daily.)

TIP

Sarah (62 as this book is published) credits years of yoga with enabling her to go on mounting her 16-hand Arab/thoroughbred horse from the ground – to the amazement of much younger riders who can't do the same – and to calming them both down when he has one of his cadenzas…

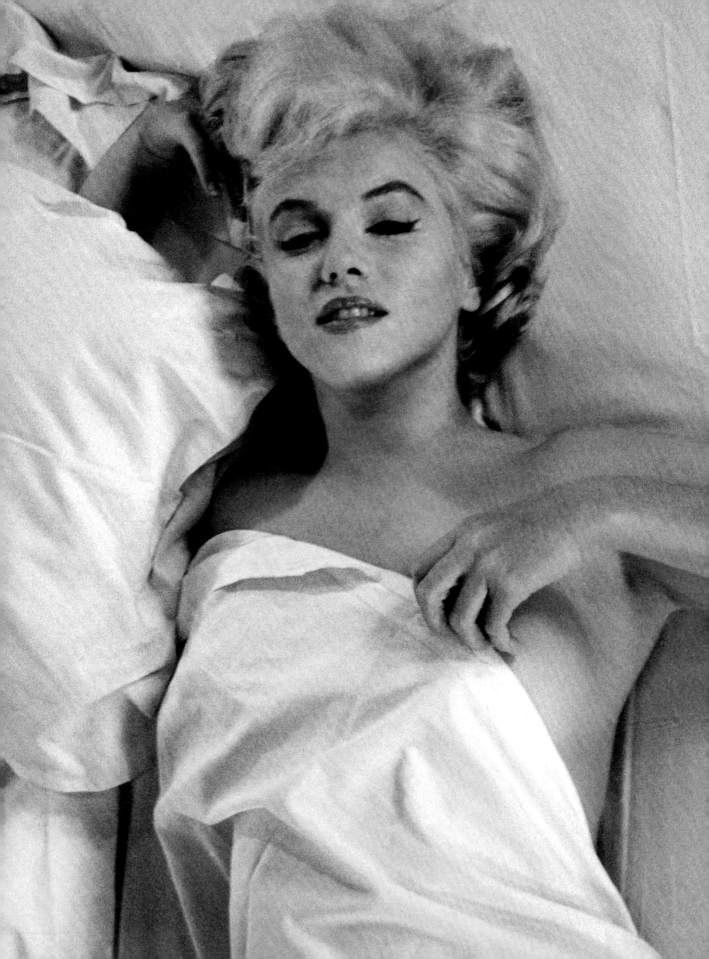

Get your Zzzzzs! How to sleep better

No doubt about it, getting enough good sleep is beautifying. And de-stressing. And energising. All-round wonderful stuff. And every good woman deserves slumber!

Trouble is we don't all get enough sleep. Especially as the years roll by. While some lucky souls can slumber through anything – from thundering traffic and snoring partners, to super-stress – others wake as a feather drops or there's the slightest ripple of anxiety. So, if it's less than restorative, how can you improve your sleep pattern?

As the queens of 'sleep hygiene', doing all the right things to optimise a good night's sleep, we are keen to pass on the stuff we know works. We're both occasionally prone to sleeplessness (and both 'larks' with a tendency to wake up at 4am in summer – or when we're fretting about something, see page 211), so when it comes to sleep aids we've been there, done that, gone to bed in the T-shirt. In other words, we know what works. First of all, get the kit. These are the 'accessories' to good sleep, and the simple steps you can take right now, in your own bedroom, to help get the zzzzzs you need. (See DIRECTORY for sources.)

If you get too hot at night, check out linen. Linen is the most amazingly cooling fabric. On a hot day, you can touch a linen pillowcase on your bed and it will be cool, whereas a cotton pillowcase on the same bed can be room temperature. If you are menopausal or peri-menopausal and you suffer from night sweats or hot flushes, at the very least treat yourself to a couple of linen pillowcases. If you can indulge yourself with linen sheets, even better. A very simple trick to cool down in the night is to flip your pillow over. We thought we were the only people who knew this, but it turns out to be so popular that there is even – we kid you not – a Facebook group called, 'I flip my pillow over to get to the cold side', with nearly one million members when we last looked. (Jo also sleeps in a French linen nightshirt, which has an equally cooling effect.)

And/or buy a Chillow. Again, if you find that you can't sleep because you're too hot at night, the Chillow is an extraordinary innovation that we've heard very good things about. (The Chillow was first brought to our attention by consultant gynaecologist Michael Dooley whose patients were raving about it for hot flushes.) It's made of a patented substance which, when activated by water (you only need to do this once), creates a memory-foam-like layer that you put between you and your pillowcase. (If you don't like the flock-y surface, you can slip it under your pillowcase – ideally linen, see left.) There's a larger version (the Chillow PLUS), originally designed for reducing fevers, which some women prefer because they can wrap it around their pillow and slip a hand underneath while they rest, getting a double cooling whammy. If you're really having a problem with hot flushes, you'll want to know about the Petite Relief Chillow which you keep in the fridge to apply when you're feeling too hot to bear. Another excellent application, for anyone who uses a laptop on their – umm, lap: put the Petite Relief Chillow under your laptop and instead of getting very hot legs, you'll feel cucumber-cool. (And lots of hospitals are now recommending Chillows for hot flushes associated with treatment for breast and prostate cancer.)

> ## 'There is no pillow so soft as a clear conscience'
> *French proverb*

And get yourself a Bucky sleep mask. Jo has road-tested just about every sleep mask known to woman, and is convinced that this is the best, the most light-excluding and the most comfortable to wear of any sleep mask out there. It's super-soft and padded, cradling the eyes without pressure. It has soft padding over the nose and cheeks, which avoids even a molecule of light peeking in. The Bucky sleep mask also Velcros around the back (so is infinitely adjustable whatever your head size). There are several designs but the one you want is Eye Shades with Ear Plugs (these are stored in a little pouch on the front). Lots of

SLEEP REGIME

This natural regime is more effective than drugs at re-establishing a sound sleep structure, says psychiatrist Dr David Servan-Schreiber. Go to bed at the same time every night including weekends but get up two hours earlier than usual. Don't nap for more than 20 to 30 minutes during the day. If you wake, get up and read a book or magazine for an hour before going back to bed. Once sleep is continuous again – which may take a few weeks – increase the time you sleep by 15 minutes every three days until you're back to your normal length.

colours, all lined with black – but we think midnight or black are the most alluring.

Have an Aromatherapy Associates Deep Relax bath before bedtime. For many years we have been slavishly devoted to Aromatherapy Associates Deep Relax Shower & Bath Oil. It is knock-out drops for us. (After you've had a few baths with this there's probably a Pavlovian response, so you only have to smell the potent blend of vetiver, chamomile and sandalwood to start to feel sleepy.) Our one caveat: if you do get toasty at night, don't have the water too hot because the effect of heating the body will linger when you slip between the sheets. We love this oil so much we give it to friends for birthdays, then they start giving it to everyone they know, like an aromatherapy chain letter.

Or pour in the magnesium flakes. Magnesium is known as 'nature's tranquilliser' and as well as taking a supplement before bed (which helps with restless legs too), we pour Magnesium Flakes in the bath so this soothing mineral can cherish aches and pains and racing minds. (There's also an oil version.) PS Researcher Dr Paula Baillie-Hamilton tells us that putting magnesium in the bath is a wonderful treatment for over-excited/hyperactive children.

Spritz your pillow. In an independent clinical study commissioned by the company, This Works Deep Sleep Pillow Spray, which features lavender, patchouli, vetiver and wild chamomile, induced 89 per cent of users to fall asleep faster. And 92 per cent said they felt more refreshed in the morning. These results amazed the formerly sceptical scientific reviewer (we know this from interviewing him). Now available in a Sleep Plus Pillow Spray formulation, which 89 per cent of testers who formerly used prescription sleep medication said they would use instead. There is a whole range to back it up, too.

Switch off the standby. There is now evidence that even the little standby light on your TV (if you have one in the bedroom) may affect your sleep pattern – not just preventing you from drifting off but interfering with the depth of your sleep. Only when the bedroom is totally dark will your body start to produce melatonin, which not only regulates sleep but also has an important role in reducing your risk of cancer. So: ditch the digital clock. Switch off any appliance that's on standby, and if you have a multi-gang plug with an orange light that tells you it's working, put gaffer tape over it.

Try a pelmet! Jo recently had a moment of absolute revelation, on a midsummer's morning when light was streaming into her bedroom before 4am: 'Ah – THAT's what a pelmet's for…' With the fashion for curtain poles rather than tracks, pelmets have very much fallen from favour – but perhaps our mothers (and grannies) knew a thing or two about keeping light out of a bedroom. If you really can't bear the look of a pelmet, try installing blackout blinds on the windows underneath, which can cover the top of the window but be half rolled up in the night, allowing air in. Meanwhile, if you have to sleep in a house where someone needs the landing light on, we suggest putting a rolled-up towel or a draught excluder at the bottom of the door, to prevent light seepage there.

Invest in a truly fabulous bed. Never, ever buy a new bed without trying it in a store. Or – better still – in a hotel: by popular request many hotels nowadays are offering for sale the actual beds that guests slumber peacefully in. (Jo is right now building up to buying one of the beds from her favourite London sleeping spot, The Langham hotel, where she gets a night's sleep like no other.) The beds with the best reputations are Hästens (made in Sweden out of bundles of horsehair, cotton, flax and pure new wool), and Hypnos (who make beds for the Queen, upholstered with cashmere, silk and lambswool). We are also impressed with the organic beds by Abaca. Some of these are very far from cheap. However, considering we spend one third of our lives in bed, we feel that investing in a great bed is probably as important as choosing a safe car as both are so essential to life.

Treat yourself to good pillows, too. It's up to you whether you like hard or soft, but make sure you replace them regularly. Do 'the pillow trick': hold out your arm, place the pillow over it – and if it flops down either side, it's definitely overdue for replacement. By reputation, the very best pillows are Hungarian or Siberian goose down, which are both very soft. Personally, we've always been impressed with Ikea pillows (they know a thing or two about sleep in a country with such long winter nights), although annoyingly they aren't quite the same size as standard UK pillows. Close enough to fudge it, though. When you want to treat yourself, try www.thebestbedlenintheworld.com for pillows: Jo's came from Claridge's (a generous gift from Clarins – she didn't nick them!), and are – as she puts it – 'like a blissful firm cloud…'.

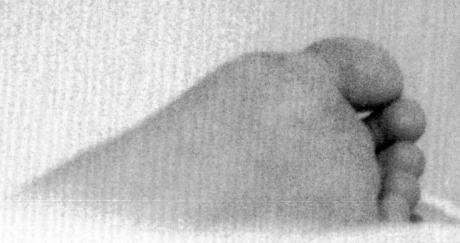

WHAT TO DO IF YOU WAKE UP IN THE WEE SMALL HOURS

Many older women get off to sleep fine but then wake between 3am and 5am. Often they can't get back to sleep; if they do, it's usually not restful slumber. Whatever the cause – and some swear it can be the phases of the moon – the result is a loss of energy and focus, and a feeling of having to drag yourself through the day until the next broken night. As well as the general advice on the previous pages, experts suggest the following ways to woo sleep; we've tried their advice and it works.

● Relax in the evening; don't drink coffee, tea or cola after 6pm and avoid fatty or sugary foods and excess alcohol which your body has to process during the night; cool your body by walking barefoot, opening a window, wearing light night clothes and having a warm bath.

● Dim lights through the evening: until electric lighting became commonplace, people naturally downshifted with the onset of dusk. Today, the light assault continues until we go to bed and we still expect to fall asleep immediately. Which is dotty since the sleep hormone melatonin needs darkness to switch it on. Last thing at night, spend a few moments gazing at the vast velvet darkness of the night sky.

● Try this delicious drink to calm the nervous system. Stir together over gentle heat: 250ml organic full-fat cow's milk or almond or rice milk, 2 teaspoons organic ground almonds, 2 cardamom pods, 5 strands saffron and a pinch of nutmeg. Strain and add one teaspoon honey, Manuka if possible.

● Take one to two capsules of Valerian and Ashwagandha Formula by Pukka Herbs before bed. Keep a capsule handy to take if you wake.

● And if you do wake up, refuse to fret about missed sleep: until recently, people took it for granted they'd wake in the long periods of natural darkness and talk, make love, tell stories or let their minds roam. Lie there and think of all the nice things you've done this year.

● Breathe: lie flat on your back, eyes closed, one hand on your chest. Inhale for a count of four, hold for seven, then exhale slowly to eight: visualise waves shimmying up a beach, hovering for a moment, then receding gently… slowly… into the sea.

● Low blood sugar may rouse you, so have a small banana and/or a small pot of organic natural yoghurt (plus teaspoon!) by your bed, also a glass of still water with a few drops of Bach Rescue Remedy in it (dehydration can lead to poor sleep and bad dreams).

● If anxieties beset you, remember that around 4am is the 'dark hour of the soul' when your brain can't process worries – thus the jangling cacophony in your head. Keep a pen and paper by your bed, and write them down.

● If you toss and turn for more than 15 minutes, turn on the radio (we love the BBC World Service), read a trashy novel (nothing stimulating), do the ironing or washing-up (nothing energetic).

Z Instant face revivers: *our award winners*

Sometimes, what you really want is to LOOK GOOD RIGHT NOW – the instant confidence-boost of a product that perks up your skin, makes you look radiant, peels back the years – especially after a short or disturbed night, before a Big Night Out, or if you've been poorly. Masks are pretty brilliant – see page 82 – but there are also serums, spritzes, gels and even gadgets which make you look as if you've had eight hours' peaceful and restorative slumber. We know some of them work (see our favourites in We Love…) and our testers do too now!

AT A GLANCE

Clarisonic Plus

Clarins Beauty Flash Balm

Liz Earle Superskin Concentrate

Nourish Radiance Rejuvenating Peptide Serum

REVIEWS

Clarisonic Plus

8.69/10 We're selfishly delighted this sonic, vibrating, massaging, brush-headed (and pricey) skin gizmo's done so well – because now when we're bombarded with questions as to whether Clarisonic really works, we can say definitively: 'yessssss!'. They sent us the Face & Body kit (with two heads) and the accompanying Refining Skin Polish, but we asked panellists to try it with their regular products. (See also Award-winning Anti-Ageing Eye Creams, pages 52–53.) NB: Most testers reported long-term, not just instant, skin improvements.

Comments: 'Unprompted and without knowing I've been using something different, friends have commented on how fresh I look lately even on days when I start at 6am.' • 'I've absolutely fallen in love with this and am raving about it to everyone I know – the first thing I noticed was how soft and smooth my skin looked, with a definite bloom' • 'skin definitely "de-aged"' • 'complexion definitely more radiant after each use' • 'gave a glow and face felt more radiant after use – and oooh, the extra pleasure of feeling I'm cleansing away all the dirt!'.

Clarins Beauty Flash Balm

8.56/10 Well, what do you know? Clarins invented this beauty category with the creation of Beauty Flash Balm over 30 years ago, winning countless awards before this one.

According to our testers, it's still a wow, living up to its reputation as 'Cinderella in a tube'. With radiance-boosting ingredients, Beauty Flash Balm 'sets' to a comfy, firming film which makes skin look instantly fresh and gorgeously glowy.

Comments: 'My skin felt lovely instantly, no tautness, make-up went on with no sliding or greasiness, there's nothing to compare to this' • 'skin looked brighter and plumper, fresher and more radiant, and it evened out skintone; fantastic product' • 'slight tingling sensation at first, which felt invigorating; very effective, quite a few people remarked on how bright and radiant my skin was' • 'skin looked dewy, glowy and radiant, lovely!'.

Liz Earle Superskin Concentrate

8.39/10 We'll admit that we hadn't thought of using this facial oil as an instant face-saver until the brand put it forward for this category. But now we have, we're impressed at how this aromatic blend of vitamin E and plant oils (avocado, rosehip, argan) does speedily revive the skin. (The chamomile, neroli and lavender fragrance is especially lovely.) If you wanted to use this before going out, we'd suggest applying, leaving to sink in, then blotting firmly with a tissue before applying make-up. Most testers loved it so much they chose to use it every night!

Comments: 'Top marks, made my skin really soft and plump, face uplifted and spirits too! I've been recovering from a hysterectomy and this has really balanced and evened out my skin, people say I

TIP

'To brighten your skin, fill a basin with warm water and add several drops of lavender essential oil. Dip a face cloth in the water then lay over your face for a few moments. Repeat five times.' – Ole Henriksen

look really well and healthy' • 'I was worried about using an oil on a spotty area, but it has really cleared my skin and sorted out the dry areas, it's done wonders' • 'skin felt gorgeous!' • 'made skintone perkier and more even, skin felt comfy but supported – like Spanx for the face…' • 'wore this just with some concealer and blush'.

Nourish Radiance Rejuvenating Peptide Serum ❀ ❀ ❀

Dull tired skin needs hydration fast for starters and research shows that this good value, rose oil-infused product instantly hydrates the skin – by 80 per cent, they say. From a range created by Dr Pauline Hili, a specialist in organic skincare, this new award winner also contains our favourite hyaluronic acid to help plump out wrinkles, with tripeptide 5 to repair damage while boosting collagen synthesis. Our testers were impressed.

Comments: 'Immediately skin looked smoother and fresher; make-up was easier to apply and stayed on for longer' • 'leaves a subtle sort of luminescence, certainly perked up my skin and also made open pores look better' • 'lovely to apply and sank in immediately; texture and general appearance improved; make up went on better; I loved the effects and would buy' • 'skin felt fresher and uplifted straight away, skin tone more even: makes a difference even on fairly young skin'.

Directory

The following includes stockist contacts for the brands featured in these books. We would also like to suggest that you might enjoy our website, www.beautybible.com, which is really a magazine online. We call it 'your path through the beauty jungle' – just like our books. Every day on www.beautybible.com, you will find different tips, the new products and treatments we love and features on beauty, wellbeing and health. There is a weekly prize draw with truly fab prizes, and our Q&A section called Beauty Clinic, which answers readers' queries of all kinds. (You can submit questions about your beauty dilemmas on the site.) You can also sign up to Beauty Bible BUZZ, our newsletter which headlines what's on the site every week.

All the supplements mentioned in this book, plus advice and information, are available from Victoria Health, tel: 0800 3898 195, www.victoriahealth.com

001 Skincare, www.001skincare.com

A

Abaca, tel: 01269 598491, www.abacaorganic.co.uk

AD Skin Synergy, tel: 01495 325284, www.adskinsynergy.com

Aerin, tel: 0800 0542 444, www.esteelauder.co.uk

Aerosoles, available via www.aerosoles.com and from stores in Paris

A'kin, www.akinbeauty.co.uk

AloeDent, from Victoria Health, tel: 0800 3898 195, www.victoriahealth.com

Alpha-H, www.alpha-h.com

Alterna, from www.lookfantastic.com

Amanda Lacey, www.amandalacey.com

Dr Andrew Markey, the Lister Hospital, tel: 020 7730 1219, www.thelisterhospital.com

Dr Andrew Weil, www.drweil.com

Andy Wadsworth, My Life Personal Training, tel: 07889 940888, www.mylifept.com

Annee de Mamiel, tel: 07516

099010, www.demamiel.com

Antipodes, available at Selfridges, www.selfridges.com

Aquafresh, www.aquafresh.co.uk

Argan Organics, www.arganorganics.co.uk

Argan+, www.arganplus.co.uk

Aromatherapy Associates, from Victoria Health, tel: 0800 3898 195, www.victoriahealth.com

Aurelia, tel: 0207 7510022, www.aureliaskincare.com

Aveda, tel: 0800 0542 979, www.aveda.co.uk

Avène, www.avene.co.uk

B

B. Flawless, tel: 03456 710 709, www.superdrug.com

Balance Me, www.balanceme.co.uk

Barefoot Botanicals, from Victoria Health, tel: 0800 3898 195, www.victoriahealth.com

BareMinerals, tel: 0800 6523 362, www.bareminerals.co.uk

Bastien Gonzalez, www.bastiengonzalez.com

Beauty Bible Lip Balm,

from Victoria Health, tel: 0800 3898 195, www.victoriahealth.com

Benefit, tel: 0800 2794 793, www.benefitcosmetics.co.uk

Beverly Hills Formula, www.boots.com

Bio-Oil, www.boots.com

Bio Effect, tel: 0844 8158 456, www.bioeffect.co.uk

Bliss, tel: 0808 1004 151, www.blissworld.co.uk

Blood test (at home): Ideal Omega 3 Test Kit, www.yourhealthy.co.uk

Bobbi Brown, tel: 0800 054 2988, www.bobbibrown.co.uk

BOCA, www.boca.co.uk

The Body Shop, tel: 0800 0929 090, www.thebodyshop.co.uk

Botanicals, tel: 01664 464472, www.botanicals.co.uk

Bourjois, tel: 0800 269836, www.bourjois.co.uk

Bowen Technique, tel: 01373 461812, www.thebowentechnique.com

Bucky, www.amazon.co.uk

Burt's Bees, tel: 0808 2341 423, www.burtsbees.co.uk

By Terry, www.byterry.com

C

CACI, tel: 020 8731 5678, www.caci-international.co.uk

CCS, www.ccsfootcare.co.uk

Chanel, www.chanel.com

Professor Charles Clark, tel: 0207 636 7661, www.thefineclinic.com

Charlotte Tilbury, www.charlottetilbury.com

Chie Mihara, tel: 00 3 496 698 0415 www.chiemihara.com

Chillow, tel: 0870 0117174, www.chillow.co.uk

Chinese herbal medicine: Register of Chinese Herbal Medicine, tel: 01603 623994, www.rchm.co.uk

Circaroma, tel: 01308 488 955, www.circaroma.com

Clarins, tel: 01279 774215, www.clarins.co.uk

Clarisonic, tel: 0800 0286 874 www.clarisonic.co.uk

Clarks, tel: 0844 4995 544, www.clarks.co.uk

Clinique, tel: 0800 0542 666, www.clinique.co.uk

Cosmetic surgery: helpful organisations (see also Wendy Lewis, under 'W')

● British Academy of Cosmetic Dentistry, www.bacd.com

● The British Association of Aesthetic Plastic Surgeons, www.baaps.org.uk

● The British Association of Dermatologists (www.bad.org.uk)

● British Association of Oral and Maxillofacial Surgeons, www.baoms.org.uk

● The British Association of Otorhinolaryngologists, www.entuk.org

● British Association of Plastic,

Reconstructive and Aesthetic Surgeons, www.bapras.org.uk

● British Oculoplastic Surgery Society, www.bopss.co.uk

● The Care Quality Commission, www.cqc.org.uk

● The European Academy of Facial Plastic Surgery, www.eafps.org

● European Association of Plastic Surgeons, www.euraps.org

● European Society for Laser Dermatology, www.esld.org

● European Society of Plastic, Reconstructive and Aesthetic Surgery, www.espras.org

● General Medical Council, www.gmc-uk.org

● International Society of Aesthetic Plastic Surgery, www.isaps.org

● The Royal College of Anaesthetists, www.rcoa.ac.uk

Cosmetics à la Carte, tel: 020 7622 2318, www.alacartelondon.com

Cowshed, tel: 020 7534 0870, www.cowshedonline.com

Crème de la Mer, tel: 0800 0542 661, www.cremedelamer.co.uk

Crystal Clear, tel: 01517 097227, www.crystalclear.co.uk

D

Daniel Galvin, tel: 020 7486 9661, www.danielgalvin.com

Darphin, tel: 0800 0546 071, www.darphin.co.uk

Dr David Cook, London Holistic Dental Centre, tel: 020 7487 5221, www.londonholisticdental.com

Decléor, tel: 020 7313 8787, www.decleor.co.uk

Dental Splendour, from Victoria Health, tel: 0800 3898 195, www.victoriahealth.com

Dermalogica, tel: 01372 363600, www.dermalogica.co.uk

Dermasuri, from Victoria Health, tel: 0800 3898 195, www.victoriahealth.com

Dermol 500, www.amazon.co.uk

DHC, tel: 0800 0232 425, www.dhcuk.co.uk

Diamancel, tel: 0808 1004 151 www.blissworld.co.uk

Dior, tel: 020 7216 0216, www.dior.com

Dr. Bragi, tel: 01753 758745 www.drbragi.com

Dr. Hauschka, tel: 01386 791022, www.drhauschka.co.uk

Dr. Lewinn's, available at www.boots.com, www.tesco.com and www.lookfantastic.com

E

Ecco, tel: 01865 728728, www.ecco-shoes-uk.co.uk

Electrolysis: British Institute & Association of Electrolysis, tel: 0844 5441 373, www.electrolysis.co.uk

Elemis, tel: 01173 161888, www.elemis.co.uk

Elizabeth Arden, www.elizabetharden.co.uk

Ellis Faas, www.ellisfaas.com

Emma Hardie, tel: 020 7307 2380, www.emmahardie.com

ESPA, tel: 01252 352230, www.espaskincare.com

Essie, tel: 0800 731 2119 www.essie.co.uk

Estée Lauder, tel: 0800 0542 444, www.esteelauder.co.uk

Eucerin, www.boots.com

F

Filorga, tel: 0333 014 8000, www.marksandspencer.com

FitFlops, tel: 020 7751 3694 www.fitflop.co.uk

G

Garnier, tel: 0800 0854 376, www.garnier.co.uk

Gielly Green, tel: 020 7034 3060 www.giellygreen.co.uk

Gillette Venus, www.gillettevenus.co.uk

Giorgio Armani, www.giorgioarmanibeauty.co.uk

Goldfaden MD, from Space NK, tel: 020 8740 2085, www.uk.spacenk.com

Gosh, www.goshcosmetics.com

Gossypium, www.gossypium.co.uk

Guerlain, www.guerlain.com

H

Hästens, www.hastens.com

HealGel, from Victoria Health, tel: 0800 3898 195, www.victoriahealth.com

He-Shi, tel: 0845 0755 842, www.he-shi.eu

Holistic Dental Tooth Powder, from Victoria Health, tel: 0800 3898 195, www.victoriahealth.com

Hypnos, tel: 01844 348200, www.hypnosbeds.com

I

Ikea, www.ikea.co.uk

Ila, tel: 01608 677676, www.ila-spa.com

In Fiore, from Victoria Health, tel: 0800 3898 195, www.victoriahealth.com

Inika, www.inikacosmetics.co.uk

J

Jane Iredale, www.janeiredale.com

Jenny Jordan Eyebrow and Make-up Clinic, tel: 020 7483 2222, www.jennyjordan.co.uk

Jessica/Jessica Vartoughian, www.jessica-nails.co.uk

JetRest eye masks, www.thejetrest.com

Jo Hansford, www.johansford.com

John Frieda, tel: 0800 6521 496, www.johnfrieda.com

John Scurr, tel: 020 7730 9563, www.thelisterhospital.com

Joico, available from salons nationwide, www.joico.com

Professor Jon Kabat-Zinn, Mindfulness-Based Cognitive Therapy, www.mbct.com

Jurlique, www.jurlique.co.uk

K

Dr Karen Burke, tel: 00 1 212 594 5351, www.empowereddoctor.com

Kérastase, www.kerastase.co.uk

Keromask, tel: 01634 893 891 www.keromask.com

Kevin Murphy, tel: 01179 270434, www.kevinmurphystore.com

Kiehl's, tel: 0800 5870 830, www.kiehls.co.uk

Kiss The Moon,

www.kissthemoon.com

Korres, www.boots.com

L

Lancôme, www.lancome.co.uk

Lanolips, from Victoria Health, tel: 0800 3898 195, www.victoriahealth.com

La Prairie, www.laprairie.com

Laura Mercier, from Space NK, tel: 020 8740 2085, www.uk.spacenk.com

Lee Stafford, www.leestafford.com

Legology, www.legology.co.uk

Léonor Greyl, available from Selfridges, Urban Retreat at Harrods and Net-a-Porter online

Lipstick Queen, from Space NK, tel: 020 8740 2085, www.uk.spacenk.com

Liz Earle Naturally Active Skincare, tel: 01983 813913, www.lizearle.com

L'Occitane, tel: 020 7907 0301, www.loccitane.com

L'Oréal, tel: 0800 0304 032, www.loreal-paris.co.uk

Lotus Journeys, www.lotusjourneys.com

Louise Galvin, tel: 020 7835 0453, www.louisegalvin.com

Lulu, www.qvcuk.com

Lumosity, www.lumosity.com

M

MAC, www.maccosmetics.co.uk

Manuka Doctor, www.manukadoctor.co.uk

Margaret Dabbs, tel: 020 7487 5510, www.margaretdabbs.co.uk

Marie Veronique Organics, www.pureshopskincare.com

Mason Pearson, tel: 020 7491 2613, www.masonpearson.com

McTimoney Chiropractic, tel: 01491 829211,

www.mctimoneychiropractic.org

Michael Dooley, The Poundbury Clinic, tel: 01305 262626, www.thepoundburyclinic.co.uk

Micro Pedi, tel: 0845 399 0042 www.micropedi.co.uk

Monu, tel: 0870 2209 094, www.monushop.co.uk

Moroccanoil, tel: 020 3514 5361, www.moroccanoil.com

Dr Mosaraf Ali, The Integrated Medical Centre, www.drmali.com

Murad, from Victoria Health, tel: 0800 3898 195, www.victoriahealth.com

MV Organic Skincare, from Cult Beauty, tel: 02456 529521 www.cultbeauty.co.uk

N

Nadia Brydon, practitioner of Western and Chinese herbal medicine, acupuncture and homeopathy, email: nadia@chanters.fsnet.co.uk

Nail Magic, tel: 020 8979 7261 www.jica.com

Nails Inc, tel: 020 7529 2340, www.nailsinc.com

Neal's Yard Remedies, tel: 0845 2623 145, www.nealsyardremedies.com

New CID Cosmetics, www.newcidcosmetics.com

Dr Nick Lowe, The Cranley Clinic, tel: 020 7499 3223, www.drnicklowe.com

Nivea, www.nivea.co.uk

No7, available from Boots www.boots.com

Nourish, www.nourishskinrange.com

O

Ogario tel: 0844 556 4393, www.ogariolondon.com

Ojon, tel: 0800 0884 165, www.ojon.co.uk

Ole Henriksen, www.olehenriksen.com

OPI, tel: 01923 240 010 www.opiuk.com

Origins, tel: 0800 0542 888, www.origins.co.uk

The Organic Pharmacy, tel: 0844 8008 399 www.theorganicpharmacy.com

Orly, tel: 01827 280080, www.orlybeauty.co.uk

OV Naturals, www.ovnaturals.co.uk

P

Paul & Joe, www.paul-joe-beaute.com/en

Paul Mitchell, tel: 0845 6590 011, www.paul-mitchell.co.uk

Percy & Reed, www.percyandreed.com

Per-fékt, www.perfektbeauty.com

PerioBrite, available at Amazon UK, www.amazon.co.uk

Pevonia, tel: 01449 727000 www.pevonia.co.uk

Philip B, www.philipb.com

Philosophy, available from Boots, www.boots.com

Phyto Phytobaume, www.feelunique.com

Phylia de M., from Victoria Health, tel: 0800 3898 195, www.victoriahealth.com

Pilates:
● **The Pilates Foundation**, tel: 020 7033 0078, www.pilatesfoundation.com

● **Body Control Pilates**, tel: 020 7636 8900, www.bodycontrolpilates.com

Pinks Boutique, tel: 01332 411588, www.pinksboutique.com

prAna Yoga Mats, from www.yogastudio.co.uk

Provenance, from Victoria Health, tel: 0800 3898 195, www.victoriahealth.com

Prtty Peaushun, www.prttypeaushun.com

Pukka, tel: 0845 375 1744, www.pukkaherbs.com

Pureology, tel: 020 8762 4121, www.pureology-uk.com

R

Radical Skincare, available from SpaceNK www.uk.spacenk.com

REN, tel: 020 7724 2900, www.renskincare.com

Repêchage, www.repechageuk.com

RéVive, www.reviveskincare.com

Revlon, tel: 0800 085 2716, www.revlon.com

Rigby & Peller, tel: 0845 0765 545, www.rigbyandpeller.com

Rimmel, www.rimmellondon.com

Roja Dove, www.rojadove.com

S

Sanctuary, www.sanctuary.com

Santhilea, www.santhilea.com

Sarah Chapman, www.sarahchapman.net

Sebastian Professional, www.sebastianprofessional.co.uk

Sensodyne, www.sensodyne.co.uk

Serious Readers lamps, tel: 0800 028 1890, www.seriousreaders.com

Seven Wonders, from Victoria Health, tel: 0800 3898 195, www.victoriahealth.com

Shavata, www.shavata.co.uk

Shiffa, from Selfridges, tel: 0800 123 400,

www.selfridges.com

Shoe Therapy, www.shoetherapy.com

Shower water filters:
- www.amazon.co.uk
- Pure Showers, tel: 0800 6127 174, www.pureshowers.co.uk

Shu Uemura, tel: 0844 8920 146, www.shuuemura.co.uk

Sisley, available from John Lewis, www.johnlewis.com

Smashbox, www.smashbox.co.uk

Soap & Glory, www.soapandglory.com

Soapsmith, tel: 0203 233 0009, www.soapsmith.com

Spa Find, www.musthave.co.uk and www.amazon.co.uk

Space NK, tel: 0208 740 2085, www.uk.spacenk.com

Spotner, www.spotner.com

St Tropez, tel: 020 7845 6330, www.st-tropez.com

Steve Mason, tel: 01273 771441, www.brightonacupunctureand-massage.co.uk

Su-Man Hsu, tel: 0203 086 9856, www.su-man.com

Superdrug, tel: 03456 710 709 www.superdrug.com

Suqqu, www.suqqu.com

Susan Posnick, www.susanposnick.com

Suzie Mitchell, tel: 01424 430389, www.spaghetti-tree.com

T

T'ai chi:
The UK T'ai Chi Association, tel: 020 7407 4775, www.taichiuk.co.uk

Taryn Rose, from Footwise, www.tarynrose.com

Temple Spa,

www.templespa.com

Terra Plana, www.vivobarefoot.com

Thalgo, www.thalgo.com

This Works, tel: 020 8543 3544, www.thisworks.com

Tim Hutchful, The British Chiropractic Association, tel: 01189 505950, www.chiropractic-uk.co.uk

Tisserand, www.tisserand.com

Tom's of Maine, www.tomsofmaine.com

Tri-Aktiline, www.amazon.co.uk

Trilogy, www.trilogyproducts.com

Tweezerman, www.tweezerman.co.uk

U

Ugg, tel: 0808 2340 990, www.uggaustralia.co.uk

Una Brennan, www.boots.com

UrbanVeda, www.urbanveda.co.uk

V

Valerie Beverly Hills, www.valeriebeverlyhills.com

Vaseline Intensive Care, www.vaseline.co.uk

Vichy, tel: 0800 169 6193, www.vichyconsult.co.uk

Viscotears, widely available at chemists

Vitage, from Cosmeceuticals, tel: 0845 555 2121, www.skinbrands.co.uk

W

Weleda, from Victoria Health, tel: 0800 3898 195, www.victoriahealth.com

Wendy Lewis, tel: 00 1 212 861 6148, www.wlbeauty.com, email: info@wlbeauty.com, Wendy Lewis Beauty Forum: www.beautyinthebag.com,

www.facebook.com/WendyLewisCo, twitter.com/knifecoach

Wild about Beauty, www.wildaboutbeauty.com

X

Xyliwhite, www.amazon.co.uk

Y

Yes to Carrots, from Victoria Health, tel: 0800 3898 195, www.victoriahealth.com

Yes to Tomatoes, from Victoria Health, tel: 0800 3898 195, www.victoriahealth.com

Yoga:
British Wheel of Yoga, tel: 01529 306851, www.bwy.org.uk

Youngblood, tel: 0845 2464 666, www.ybskin.co.uk

YSL, www.ysl.com

Z

Zelens, tel: 0207 6313212 www.zelens.com

Zoya,www.lovelula.com, www.naturisimo.com, www.amazon.co.uk

ANTI-AGEING BOOKSHELF

Food Rules by Michael Pollan (Penguin)

Healing Without Freud or Prozac by Dr David Servan-Schreiber (Rodale International)

I Feel Bad about My Neck by Nora Ephron (Black Swan)

The Lowdown on Facelifts and Other Wrinkle Remedies by Wendy Lewis (Quadrille)

Plastic Makes Perfect by Wendy Lewis (Orion)

The New Yoga for People Over 50 by Suza Francina (Health Communications)

Yoga and the Wisdom of Menopause by Suza Francina (Health Communications)

Yoga Builds Bones by Jan Maddern (Element)

The Yoga Facelift by Marie-Véronique Nadeau (Conari Press)

The Ultimate Natural Beauty Book by Josephine Fairley (Kyle Cathie)

DVD:
Yoga for Beginners by Patricia Walden (from www.yogastudio.co.uk)

Index

Acknowledgements

This book is the result of decades of research. We would like to thank all the friends, colleagues and experts worldwide who have helped us so generously over the years. Also our doughty and dedicated teams of testers, without whose commitment to trialling products and writing up their findings, Beauty Bible wouldn't be here.

A vast vote of thanks to our illustrator David Downton (who's also included in the dedication), who has surpassed himself – and made us laugh a lot too: our Beauty Bible publications would not be so stylish and beautiful without his support and super-talented input.

Particular thanks to:

Maggie Alderson
Bobbi Brown
Nadia Brydon
Dr Karen Burke
Sarah Chapman
Professor Charles
 Clark
Dr David Cook
Margaret Dabbs
Barbara Daly OBE
Shabir Daya

Carmen dell'Orefice
Michael Dooley
Roja Dove
Liz Earle MBE
Mary Greenwell
Terry de Gunzburg
Newby Hands
Tim Hutchful
Eve Lom
Dr Nick Lowe
Lulu
Trish McEvoy
Lorna McKnight

Annee de Mamiel
Dr Andrew Markey
Laura Mercier
Suzie Mitchell
Marie-Véronique
 Nadeau
Tim Petersen
Philip B
Kathy Phillips
John Scurr
Gill Sinclair
Dr Andrew Weil
Andreas Wild

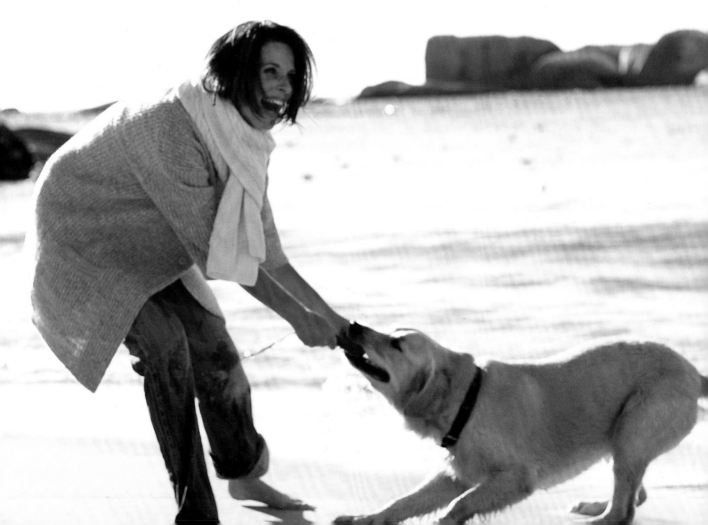

Photo acknowledgements

We would also like to thank a raft of beauty PRs who supported us so efficiently with our project but would need an extra book to include them all. But special thanks go to Emma Dawson and her team at L'Oréal; Sarah Griffiths and her team at Estée Lauder Companies; Julietta Longcroft and Tom Konig Oppenheimer at TCS (who went so far as to appoint a special 'Beauty Bible Liaison Officer', Ellie Howden, who we also thank); Nancy Brady and all at NBPR; Jenny Halpern and her crew at Halpern PR; Jo Fox Tutchener and Michelle Boon at Beautyseen; Rick Havemann at www.avea.co.uk; Fiona Dowal, Owen Walker, Max Flower and the team at Modus Dowal Walker; Phily Keeling at Chanel; Lesley Chilvers at Bourjois; Kate Hudson and Helen Mitchell at Guerlain; Jazz Kaur at Benefit (who helped us with this book wearing her former Guerlain chapeau); Aude Chatelin at Dior; Carri Kilpatrick and the Kilpatrick PR team; Kelly Marks and all at Pure PR – plus everyone at Liz Earle (especially Kim Buckland, who set up Liz Earle Naturally Active Skincare with Liz herself).

Thanks to our publisher Kyle Cathie, as ever, and to our colleagues at YOU magazine, Sue Peart, Catherine Fenton and Rosalind Lowe.

And, of course, to our wonderful Beauty Bible team (see dedication).

Title page Plainpicture/beyond
p7 Adrian Peacock, Charlotte Murphy
p9 Icon Photo/C.Watts
p10-11 Kellie Hindmarch
p14-15 Photolibrary/D&L Jacobs
p20 www.urbanlip.com
p22 Photolibrary
p26 Rex Features/T.Logan
p32 Getty/E.Estabrook
p35 Camera Press London/Brigitte
p36 Plainpicture/Ableimages
p39 www.urbanlip.com
p40 www.urbanlip.com
p45 Camera Press London/B.Coster
p46-47 www.urbanlip.com
p50-51 Photolibrary/Photoalto
p52-53 Photolibrary/B.Lark
p54 Photolibrary/Superstock Inc
p57 www.urbanlip.com
p58 Corbis/S.Prezant
p61 Trunk Archive.com/A.Bettles
p63 Getty/Superstudio
p65 Photolibrary/Imagesource
p66 Getty/J.Tisne
p67 Getty/B.Yee
p69 Photolibrary/M.Constantini
p71 Photolibrary/Photoalto
p75 Photolibrary/S.Zulawinski
p79 www.urbanlip.com
p81 Photolibrary/J.Feingersh
p83 Photolibrary/B.Vogel;
p86 Camera Press London/*Journal für die Frau*
p92 Getty/P.de Villiers
p94 Photolibrary/C.Sharp
p97 Photolibrary/T.Kruesselmann
p98 Plainpicture/applypictures
p106 Trunk Archive.com/H.Salinas
p106 Camera Press London/J.Veysey
p106 Corbis
p106 Photolibrary/Z.Smith
p106 Getty/A.Mo
p107 Rex Features/Col Pics/Everett
p107 Camera Press London/J.Veysey
p107 Camera Press London/C.Djanogly

p108 Getty/Tedfoo
p115 Trunk Archive.com/Pamela Hanson/Hair: Julien d'Ys/Make-up: Stephane Marais
p122 Photolibrary/It Stock RF
p125 Photolibrary/F.Wirth
p129 Photolibrary/B.Erlinger
p132 Photolibrary/A.Oliel
p133 www.urbanlip.com
p139 Photolibrary/Photoalto
p140 Photolibrary/B.Lark
p143 Getty/Dorling Kindersley
p144 Photolibrary/R. Kaufma/L. Hirshowitz
p146 Photolibrary/Radius Images
p151 www.urbanlip.com
p153 Photolibrary/M.Burkhart/Corbis
p154 Photolibrary/Stockbrokerxtra images
p158-159 Photolibrary/Fancy
p161 Photolibrary/Fotosearch
p165 Getty/B.Fraker
p166 Tim Petersen
p168-169 Photolibrary/Pixtal Images
p171 Photolibrary/Corbis
p173 Photolibrary/F.Cirou
p177 Camera Press London/Titti Fabi
p178 www.urbanlip.com
p179 Photolibrary/J.Klee
p181 Getty/A.Rohmer
p182-183 Photolibrary/Tetra Images
p185 Photolibrary/C.Chiossone/Photex
p186 Magnum Photos/Robert Capa/International Centre of Photography
p189 Getty/T.Barwick
p191 www.urbanlip.com
p193 Photolibrary RF
p194 Photolibrary/Uppercut Images
p196 Photolibrary/M.Anderson
p201 Photolibrary/Emotive Image
p202 Photolibrary/P.Leonard;
p204-205 Photolibrary/Innerhofer Photodesign
p207 Getty/LaCoppola-Meier
p208-209 Magnum Photos/Eve Arnold
p210-211 Arcangel/R.Musyhiar
p213 www.urbanlip.com
Acknowledgements page www.urbanlip.com

We would like to dedicate this book to the Beauty Bible 'team' who worked so hard to help us make it happen: Sally Cole, David Downton, Amy Eason, David Edmunds, Jessie Lawrence, Ben Lovegrove, Liz Murray, Jenny Semple, and also to our divine agent Kay McCauley, who we want to be like – and look as good as – when we grow up...

This edition first published in Great Britain in 2016
by Kyle Books
an imprint of Kyle Cathie Ltd
192–198 Vauxhall Bridge Road
London, SW1V 1DX
email: general.enquiries@kylebooks.com
website: www.kylebooks.com

First published in hardback in 2011 by Kyle Cathie Ltd
First published in paperback in 2012 by Kyle Books

10 9 8 7 6 5 4 3 2 1

ISBN: 978 0 85783 317 4

Josephine Fairley and Sarah Stacey are hereby identified as the authors of this work in accordance with Section 77 of the Copyright, Designs and Patents Act 1988

A Cataloguing in Publication record for this title is available from the British Library

Design: Jenny Semple
Illustrations: David Downton
Editor: Vicky Orchard
Editorial assistant: Amberley Lowis
Copy editor: Liz Murray
Picture researcher: Sally Cole, Perseverance Works Ltd
Production: Gemma John, Sheila Smith and Nic Jones

Colour reproduction by Scanhouse
Printed and bound in China by C&C Offset Printing Company Ltd